Diseases of Dogs

The Encyclopedia for the Small Animal Practitioner
covering both Medical and Surgical Problems of Dogs

Diseases of Dogs

The Encyclopedia for the Small Animal Practitioner
covering both Medical and Surgical Problems of Dogs

Revised by

Horst-Joachim Christoph

Professor of Small Animal Surgery and Experimental Surgery,
Director of the Clinic and Outpatients' Department for Small
Domestic Animals in the Karl Marx University of Leipzig

PERGAMON PRESS

OXFORD · NEW YORK · TORONTO · SYDNEY · BRAUNSCHWEIG

PERGAMON PRESS LTD.,
Headington Hill Hall, Oxford, OX3 0BW

PERGAMON PRESS INC.,
Maxwell House, Fairview Park, Elmsford, New York 10523

PERGAMON OF CANADA LTD.,
207 Queen's Quay West, Toronto 1

PERGAMON PRESS (AUST.) PTY. LTD.,
19a Boundary Street, Rushcutters Bay, N.S.W. 2011, Australia

PERGAMON PRESS GMBH,
Burgplatz 1, Braunschweig 3300, West Germany

First English edition 1975
Library of Congress Catalog Card No. 71 - 163386
Printed in Great Britain
ISBN 0 08 015800 5

Title of the original German edition:
Abriß der Klinik der Hundekrankheiten 2. Auflage 1962
© VEB Gustav Fischer Verlag, Jena, 1960

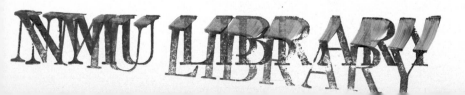

Erfüllte Pflicht empfindet
sich immer noch als Schuld,
weil man sich
nie ganz genug getan.

GOETHE (1829)

Contents

Preface to the First German Edition

When I was asked to write a book on Diseases of Dogs, I readily agreed although it was obvious that it would be impossible for me to deal in detail with all the diseases to which the dog is heir. The book is therefore described as an outline and it represents mainly our experience in the Leipzig Clinic. The work cannot claim to be comprehensive as some diseases only occur in certain geographical locations and in the clinic we are interested in certain fields. Those sections dealing with conditions which have not been studied extensively in Leipzig have been critically appraised by a colleague experienced in the particular condition. This outline, therefore, should not be regarded as a complete textbook on the subject, but it is hoped that it will prove an encouragement and a guide to the practising veterinarian and, above all, to the student.

The material comprising the book can be divided into two main parts. The first part deals with such matters as the systematic examination of the patient, estimation of age, methods of restraint and therapeutic techniques. A separate chapter is devoted to the treatment of bacterial infections, in which the actions and dosages of the various therapeutic agents in common use are described, in order to avoid repetition in the text. Similarly, a special chapter describes methods of analgesia and anaesthesia. In the second part of the book, diseases are dealt with according to the organ system involved. The functions of our Clinic include the performing of certain cosmetic operations, such as docking of the ears, correction of the carriage of the ears and tail, etc., the techniques of which are described in the relevant chapters. Most of the operations described are designed for use under the conditions pertaining to general veterinary practice. With regard to surgery and ophthalmology we follow the precepts of the Vienna School (of Prof. Dr. O. ÜBER-REITER).

In Part III, I have compiled a list of drugs giving details about the manufacturers and packaging, which should facilitate the dispensing of these products. This list contains the drugs which are mentioned in the text and which are available as preparations ready for use, but should not be regarded as being fully comprehensive.

Effective illustration of the text has been given special consideration. The material for these illustrations has been drawn from the rich collections of photographs and radiographs in the Clinic. Some of these pictures have already been published in the literature but no acknowledgement has been made in their captions. Most of the photographs (89) were taken under my direction by Messrs. H. Lachmann, Leipzig. For the supply of individual photographs my thanks are due to my Colleagues, Notscheff, Sofia (2), Vöhringer, Halle (4) and Thiele, Leipzig (2). I am grateful to the State Secretariat for University and Technical Schools of the

German Democratic Republic for their financial support in the preparation of the illustrations.

Finally, my special thanks are due to my Colleagues and Staff of the Clinic. The VEB Gustav Fischer Verlag, Jena, have conformed to my wishes in regard to the printing of the book in every way. I am very grateful for their advice and for the high standard of presentation of the book.

Leipzig, February, 1959   H. J. Christoph

Preface to the Second German Edition

Since the first edition of this book was sold out, it has became necessary to revise and add to the original text to form the second edition.

In the first part, a chapter on "Physical Therapy" and one on "X-ray Technique" have been added. Most small-animal practitioners are equipped with apparatus for the various forms of physical therapy and radiography, so these chapters were considered essential. The present senior scientific assistant of the Clinic, Dr. S. Schlaaff, has kindly written the chapter on X-ray Technique. The second part of the book has been thoroughly revised and the additions need not be summarised in detail. Some of the less effective illustrations, especially the line drawings, have been replaced by photographs, some of them coloured, and new material has been added. For their assistance with the illustrations, I am grateful to the chief of the Clinical Laboratory, Fraulein Chr. Weber, the ladies of the University Illustration (Bildstelle) Department and to Herr Lachmann. My sincere thanks are due to all Colleagues who made valuable suggestions and gave encouragement for the work on the new edition.

The publisher has again fully supported the completion of the second edition, not only in the matter of printing technique, and I feel this fact deserves special acknowledgement.

Leipzig, October, 1960   H. J. Christoph

I. General Part

1. Clinical examination

A general clinical examination should always be made as a routine procedure whenever a dog is presented for the first time. Frequently diseases, which the owner believes to be confined to a particular organ or system, are only correctly diagnosed after a thorough general examination has been made. It is advisable to examine the patient according to a set routine otherwise omissions may occur.

A complete case history is essential for a correct diagnosis and treatment. The owner should be encouraged to give a chronological description of the symptoms which have caused him to seek professional advice, and also to give details of any lay treatment which has been given. Quite often in the larger towns, a succession of veterinarians are consulted about the same case and it is imperative that any treatment prescribed should be revealed, as certain drugs may have a cumulative or synergistic effect. Often the owner is unable to give an articulate description of the symptoms and one is obliged to make a searching, but patient enquiry in order to elicit a comprehensive histroy. Occasionally the dog is presented by friends or relatives of the owner who know little or nothing of the history of the case. In such instances one should decline treatment until a good history can be obtained. The case history should include details of any past illnesses as well as the present condition. The diet, management, and the general environmental conditions of the dog should be elicited. In the case of bitches, details of the previous oestrus cycles and reproductive history must be obtained.

Once a full history has been obtained, the clinical examination can commence. Before a systematic examination is performed, the temperature, pulse and respiration must be ascertained. There may be quite considerable variation in these in nervous or highly strung animals. The temperature may be taken whilst the case history is being established. Experienced owners often take the dog's temperature at home and thus get a more reliable reading than in the strange surroundings of the consulting room. The internal body temperature is measured with a clinical thermometer, marked with the Centigrade or Fahrenheit scale. The mercury is shaken down and the thermometer, lubricated with a little vaseline, is inserted for half its length into the rectum and retained there for two to three minutes. The base of the tail is held with one hand and the thermometer inserted with the other (Fig. 1). This procedure avoids the danger of the dog suddenly sitting down and breaking the thermometer. The normal internal temperature lies between 37.5° and 39.0 °C (100.0°–102 °F), but there is a good deal of variation between small and large breeds and between puppies and older dogs. In young dogs or small breeds, e. g. Pomeranians, a temperature of 39.2 °C would be considered normal, whereas in older dogs or large breeds, e. g. St. Bernard, the normal temperature might be 37.5 °C or slightly lower. Apart from these differences of age

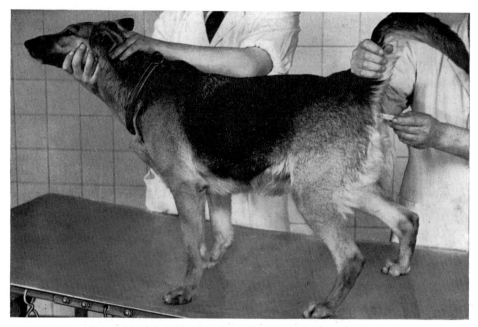

Fig. 1. Taking the temperature of a dog.

and breed, the temperature is subject to daily fluctuations and male dogs have a lower temperature than bitches. The lay idea that the body temperature is reflected in the dog's nose is not very accurate, as the warmth of the nose depends on the secretion of its glands (viz. cold due to evaporation).

While the case history is being taken, a general impression of the animal is obtained, viz. its breed, sex and age. The dog's bearing, temperament and body movements are noted as soon as it enters the consulting room. Individual examination begins with an estimation of the dog's state of nutrition, whether it is obese (Fig. 2) or cachectic (Fig. 3). Palpation will indicate the condition of the bones, joints and musculature, and may reveal muscle atrophy, paralysis or spasms.

After this general impression of the patient is obtained, the examination is extended systematically to the individual organs. It is best to begin with the skin and hair. If the history has indicated ear disease, the ear should be given a detailed examination. Examination of the visible mucosae may suggest serious internal diseases. The eyes should be examined and often they reveal conditions (e. g. follicular conjunctivitis) of which the owner was unaware.

The respiratory system is investigated, beginning with the nose and then the larynx, trachea and lungs. The whole thorax is examined; the frequency, depth and type of respiration may give valuable clues to certain diseases and to the condition of the respiratory tract. Percussion is of limited value in the dog and radiography is much more useful. A thorough auscultation of the heart is performed, and at the same time the quality and frequency of the pulse may be assessed by palpation of the femoral artery.

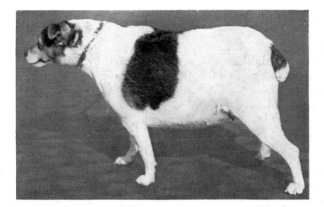

Fig. 2. Adiposity.

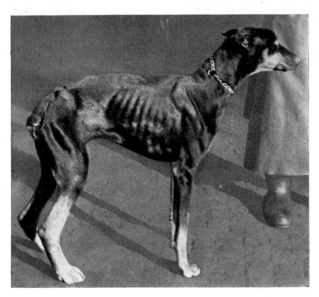

Fig. 3. Cachexia. Abscess in the right gluteal muscle.

Investigation of the digestive system should commence with the buccal cavity and includes the tongue, salivary secretion, the condition of the teeth, the tonsils and pharynx. The oesophagus may be palpated in its cervical portion, and abdominal palpation may reveal abnormalities in the stomach, the intestines, the liver and spleen. Various radiographical techniques (inflation with air, pneumo-peritoneum, and the use of contrast media) may be required for a thorough examination. The anus and its related glands should be inspected and the rectum may be investigated by digital exploration. Laboratory examination of the faeces should be performed where possible.

The kidneys and the bladder may be palpated through the abdomen or the latter per rectum. Laboratory examination of the urine yields most valuable information about the state of the urinary system. Sometimes the blood urea must be determined before a firm diagnosis of renal disease can be made.

In the examination of the genital system of the male dog, palpation of the prepuce, penis, penile bone, testes and epididymis may reveal certain lesions. The prostate may be palpated per rectum or, if enlarged, by abdominal palpation. In the bitch, the vulva and the vagina may be inspected visually, the vagina by the use of a speculum. In the large breeds, or in fat bitches it may be difficult to palpate the uterus through the abdomen, and it is situated too far forward to reach per rectum. In these cases it may be necessary to employ special radio-graphical techniques to visualise the uterus. The mammary glands should be inspected and palpated.

The general examination of the patient may be concluded with an examination of the central nervous system.

As stated in the introduction, it is important that the first examination of the patient should be as comprehensive as possible. Many diseases involve a variety of organs and the correct diagnosis may only be reached through a thorough general examination.

2. Estimation of age

The veterinarian is often asked to give an opinion as to the approximate age of a dog, e. g. in legal cases, or in stray dogs which have been found a new home, etc. The dentition provides the most important evidence for estimation of age, either by the eruption of the teeth, signs of wear, or loss of teeth. One must also take into account the facial expression, the dog's bearing, greying of the hair of the head, opacity of the crystalline lenses and dilatation of the pupils in older animals.

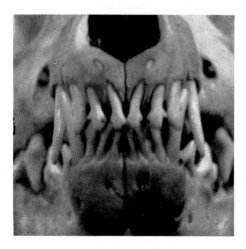

Fig. 4. Age: 2 months. The incisor teeth are already set wide apart. Wearing of the main lobes has not yet commenced.

The incisor teeth are especially useful in the estimation of age. They can be divided, according to their position, into central, medial and lateral or corner teeth. The incisors of the upper and lower jaws show certain differences in shape. In the upper jaw the incisors are longer and the crown is trituberculate, so that beside the large central lobe there are two small lateral lobes. One speaks of the lilylike appearance of the teeth because the crown resembles a fleur-de-lys. These three lobes have sharp external edges, which arise from the wall-like base of the crown. In the lower jaw the incisors are rather smaller and their inner borders are not lobed, i. e. they are bi-tuberculate. Wear of the teeth results in various contact surfaces or tables being formed, which appear oval, rounded or inverted oval in shape.

As in other domestic animals, the milk teeth of the dog erupt first and are replaced later by the permanent dentition. The milk incisors are distinguished from the permanent incisors in that they are smaller, and pointed, bluish-white in colour, and the lily shape is more evident. The canines, also called fangs or dog teeth, are large and conical and curved with a forward convexity. The lower canines fit directly on to the lateral incisors; those of the upper jaw lie somewhat further back, so that there is a space into which the lower canine fits when the bite is closed.

The following changes in the bite of teeth can be used for the estimation of age: (1) The eruption and wearing out of the milk teeth. (2) Changes in the teeth. (3) Changes in the shape of the teeth due to wear. (4) Falling out of teeth.

Puppies are born without teeth, but at the age of 3 to 4 weeks the milk cutting teeth erupt. Usually the canines appear first, and then in rapid succession the incisors (first in the upper and then in the lower jaw). As the incisors at this age are not subject to wear, they are fairly sharp. As the dog grows older the spaces in between the incisors widen, signs of wear can be detected, and they become loosened so that they may be arranged in a sloping manner (2 to 4 months old, Fig. 4). The age at which the milk teeth are replaced varies with the breed, thus they are replaced earlier in the larger than in the smaller breeds. The incisors

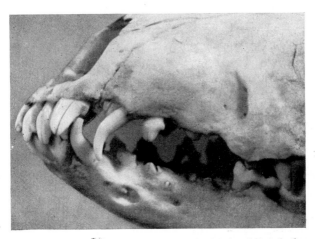

Fig. 5. Age: 5 months. The permanent canine begins to break through.

are replaced almost simultaneously, the process beginning at $3\frac{1}{2}$ to 4 months and is usually complete at 5 months, although the permanent lateral incisors are usually not fully developed at this age.

The canine teeth are replaced at the age of 5 to 6 months (Fig. 5) and quite often the milk and permanent canines are present together, but are of different lengths. A dog with such double canines can be estimated as being 6 to 7 months old. In the lower jaw the permanent canine erupts medially to the temporary canine, whereas in the upper jaw it lies in front of the milk tooth (Fig. 6).

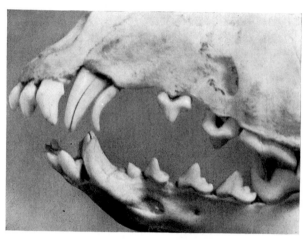

Fig. 6. Age: 7 months. The milk and permanent canines are still present in both the upper and lower jaws.

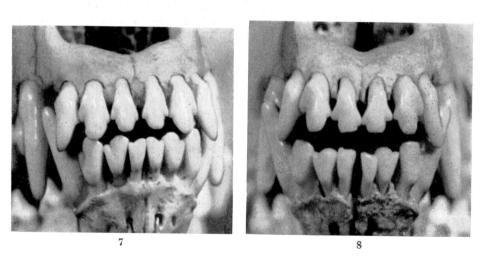

7   8

Fig. 7. Age: 6 months. Wearing of the main lobes still not present.

Fig. 8. Age: $1\frac{1}{2}$ years. The main lobes of the incisors of the lower jaw are worn away.

By 6 months of age, the permanent incisors have completed their eruption and are fully formed. They appear porcelain white and show no traces of wear (Fig. 7). The central lobes show the first signs of wear and when this lobe is completely worn away, the lateral lobes commence to wear, so that the appositional surface of the tooth is quite extensive.

Wear of the central, medial and lateral incisors usually proceeds at fairly regular intervals. At 6 months of age, the central incisors of the lower jaw begin to wear and by 18 months the main lobes are worn away (Fig. 8). From 1½ to 2 years wearing of the medial incisors of the lower jaw also begins and is complete at about 2½ years (Fig. 9). Between 2½ to 3 years the main lobes of the central incisors of the upper jaw commence wearing, and at 3½ years this process is complete. The tables of the lower lateral and medial incisors are now square shaped (Fig. 10). At 3½ to 4 years the wearing down of the main lobes of the medial incisors of the upper jaw begins and is complete at 4½ years (Fig. 11). Between 4½ to 5 years the lower lateral incisors come into wear (Fig. 12), and by 5½ years their main lobes are completely worn down (Fig. 13). The shape of the tables of the lower central medial incisor is still square. Sometimes a yellow star can be seen on the table. About this age the canines also begin to show signs of wear. At 6 years the main lobes of the upper lateral incisors have been worn away, but because the apposition of the lateral incisors is not absolutely perfect, there may be a less regular wearing process here than in the other incisors. After 6 years of age signs of wear are not so evident and one now has to take note of the so-called "inverted oval" of the tables of the various pairs of teeth. By 7 years the table of the lower central incisor is an inverted oval (Fig. 14), at 8 to 9 years on the lower medial incisors (Fig. 15), and at 9 to 10 years on the upper central

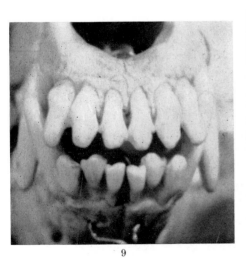
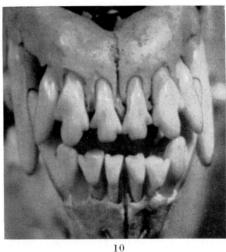

9

10

Fig. 9. Age: 2½ years. The main lobes of the medial incisors of the lower jaw are markedly worn away, conforming to the rather faulty arrangement of the teeth.

Fig. 10. Age: 3 years. Wearing has begun on the main lobes of the incisors of the upper jaw.

2*

incisors (Fig. 16). At 8 years the table on the lower central incisors broadens anteriorly against the labial surface. At 9 years, all the lower incisors undergo a crumbling of their anterior surfaces which is ascribed to the gnawing of hard objects with the blunt, truncated teeth.

The canines commence to show signs of wear at 5 years old. By the age of 7 to 8 years they are blunt, laterally displaced and often covered with tartar. With the passing of the years, they become blunted and shorter and the formation of tartar increases.

There is also a regular progression in the process of falling out of teeth. At the age of 10 to 12 years the lower central incisors fall out, followed shortly by the upper

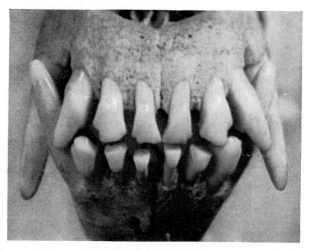

Fig. 11. Age: 4½ years. Wearing away of the main lobes of the medial incisors of the upper jaw is complete and corresponds to the arrangement of the teeth.

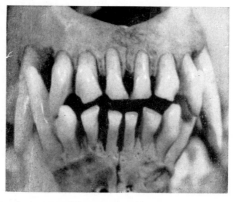

Fig. 12. Age: 5 years. Wearing away of the main lobe of the lateral incisors of the lower jaw has begun.

centrals. The other incisors fall out between 12 and 16 years and the canines between 16 to 20 years.

The prerequisite for the regular wear of the incisors is that there should be perfect apposition of the upper and lower jaws. Ideally the bite should act like a pair of shears, i. e. the lower incisors should lie a little behind those of the upper jaw and be in contact with them. Where the jaws are so formed that the teeth meet ("forceps bite") or where the lower incisors lie anteriorly to the upper ("reversed shears"), the signs of wear may differ considerably from the process described

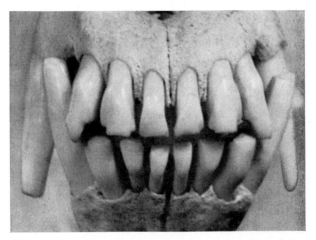

Fig. 13. Age: 5½ years. The main lobes of the lateral incisors of the lower jaw are completely worn away.

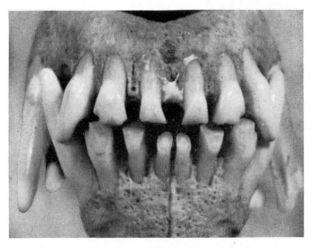

Fig. 14. Age: 7 years. The frictional surfaces of the incisors of the lower jaw have the shape of a reversed oval.

above. They are quite irregular in the condition of **Brachygnathia superior** ("Over-shot"), an anomaly of the bite which shows an hereditary shortening of the upper jaw (Fig. 17). This is typical of many breeds such as the German Boxer, French Bulldog, British Bulldog, Pekingese, etc.

The counterpart of this is **Brachygnathia inferior** ("Undershot") (Fig. 18). This is an hereditary shortening of the lower jaw and is often seen in the Dachshund, Collie, etc.

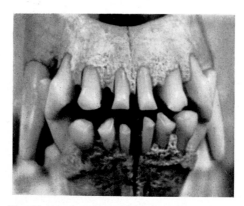

Fig. 15. Age: 8–9 years. The frictional surfaces of the medial incisors of the lower jaw have the shape of a reversed oval.

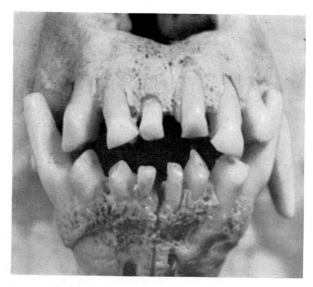

Fig. 16. Age: 9–10 years. The frictional surfaces of the incisors of the upper jaw have the shape of a reversed oval.

When estimating age by dental wear one must take into account the relative hardness of the teeth. In large breeds (St. Bernard, Great Dane, Borzois, etc.) the teeth are softer than in the smaller breeds (Dachshund, Pomeranian, Pinscher, etc.). When estimating age in the former breeds, therefore, we should estimate rather younger, and in the latter breeds, rather older ages, than the signs of wear

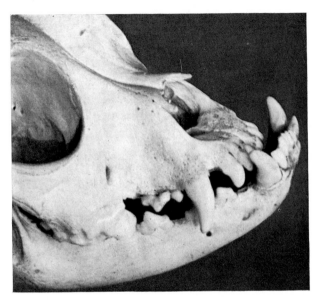

Fig. 17. Superior Brachygnathia. There can be no wear of opposing teeth due to lack of apposition.

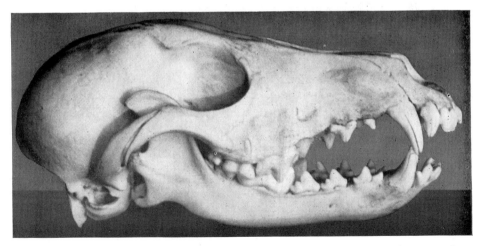

Fig. 18. Inferior Brachygnathia. Normal wear of the opposing teeth cannot be expected.

appear to suggest. Dental wear is also influenced by differences in the use of the teeth (dogs eager to retrieve and carry objects), the mode of life (lap dogs) and especially the type of diet.

In estimating age we must also take into account the facial expression and general comportment of the dog, greying of the hair and changes in the eyes.

The facial expression. A young dog (about 1 year old) has an alert expression with a bright lively look: at the age of 2 to 4 years, and according to the breed and individual temperament, it is still lively and alert, but in older animals (over 7 years old) it is more phlegmatic and sober in mien.

Comportment. In the young dog, the bearing of the body is not very expressive, the animals showing the awkwardness of youth in their movements. At 2 to 5 years old a certain poise is apparent in their bearing, whilst the old dog (over 10 years) is slower and more deliberate in its movements, often shows a downward curvature of the back and walks heavily with a stoop.

Greying of the hair. In many dogs (white haired, yellowish white or white and coloured) a few grey hairs may be indistinguishable from other similar hairs. Furthermore, certain breeds, e. g. black poodles, spaniels, Newfoundlands, etc., do not show grey hairs when they age. Usually one finds the first grey hairs, at first sparse, but later more abundant, around the lips and chin, then on the back and around the nose, then the eyelids and eyebrows, the forehead and ears until finally the whole head may be grey. Isolated grey hairs on the chin and lip areas may well become apparent at $4\frac{1}{2}$ years and are obvious at 5 to 6 years. Greying of the hair increases at intervals of $\frac{1}{2}$ to 18 year so that usually a dog over 10 years old shows numerous grey hairs around the eyes and on the forehead. A completely grey head is mainly seen in dogs over 13 years old. Greying of the hair may occur earlier in dogs suffering from chronic debilitating diseases. Quite often in very old dogs the grey hairs extend also over the neck and chest and the extremities.

Ocular changes. About 12 to 18 months before the development of true senile cataract, inspection of the eyes will reveal a grey light reflex, the so called age reflex. This reflex is due to differences in refraction caused by commencing sclerosis of the perinuclear layers and the nucleus of the crystalline lens. If a light is shone into the eye, it is reflected in the form of greenish-blue concentric rings. The age reflex is first seen at about 7 to $7\frac{1}{2}$ years of age, and transient variations may appear from time to time. It is most evident when the dog is between $7\frac{1}{2}$ to $8\frac{1}{2}$ years old.

The change from the age reflex to the formation of a cataract becomes noticeable between $8\frac{1}{2}$ and 9 years of age on an average. The cataract formation is always bilateral and is perinuclear in situation. On examination of the eye by reflected light in the early stages, one sees a circular, central and pericentral, light grey turbidity with a clearly distinguishable brilliant green reflex, especially at the circumference of the turbidity. Using transmitted light, the lesion appears as a disc-shaped, darker opacity. The fundus can still be seen, but it appears somewhat distorted. As the condition progresses, the turbidity seen by reflected light becomes more opaque and is clearly demarcated from the unchanged and transparent marginal zone, along the equator of the lens capsule. Examination by transmitted light often reveals numerous small, dark dots, close to one another in the region of the cataract, which represent small fissures or spaces filled with turbid fluid. More rarely in very old dogs there may be variable numbers of small, radially arranged, wedge-shaped striations in the zone of the equator, rather like the spokes of a wheel. In the rarest cases there may be complete turbidity of the perinuclear zone. Incipient senile cataract usually appears about nine years of age and is present in most dogs of ten years. The condition remains unchanged for a very long time and appears to cause little disability. True senile cataract, with more pronounced turbidity and dense opacity, may be seen sporadically at $9\frac{1}{2}$ years old, but may occur from $6\frac{1}{2}$ to 11 years of age. Again the condition usually remains unchanged for several years and seldom leads to total blindness.

3. Methods of restraint

In order to handle and examine patients, many of whom are of uncertain temperament, it is essential that one should be familiar with methods of control and restraint. The dog should be approached quietly while speaking in a calm, coaxing voice, and the back of the closed hand should be extended towards the animal. If there is no aggressive response the dog can be gently stroked on the back and

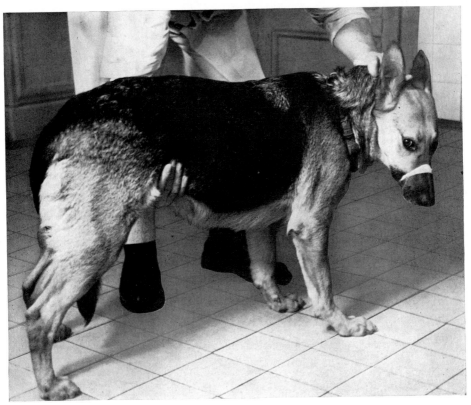

Fig. 19. Lifting a big dog on to the table.

sides of the chest working up to the head. To lift the animal on to the examination
table, the scruff of the neck is gripped with one hand, close to the occiput and the
free arm is bent under the abdomen in larger dogs (Fig. 19), or the hand placed
under the chest in the smaller breeds (Fig. 20). Small dogs should not be lifted by
the forelegs as this may cause strain of the shoulder muscles. Never rely on the

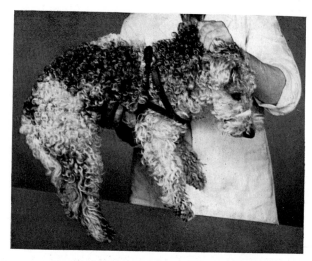

Fig. 20. Lifting a small dog on to the table.

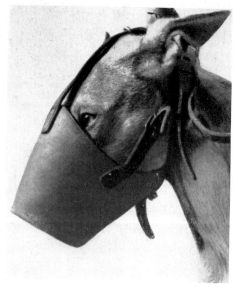

Fig. 21. "Box muzzle." It can also be used to prevent the dog licking certain parts of the body.

owner's assurance that the dog does not bite; it is always safer to apply a tape or a box muzzle (Fig. 21) before proceeding with any treatment. A tape muzzle may be applied by looping a piece of tape or bandage (1–2 cm width) around the jaws with one hitch on the bridge of the nose, returning the loop under the mandible with another hitch, passing the tape behind the ears and tying (Fig. 22). If the dog is

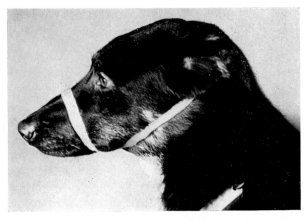

Fig. 22. Dog with tape muzzle applied.

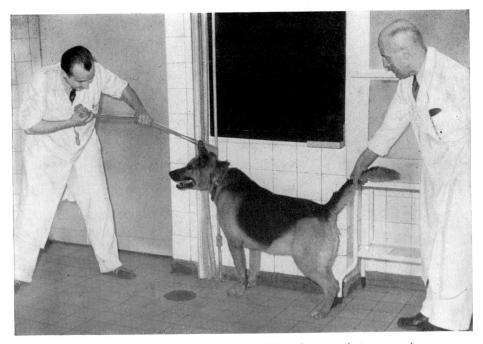

Fig. 23. Securing a snappy dog to the wall in order to apply tape muzzle.

so aggressive as to be unapproachable, the leash is passed through a ring (or a hot water pipe) on the wall and pulled tight, so that the head is brought close to the ring. An assistant holds the dog by the tail, so that both ends of the body are controlled (Fig. 23). The dog can now be grasped by the scruff of the neck and held whilst the tape muzzle is applied. To lay the dog on its side, the legs on the far side of the body are grasped and pulled from under the animal (Fig. 24), the head being supported by the owner so that it does not come down too heavily. To restrain the dog in this position, the assistant leans over the animal's back and grasps

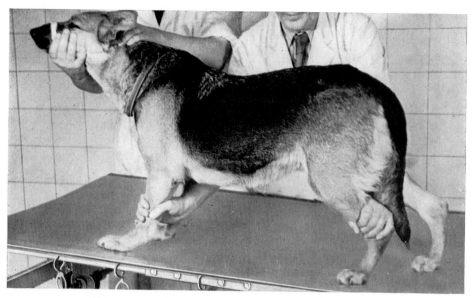

Fig. 24. Gripping a dog by the limbs of the opposite side in order to lay it down on its side.

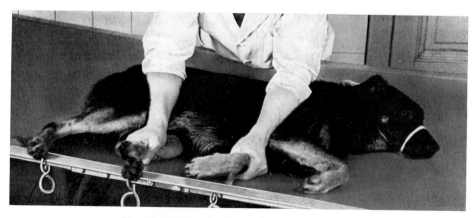

Fig. 25. Holding the dog in the lateral position.

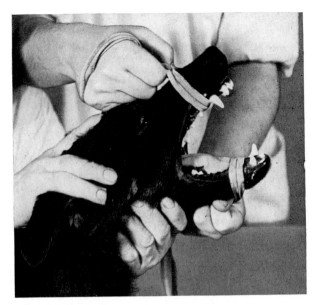

Fig. 26. Opening the jaws with tapes.

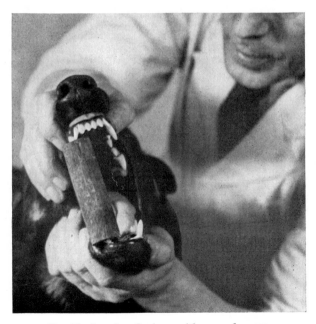

Fig. 27. Opening the jaws with a wooden gag.

the two underneath legs (Fig. 25). When the interior of the mouth has to be examined, the neck and lower jaw grip is used (Fig. 26). The thumb and index finger of the hand holding the lower jaw presses the dog's lip between the teeth, thus compelling the animal to open its mouth. If any manipulation is to be performed in the

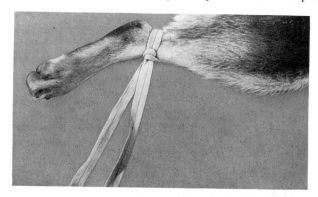

Fig. 28. Simple sling for the hind limb.

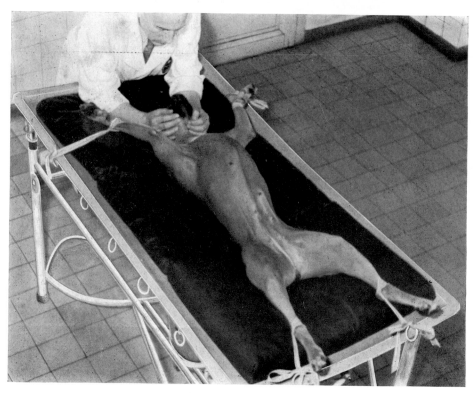

Fig. 29. A dog tied down on its back.

mouth it will be necessary to pass a loop behind the canines of both upper and lower jaws, so that the mouth can then be held open by an assistant. This should not be done by two people as the feel of the maximum opening of the jaws cannot be appreciated and luxation of the jaws might result. Another method, which has been recommended, is to place a wooden biting stick between the two canines of one side and then close the jaws on to this by means of a tape loop or with the hand (Fig. 27).

For surgery the dog has to be secured on its side by means of a double noose placed round the limb, proximal to the carpus on the forelegs and to the hock joint on the hind legs (Fig. 28). When the dog is restrained on its back, the limbs should be extended as much as possible (Fig. 29). When the dog is restrained on its side it is tied diagonally (Fig. 30), both pairs of limbs being secured together with a loop. The leg is tied with a double loop, the ends of which are passed around the second leg and then between the two limbs on the proximal side (Fig. 31). Whenever a dog is tied down, all knots must be of the quick release type in case of emergency. For operations in the perineal area, the dog is tied on its side with the upper leg drawn forward to expose the operation site (Fig. 32). The dog may be fixed on its sternum for certain operations (Fig. 33).

The subject of restraint is also concerned with the prevention of self inflicted trauma by licking, biting or scratching. The box muzzle already mentioned (see Fig. 21) prevents the dog from licking or biting, but injury may be produced by rubbing with the leather muzzle. In this case the Elizabethan collar (Fig. 34) offers the best means of protection.

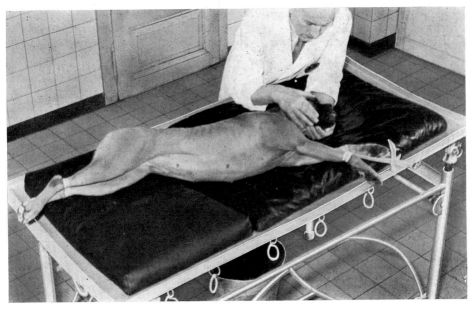

Fig. 30. A dog tied down diagonally in the lateral position.

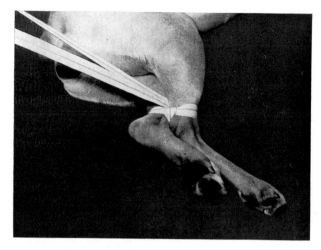

Fig. 31. Putting a double sling on the hind limb. After tightening the second sling, the sling is drawn distally.

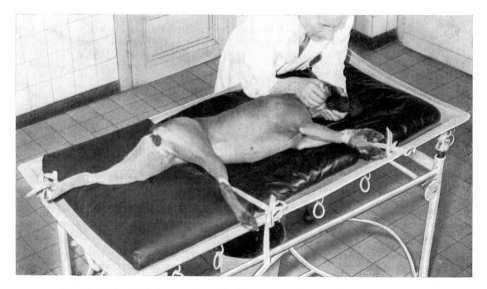

Fig. 32. A dog tied down on its side for an operation on the perineal region.

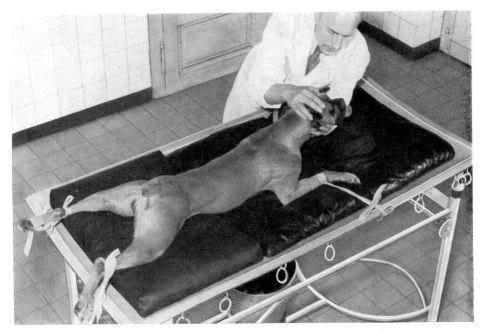

Fig. 33. A dog tied down in the ventral position.

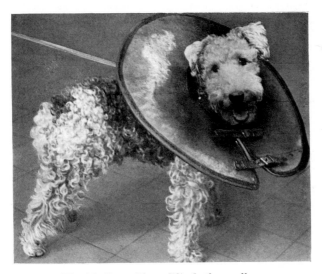

Fig. 34. Dog with an Elizabethan collar.

4. Techniques of administration of medicaments

To administer a tablet or a capsule the jaw is opened as described above, the tablet is placed behind the swelling formed by the tongue with the aid of curved dressing forceps (Fig. 35), and the jaws held closed. Swallowing can be encouraged by light pressure on the larynx. Where a fluid is being given, the dog's head is tilted upwards, the lips on one side are drawn back, so that a pouch is formed into

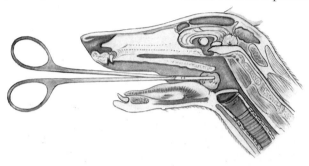

Fig. 35. Administration of solids.

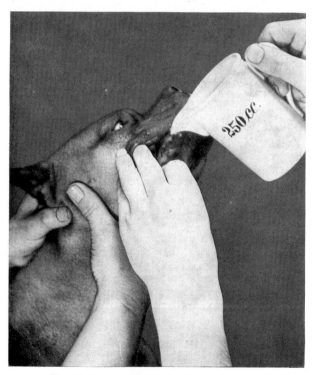

Fig. 36. Pouring fluid into the cheek pouch.

which the fluid is poured carefully (Fig. 36). The fluid passes around the back of, and through the molar teeth and into the pharyngeal area, thus stimulating the swallowing reflex in most dogs. When the animal is obstinate, light stroking of the larynx or holding the nostrils firmly closed will usually make the dog swallow. If accurate doses of liquid medicine have to be administered, or if the dog is very troublesome, it is best to use a stomach tube. A perforated wooden block is inserted between the incisors and the jaws are then firmly closed by the neck and lower jaw grip. The head is tilted backwards and the stomach tube is passed through the hole in the block into the oesophagus (Fig. 37). If the tube enters the trachea, violent coughing usually results and respiratory sounds can be heard through the tube. Apart from the administration of medicine, the stomach tube can also be employed for gastric lavage, or to siphon off the stomach contents for examination. Water at body temperature is passed into the stomach tube, the funnel end of the tube is lowered below the stomach level, and the fluid is then siphoned out of the

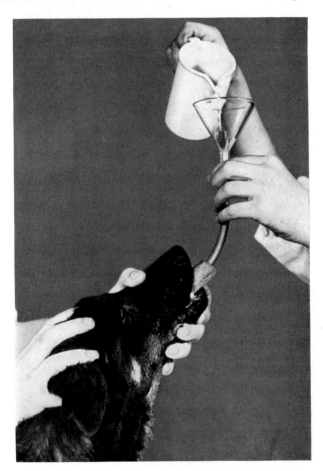

Fig. 37. Administration of fluid by means of a stomach tube.

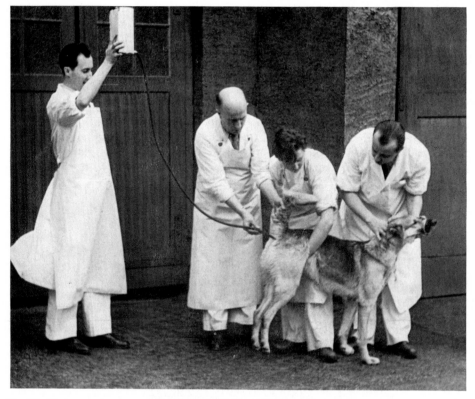

Fig. 38. Giving a pressure enema with the dog's hind end raised. Epidural anaesthesia is necessary because of marked straining.

stomach. Stomach contents may also be sucked out by connecting the stomach tube, via a vacuum collecting flask to a water siphon.

Drugs may also be administered by the rectal route. If the dog is highly strung or snappy, the drug is best given in the form of a suppository and usually the owner can manage the procedure quite easily. Small amounts of liquid may be given in the form of a rectal infusion or enema. The rectum is first cleared with a normal enema or the procedure is performed after a normal bowel evacuation. The fluid should be at body temperature and is given slowly, otherwise it will be expelled. Advantages of this route are: (a) the drug, although incompletely absorbed, will pass directly via the portal vein to the liver and is not altered by the action of the stomach secretions; (b) drugs, which are gastric irritants and would cause vomiting or anorexia, can be given per rectum. To give an absorption enema of this kind, a Janet or a Schimmelbusch syringe, attached to a rubber tube, is used. Enemas may also be used to clear the lower bowel or to flush out the alimentary tract in reverse. To do this a large enema can (about 2 litres) with a long tube to increase the pressure is used (Fig. 38). The dog may be held with the hindquarters

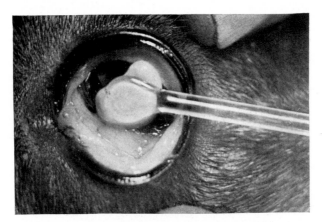

Fig. 39. Introduction of ointment into the eye.

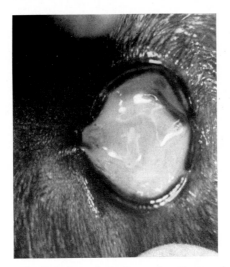

Fig. 40. The ointment is distributed evenly in the conjunctival sac by massage of the lids.

raised and fluid introduced until vomiting occurs. If the dog strains excessively epidural anaesthesia may be induced to eliminate the straining.

In ophthalmic work, drugs often must be introduced into the conjunctival sac. Eye drops may be instilled with a dropper with the lower lid drawn down. Eye ointments may be squeezed directly from the tube on to the eyeball, or smeared on a glass rod, which is applied so that the ointment adheres to the cornea (Fig. 39), or the lids are closed over the rod which is then withdrawn and the ointment evenly distributed over the conjunctival sac by gently massaging the eyelids (Fig. 40).

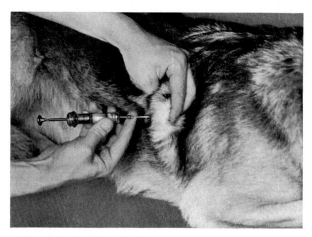

Fig. 41. Subcutaneous injection.

Administration of drugs by injection is said to be parenteral, i. e. it by-passes the digestive tract, and may be subcutaneous, intramuscular, intravenous, intraperitoneal, or intratracheal. The advantage of parenteral over peroral or enteral administration is that the drug passes rapidly into the bloodstream and without alteration or dilution by the intestinal contents, thus achieving a higher blood level. A possible disadvantage is that the excretion of the drug or its by-products by the kidneys occurs more rapidly than when given by the mouth. According to the drug or the method used, the injection can have either a general effect on the whole body, or only a local action. For every type of injection, the following conditions must be rigorously followed. The syringe must be sterile, the needle must be of a suitable size and the solution should be at body temperature. The injection site must be clean and disinfected. For a subcutaneous injection, unfortunately, one cannot always cut the hair short because the owner is usually not agreeable to this. The injection must always be given slowly.

Subcutaneous injections. We give subcutaneous injections into the side of the chest, although many practitioners inject under the loose skin of the neck. The disadvantage of this site is that if an abscess forms, due to a reaction to the drug injected, it is more difficult to treat, as in this position pouching or pocketing of pus can occur. To make a subcutaneous injection, a fold of skin is lifted and the needle is pushed through the skin with a short thrust (Fig. 41). By moving the needle back and forward in a short arc, one can determine whether the needle is freely movable and whether in fact it is under the surface skin and not in the fascia or even in the thorax. After the injection has been made, the site is lightly massaged to distribute the fluid under the skin. This facilitates and hastens the absorption. To increase the rapidity of the absorption a hyaluronidase preparation is recommended. Hyaluronidase increases the ability to absorb water, reduces surface tension and thus decreases viscosity and increases permeability. One can give hyaluronidase together with the drug in a single injection as long as the pH is between 4.0 and 7.5. Outside this pH range the hyaluronidase is inactivated.

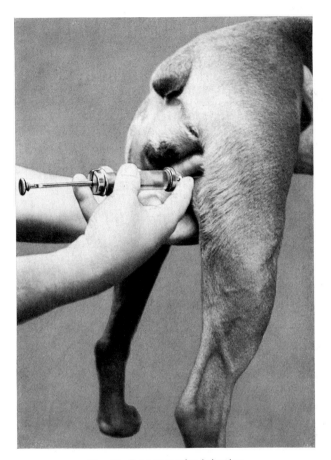

Fig. 42. Intramuscular injection.

We first inject the hyaluronidase preparation, leave the needle *in situ* and then shortly afterwards give the required drug through the same needle. About 3–10 VRE (viscosity reduction units) are injected. It is necessary to take care with this method as the acceleration of absorption may also increase the toxicity of the drug.

Intramuscular injection. Intramuscular injection in the dog is given into the muscle of the hindquarters, the muscles being the biceps femoris, the semi-tendinosus, or the semimembranosus. The needle is thrust vertically and deep into the muscle (Fig. 42). Before making the injection it is advisable to withdraw the plunger of the syringe, so that, if a blood vessel has been punctured, blood will be drawn into the syringe. The position of the needle can then be altered and the injection given in another site.

Intravenous injection. Intravenous injection is given into the small saphenous vein, the jugular vein or the cephalic vein. The hair over the site is clipped, or in long-haired luxury dogs the hair can be parted. The injection site is then well

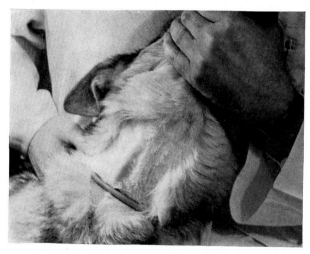

Fig. 43. Compression of the jugular vein to make it stand out.

moistened with spirit or water in order to fix the small particles of dirt in the hairs and to disinfect the skin. Intravenous injection into the jugular vein is not very often used in the dog (Fig. 43). This site is mainly used for taking blood, and for this purpose a relatively large needle is used. The dog is restrained on its sternum, the assistant raises the head as far as possible with one hand and with the other tightens a tourniquet placed round the neck, so that the jugular vein is compressed (Fig. 44). Intravenous injection into the small saphenous vein is performed with the dog lying on its side. The hind legs must be well compressed so that the vein becomes evident (Fig. 45). To make the injection easier the raised vein should be first lightly tapped with two fingers, employing a wrist action, in order to stimulate the muscle of the vein to contract. Some breeds, e. g. Chow-chows, often have what are called "roller veins", which make intravenous injection extremely difficult. In order to fix such veins they are frozen with ethyl chloride spray. To insert the needle the hind leg is grasped over the hock joint with the free hand (the right leg with the left hand), the thumb and forefinger being placed alongside the raised vein. When the needle is inserted it is fixed with the thumb and fore-finger of this hand whilst the other fingers firmly enclose the hind leg (Fig. 46).

In this way the needle cannot be dislodged from the vein even if the animal struggles. If an irritant drug is accidentally injected extra-vascularly, 5–10 VRE of hyaluronidase should be injected into the site immediately, in order to avoid inflammation and sloughing of the tissues.

Intravenous injection into the cephalic vein is used in the small, fine-skinned breeds (Pinscher) and the shortlegged dogs (Dachshund). The dog is restrained on its sternum and the foreleg is compressed over the elbow joint with a rubber tourniquet or with the hand (Fig. 47). With the free hand (left hand for right leg), the leg is held so that the thumb and first finger lie alongside the vein and can be used to control the needle in the vein as in the hind leg (Fig. 48).

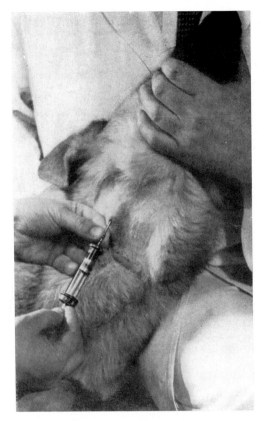

Fig. 44. Taking blood from the jugular vein.

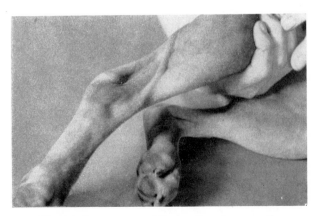

Fig. 45. Compression of the small saphenous vein.

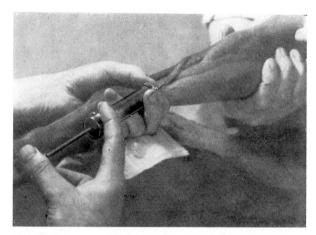

Fig. 46. Intravenous injection into the small saphenous vein.

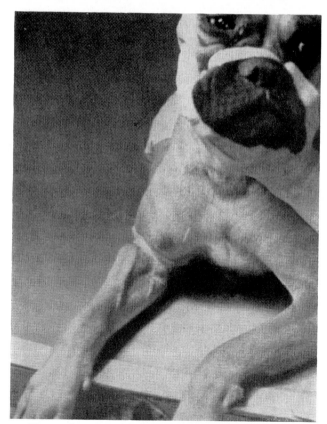

Fig. 47. Compression of the ante-brachial cephalic vein.

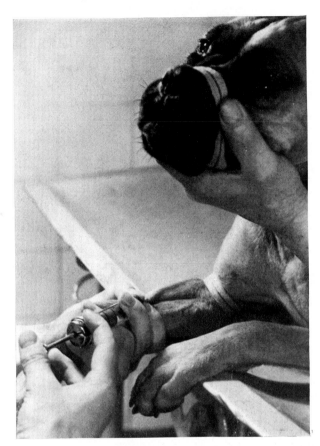

Fig. 48. Intravenous injection into the ante-brachial cephalic vein.

Before making an intravenous injection, the plunger of the syringe should be withdrawn a little to allow blood to enter the syringe, thus confirming that the needle is actually within the vein. On completion of the injection, a few drops of blood should be allowed to flow from the needle before it is withdrawn, to ensure that no irritant drug escapes into the perivascular tissues from the punctured vein. Finally the site is lightly compressed with a swab to check leakage of blood and prevent haematoma formation.

Intratracheal injection is performed by inserting the needle between two tracheal rings. The patient is restrained on its sternum with the head tilted back, the trachea is fixed with the thumb and forefinger of the free hand and the needle inserted (Fig. 49).

Intraperitoneal injection is made with the dog lying on its side, the needle being inserted at right angles to the abdominal wall, lateral and caudal to the umbili-

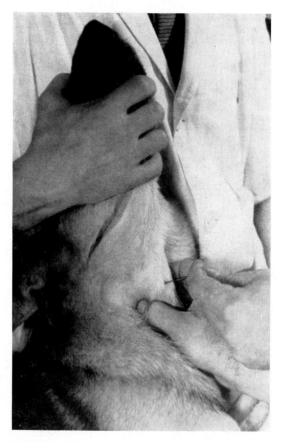

Fig. 49. Intratracheal injection. The trachea is fixed with the thumb and forefinger of the right
hand.

cus (Fig. 50). Absorption of drugs through the peritoneum is extremely rapid,
by-passing the liver barrier, so that this route is a practicable alternative to the
intravenous route, where the latter is too difficult, e. g. very small dogs or where
the veins are collapsed.

Intra-articular injection may be made into the shoulder, elbow or stifle joints
without great difficulty, but it is important that asepsis should be strictly observed.

Subconjunctival injection is used in certain ocular conditions in the dog and is
quite easily accomplished with a fine needle and the use of a surface anaesthetic.
The head must be held immobile during the injection (Figs. 51–53).

**Editor's note: Many clinicians would prefer to administer a short-acting general
anaesthetic in these cases, as a sudden movement by the dog may cause severe
damage to the eye.**

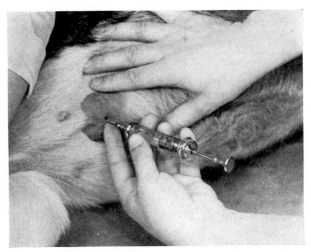

Fig. 50. Intraperitoneal injection.

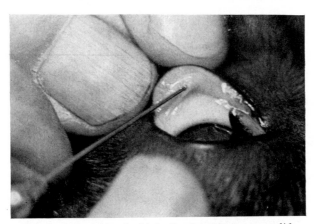

Fig. 51. Subconjunctival injection into the upper eyelid.

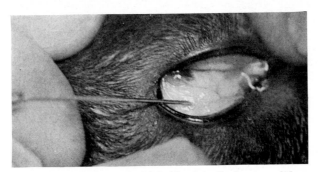

Fig. 52. Subconjunctival injection into the lower eyelid.

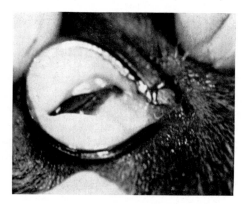

Fig. 53. Reaction to subconjunctival injection. The conjunctivae of both lids have become oedematous.

5. Physical therapy

In many diseases, physical therapy may be usefully employed as an adjunct to medical or surgical treatment. Some measures, such as massage, Priessnitz compresses, fomentations, etc., can be delegated to the owner, but more specialised techniques, such as diathermy, ultraviolet ray therapy, microwaves, etc., must be performed by the veterinarian. Some physiotherapy techniques used in human medicine, such as Sitz baths, underwater massage, etc., are rather impracticable in canine medicine. Too much emphasis should not be placed on physical therapy, which is an adjunct to, and not a substitute for, specific treatment, but it has a definite place in treatment and is not designed just to keep the owner occupied or to impress with gleaming, chromium-plated apparatus.

Massage can be given to the dog in the form of active exercise or by passive massage. Controlled exercise on a leash and in a harness is used in chronic lameness resulting from healed fractures, luxations, orthopaedic procedures, etc. The exercise should be designed to make the dog use the affected leg, e. g. by strapping up the opposite leg, first at a walk and then at a trot. The dog should not be allowed to gallop as then all four legs are subjected to an equal amount of stress. Passive massage improves the circulation of the skin or the muscles or organs lying beneath it. Commencing at the extremities, the massage is applied in the direction of the heart, thus improving the venous return and hastening the transport of metabolic wastes. The arterial blood flow is also improved and this leads to a better vascularisation of the affected area. Adhesions and fibrosis can often be broken down and dispersed by massage. Massage is usually given as a precursor to active exercise and is used in chronic disabilities following fractures, luxations, the nervous sequelae of distemper, etc. It may be used to relieve painful muscular cramps and spasms in the rheumatoid syndromes, but it is contra-indicated in very acute inflammatory conditions. In the dog, massage may be given by stroking, rubbing, kneading, tapotement or pressure with the flat of the hand or a brush with strong bristles. Sometimes oils or ointments may be rubbed into the skin after the hair has been clipped short. When a stimulant action on the circulation is required, camphor preparations such as spirits of camphor or 20 % camphor ointment may be employed.

Ultrasonic therapy can be regarded as a refined form of passive massage. Oscillations are produced by induced electrical changes in crystals with one or more polar axes. The oscillations are emitted as ultrasonic waves, focused to cover only a few square centimetres, and producing a thermal effect by their passage through the tissues. The value of ultrasonic therapy in veterinary medicine has still to be proved.

Hydrotherapy, the external use of water, not only has a local effect on the skin but also on the organs and tissues lying beneath it. The water acts as a stimulus which, according to the temperature, causes warm or cold sensations with corresponding reactions in the tissues. This effect is similar to the stimulation of the sympathetic (cold) or parasympathetic (warm) nervous systems. There is a certain temperature range (the indifferent zone), which produces neither warm nor cold stimuli. In man the zone lies between 34° and 36 °C, but for the dog it is much lower at about 15°–20 °C. Cold causes contraction of the peripheral blood vessels, substantially reducing the calibre of the capillary bed and thus producing a rise in blood pressure. If the cold stimulus is transient, there is an increase in nerve sensibility, but if it is prolonged, as with the use of ice packs, the nerves become paralysed (the principle underlying cold anaesthesia). This nervous paralysis eventually produces relaxation of the muscular coats of the constricted blood vessels and so hyperaemia results. Warmth relaxes the peripheral blood vessels, opening out the capillary bed, and producing a fall in blood pressure. Oxidative processes in the tissues are accelerated by warmth and there is a stimulation of the breakdown of albuminous substances.

Baths are mainly used for cleansing purposes in the dog and should not be given too frequently, as soaps and shampoos dissolve the fine fatty and sebaceous substances out of the hair and destroy the water-repellent properties of the coat. Antiparasitic baths should not be used as a routine measure as untoward skin reactions may occur.

Foot baths may be used in certain conditions. For example, very warm, oak bark baths may be used in interdigital eczema, and cold, oak bark baths are used for dogs with sensitive pads, or when the pads are abraded after running over frozen or rough ground.

Amongst the wet compresses, probably the most important is the Priessnitz pad, which is based on the interaction of warmth and cold. Two types of pack are used, the permeable and the impermeable. In the permeable form a linen cloth is saturated with cold water, lightly wrung out and firmly fixed around the affected part of the body. Over the wet cloth a woollen scarf is wrapped so that it overlaps the cloth in front and behind by one to three fingers' breadth. This overlapping is important as otherwise evaporation of the water occurs with a resultant chilling effect which defeats the purpose of the compress. The cold stimulus of the wet pack causes an initial vaso-constriction and consequent rise in blood pressure, but the paralysing effect of the prolonged cold soon relaxes the peripheral vessels and a reactionary hyperaemia occurs. This hyperaemia is increased by the warmth now accumulating under the woollen covering. In the impermeable form of the

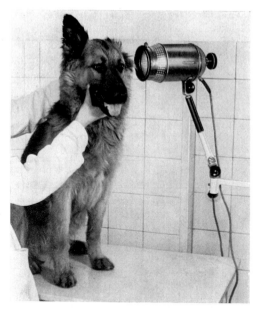

Fig. 54. Infrared treatment of the ear.

Priessnitz pack, the effect of the moist heat is accentuated, as here a waterproof layer, made of guttapercha, rubber cloth or parchment paper, is placed between the linen cloth and the woollen covering. The pack is left in position for about $1-1\frac{1}{2}$ hr, then the wet part is removed, the woollen covering remaining in place for another hour to allow the heat reaction to subside. The pack may be repeated two or three times a day, but should never be left on at night. The Priessnitz pack is indicated in acute conditions of the larynx, the pharynx, trachea and lungs, and it is recommended for the relief of acute and painful conditions of the stomach and intestines.

Cold compresses are employed to reduce heat, either in the body as a whole or at the site of a local inflammation. They are also used to produce vaso-constriction in cases of haemorrhage, haematoma formation, cerebral concussion, etc. To the stimulus of the cold water is added that of the cold due to evaporation, so that a double action is achieved. Prolonged cooling, however, will lead to a reactionary hyperaemia and thus counteract the desired effect.

Hot compresses are especially valuable where it is desirable to encourage leuco-cytosis, in addition to promoting a local hyperaemia, e. g. to hasten the ripening of an abscess. The compress is covered with an impermeable rubber or plastic cloth to limit evaporation, otherwise they soon cool. We like to use hot compresses in the treatment of keratitis, the compress being applied to the closed eye and left on for 5–7 min. The procedure should be repeated several times daily; if the compress is left on continuously it is not so effective.

Warmth can also be applied by radiant heat in the form of infrared radiation (Fig. 54). Infrared irradiation is chiefly employed in the treatment of superficial

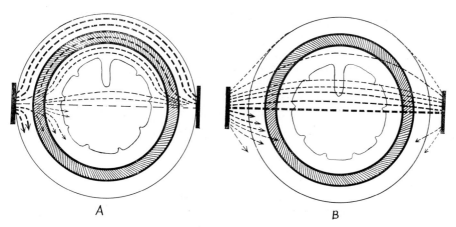

Fig. 55. Current distribution for long-wave diathermy (A) and in the short-wave field (B) in the skull, according to Schliephake. It is assumed that the current flows only in one direction from left to right. The dotted lines show the current distribution. The strength of the current is expressed by the thickness of the lines.

lesions, such as abscesses, otitis, etc., as the rapid warming of the skin which occurs prevents any really deep effect of the treatment. Infrared treatment is usually applied for 5–10 min at a session.

Warmth may also be engendered in the body by the use of electricity. Passage of electricity through the tissues produces Joule's heat, which is directly related to the resistance of the tissue components and the amount of current employed. One must differentiate between diathermy (long wave), short wave, and ultra-short wave therapy. Diathermy operates at a frequency of 800,000–1,000,000 oscillations per second, corresponding to a wavelength of 300–500 m. The dia-thermal current is an "output" current, so that the electrodes must be connected directly to the body as any interposed non-conducting material, such as air, will block the current. A similar phenomenon occurs within the body, where the current will pass around non-conductors such as bone, etc. (see Fig. 55 A). In veterinary medicine, diathermy has largely been displaced by short or micro-wave therapy, due to the technical difficulties involved in its use in animals. The electrodes must be fixed with bandages to either side of the dog, and if badly positioned may cause severe burns due to auto-overheating.

Short waves operate at a wavelength of 11–6 m; the higher their frequency and the correspondingly shorter their wavelength, the greater their effect. They can flow through non-conductors without diminution, they have a uniform action in depth and produce good temperature rises in the internal organs (Fig. 55 B). The short waves are applied by the condenser field method, whereby the capacity effect of the high frequency field is used between two condenser plates lying in a secondary circuit. Short waves are used in various stages of inflammatory or purulent conditions, especially in acute types, vascular disorders, paralyses, nervous sequelae of distemper, rheumatoid disease, etc. (Fig. 56). Certain pre-cautions must be observed during therapy if accidents are to be avoided and the

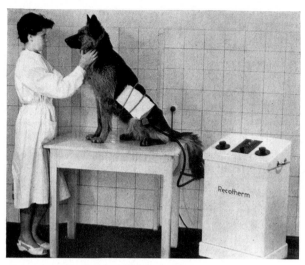

Fig. 56. Short-wave therapy.

best results attained. The dog must not be in contact with any metallic object, e. g. table, metal collar, etc., and should be lying comfortably with as little movement as possible, so that the electrical field is not appreciably disturbed. The control switch should be so adjusted that the control light is at maximum illumination. Electrodes are arranged according to the severity and site of the lesion, the greater the space between the electrodes the greater the depth of penetration of the waves. A spacing of 1–6 cm between electrodes is designed to give optimum results; if it is necessary to increase the distance, then perforated felt inserts are used. The latter, the electrodes and the skin of the patient must be kept dry. It is important to choose the correct dosage of short waves, so that no unpleasant heat sensations, evidenced by restlessness of the patient, occur. In general, in acute diseases, small doses are used in repeated daily sessions, whilst in chronic conditions larger doses are employed two or three times a week. In the initial stages of treatment sessions should be limited to 2–10 min at a time, but later these periods can be extended to 10–20 min or even longer.

In ultra-short-wave therapy, the counterpart of the condenser field system described above is the "coil field" method. In this method, heat is produced in the tissues by induction via eddy currents. An induction coil is placed around or in contact with the part of the body under treatment and is connected with a high frequency generator. The high frequency magnetic alternating current sets up eddy currents in the tissues which produce heat. If short waves are shortened still further, one can produce waves a decimetre or a centimetre long, the microwaves. Very high frequency electromagnetic oscillations (up to 3000 MHz) are generated in a magnetic field tube (Magnetron) by a stream of electrons issuing from the cathode into a heating filament arranged axially and directed through the solenoid (the magnetic field of a magnetic coil) into coiled orbits. A wavelength of 12.4 cm

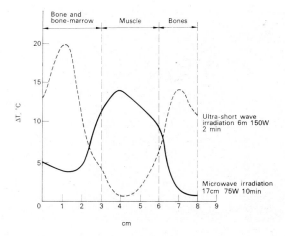

Fig. 57. Behaviour of a three-layer medium (bone with bone marrow, muscle and bone) to ultra short wave and microwave irradiation, according to Hübner.

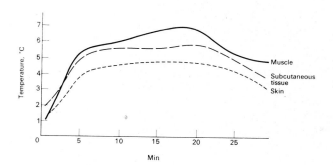

Fig. 58. Heating in human tissue in micro-wave irradiation.

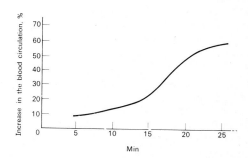

Fig. 59. Increase in the blood circulation in micro-wave irradiation.

4*

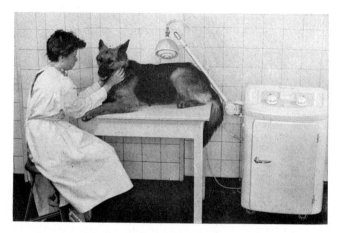

Fig. 60. Micro-wave therapy with the circular field irradiator.

(2450 MHz) has been found to be the most useful in treatment. The energy is fed through a coaxial cable to a dipole, focused by a concave mirror, and directed as free radiation on to the affected portion of the body. This system frees the technique from the limitations imposed by the two electrodes of the short wave apparatus.

When short waves are used, there is always a marked heating of the subcutaneous fat, but with microwaves absorption by bone and fat is well below that in tissues with a high water content. This means that the therapeutically desirable heat effect occurs particularly in the muscles and the other well-vascularised organs, an effect clearly shown by Figs. 57 and 58. There is a marked increase in the circulation of the region irradiated, warmth following the reddening of the skin due to active hyperaemia. This effect gradually diminishes peripherally but is effective over the whole of the irradiated area. If the dosage has been assessed correctly, the warming and reddening of the irradiated area of skin attains a maximum intensity and then remains constant, apart from small variations. Dilatation and elongation of the capillaries occurs, the circulation is speeded up with a consequent improvement in the nutrition of the tissues (Fig. 59).

Indications for microwave therapy are essentially the same as for shortwave treatment, e. g. acute and chronic inflammations (especially the ripening of abscesses, pneumonia, cystitis, intra-abdominal adhesions after laparotomies, post-operative conditions, etc.), nervous sequelae of distemper, vascular disorders, rheumatoid conditions, etc.

We use the "Radarmed" microwave machine, consisting of a round emitter for universal use (Fig. 60) and a longitudinal field emitter (Fig. 61) which is designed for use with large dogs, for radiation of the whole of the limb or the vertebral column. The emitter is placed about 15–20 cm from the organ to be treated, which means that in some cases it is only 5–10 cm from the patient's body.

Dosage must be tailored to suit the needs of the individual patient. As the dog cannot report its experiences, dosage should be tested on the operator first. As

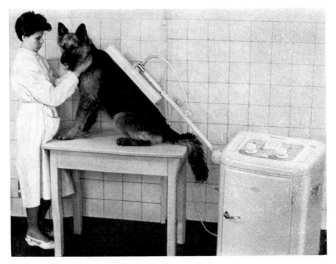

Fig. 61. Micro-wave therapy with a longitudinal field irradiator.

with short wave therapy, the more acute the disease, the lower the dose and the more frequent the treatment; chronic conditions can be subjected to higher doses at longer intervals. Depending upon the site and the condition to be treated, we start with a dose of between 20–40 W for 4–7 min, later increasing this to 80 W for about 20 min.

Electrotherapy

Under this heading, the only method used in the dog is galvanisation, i. e. treatment with direct or with low-frequency alternating current (Faradisation). The constant galvanic current produces a different effect according to the direction of the current flow. If the positive electrode (anode) is placed at the extremity of the limb and the negative electrode (cathode) near to the central nervous system, the musculature will be strongly stimulated with resultant marked muscle contractions. If the position of the electrodes is reversed, a paralysing effect occurs extending from the central nervous system, the so-called "galvano-narcosis".

The muscle-stimulating effect is sometimes used for the treatment of the flaccid paralysis of the hind limbs which occurs following distemper. The electrodes and the hair at the site of application must be thoroughly moistened with salt water to lessen the resistance. The muscles are thrown into contraction by switching the current on and off, the dosage being carefully adjusted to suit the individual patient. Dogs appear to be more sensitive to galvanic currents than do human beings. A course of treatment which does not exceed 2–3 min per session and which is repeated 2–3 times a week appears to be sufficient in most cases. Quite often owners refuse further treatment as the convulsive-like muscle contractions are rather alarming to an inexperienced observer.

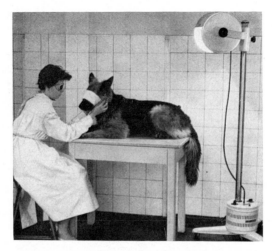

Fig. 62. Ultraviolet irradiation. The eyes of the attendants and of the patient must be protected.

Light therapy in the form of ultraviolet light is occasionally used in the treatment of rickets and sometimes prophylactically in a litter of young puppies. Other indications for ultraviolet irradiation are eczemas of various kinds, delayed healing of wounds, otitis externa, etc. The patient is irradiated with the ultraviolet rays at a distance of 80 to 100 cm for 4 to 6 min, two to three times a week. It is advisable to cover the eyes with a pair of goggles or with strips of celluloid and the operator should also wear a pair of goggles (Fig. 62).

6. Treatment of bacterial infections

Chemotherapy plays an important part in the treatment of bacterial infections and the effective use of this form of treatment was ushered in with the use of sulphonamides. Despite the widespread use of sulphonamides, certain important points must be borne in mind if the treatment is to be safe and effective. In therapeutic doses most sulphonamides are bacterio-static in action. This means that they inhibit the growth of bacteria, which are then killed by the body defences of the patient. In acute diseases therefore one can expect better results than in chronic diseases, because in the latter the body's defences may be so exhausted that they are no longer capable of offering serious resistance.

The sulphonamides soon attain a high blood level, but this unfortunately quickly falls below the effective level of 5 mg%. Many of the sulphonamides do not reach an effective blood level at all and therefore have only a local action (Fig. 63). After absorption, sulphonamides undergo acetylation (the addition of acetic acid) and form crystals which can produce irritant actions in the kidneys. In order to inhibit the formation of crystals as much as possible, it is advisable to give plenty of fluids during sulphonamide therapy so that the concentration

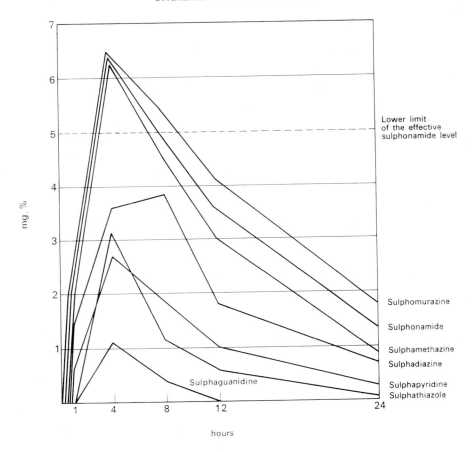

Fig. 63. Level of sulphonamides in the blood after a single oral administration of 71.5 mg per kg bodyweight to the dog. (Modified from SCHULZE, Mhefte vet. Med. **5**, 70 1950.)

of the sulphonamides in the urine is kept at a low level. In addition, oral administration should be given only on an empty stomach. In order to avoid acidosis, alkalis are advisable, e. g. sodium bicarbonate. Sulphonamides may be given internally as tablets or systemically by subcutaneous injection. As sulphonamides are aniline derivatives it is possible for them to cause haemoglobinaemia and sulphaemoglobinaemia. Sulphur, aperients, and antipyretics may assist in the formation of these substances, so they should not be given together with sulphonamides. Apparently sulphonamide treatment may produce a tendency to haemorrhage which may cause difficulties during surgery. Quite often their use locally for the treatment of raw wounds leads to post-operative bleeding, which can only be explained as due to the effect of the sulphonamides. Sulphonamides cause inhibition of micro organisms in wounds and they thus promote healing of such wounds, but one often gains the impression that the granulation of a wound is delayed by the use of these substances.

To achieve the best results with sulphonamides we must use the drugs for several days in a dosage which will give a sufficiently high blood level (5 to 8 mg%), and which lasts for about four days. If the patient's fever has not diminished within 3 days, treatment should be discontinued, because in these cases it is likely that the causative organism is not sensitive to the drug. Where a rapid fall of temperature occurs, treatment should be continued for a minimum of 4 days, otherwise a recrudescence of the infection may take place. Under-dosage or too short a dosage with sulphonamides may lead to the development of resistant strains of organisms.

The sensitivity of various organisms to sulphonamides can be seen in their spectrum of action given in Fig. 64. Where the brown divisions are only half-filled in, it implies that only certain individual sulphonamides are active or that their activity is not 100 %.

The soluble sulphonamide most commonly used in the dog is Sulphadimidine and this is usually administered by subcutaneous injection once daily. In acute infections the initial loading dose may be given intravenously and the blood level maintained by subcutaneous injections subsequently. A tablet form is also available.

To minimise the risk of crystalluria damaging the kidneys, different sulphonamides may be combined together in one tablet. In the dog, the most effective mixture contains Sulphamerazine, Sulphadiazine and Sulphapyridine. In recent years several long-acting sulphonamides have been developed which require only a single daily dose to produce therapeutic blood levels. Examples in use in canine medicine are Sulphamethyl-phenazole and Sulphamethoxypyridazine. A new antibacterial agent, Trimethoprim, has been synthesised which acts synergistically with sulphonamides by blocking a further bacterial metabolic pathway. For use in canine infections it is combined with Sulfamethoxazole, a sulphonamide which gives the most satisfactory blood levels in concert with Trimethoprim in the dog.

An unusual use for a sulphonamide was discovered accidentally during laboratory tests in rats. The substance, Sulphapyrimidine, had an apparent rejuvenating effect on the rats and the drug is now available for use in ageing dogs.

For topical treatment, powders or emulsions are used, the disadvantages of topical sulphonamide treatment having been mentioned above.

The increasing use of antibiotics is due to the fact that they have a wider spectrum of activity and therapeutically cover a much broader field, so that fewer toxic effects are to be expected than in many sulphonamides. Antibiotics are chemical substances which are produced by fermentation, or biological, or technical synthesis. In the dog the antibiotics in common use are Penicillin, Streptomycin, Tetracyclines and Chloramphenicol, whose spectrum of activity can be seen in Fig. 64. Other antibiotics used in canine medicine include Ampicillin and Neomycin.

Penicillin gives rise to practically no toxic or untoward side effects, the hypersensitive reactions seen in man not being observed in the dog. Treatment with Streptomycin (for leptospirosis) for a few days does not cause toxic symptoms, but if dosage is prolonged as it may be for tuberculosis, there is a grave risk of damage to the nervous system. This is manifested by signs of damage to the

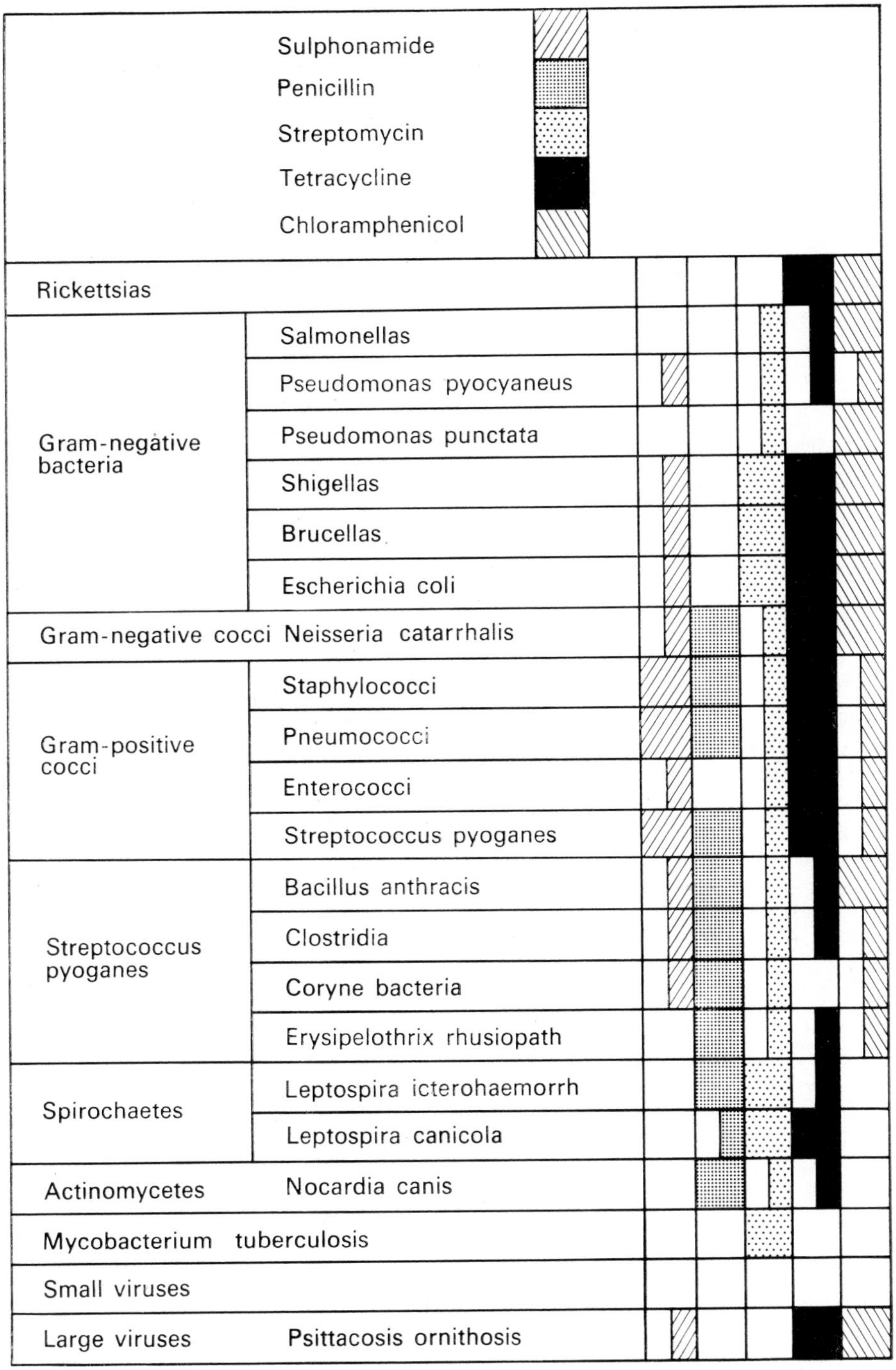

Legend (antibiotic patterns):

- Sulphonamide
- Penicillin
- Streptomycin
- Tetracycline
- Chloramphenicol

Group	Organism	Sulphonamide	Penicillin	Streptomycin	Tetracycline	Chloramphenicol
Rickettsias					■	▨
Gram-negative bacteria	Salmonellas				▨	▨
	Pseudomonas pyocyaneus	▨			■	▨
	Pseudomonas punctata					▨
	Shigellas	▨			■	▨
	Brucellas				■	▨
	Escherichia coli	▨			■	▨
Gram-negative cocci	Neisseria catarrhalis	▨				▨
Gram-positive cocci	Staphylococci	▨			■	▨
	Pneumococci	▨			■	▨
	Enterococci	▨			■	▨
	Streptococcus pyoganes	▨			■	▨
Streptococcus pyoganes	Bacillus anthracis	▨				▨
	Clostridia	▨			■	▨
	Coryne bacteria	▨				▨
	Erysipelothrix rhusiopath					▨
Spirochaetes	Leptospira icterohaemorrh					
	Leptospira canicola				■	
Actinomycetes	Nocardia canis				■	
Mycobacterium	tuberculosis					
Small viruses						
Large viruses	Psittacosis ornithosis	▨			■	▨

Fig. 64. Spectrum of the activity of the sulphonamides and antibiotics in the dog.

vestibular apparatus. Dogs suffering from nephritis should only receive a short dosage of this antibiotic, otherwise further damage to the kidney may result. Chloramphenicol may produce gastro-intestinal upsets especially where treatment is prolonged due to imbalance of the normal gut flora and an aplastic anaemia. Prolonged treatment with Chlortetracycline may lead to signs of a deficiency of vitamins K and B becoming apparent, so these vitamins should be administered during treatment with this antibiotic.

Penicillin should only be used where there are definite indications for it and not for trivial infections. Its topical application should also be restricted as there is a danger of producing penicillin-resistant strains. The antibiotic may be given by intramuscular or subcutaneous injection, or by the oral route. Penicillin G produces a rapid rise in the blood level but it is excreted rapidly so there is a rapid fall in the blood level. Conversely, Depot Penicillin produces a serum level more slowly but maintains it for 10 to 24 hr. If one combines Penicillin G and Depot Penicillin one gets the best of both worlds in obtaining rapidity of action and a longer dura- tion. The dosage of penicillin depends upon the type and the site of infection, the sensitivity of the organism involved, on the type of penicillin preparation used, the route of administration and the rate of absorption and excretion. Rapidly acting penicillins are penicillin G and sodium penicillin G. The dose of these is 10,000 international units per kilogram bodyweight at intervals of 6 hr. With the longer acting depot penicillins an injection once daily of 20,000 international units per kilogram bodyweight is usually sufficient. Both these types of penicillin may be combined to make an aqueous suspension. In this case the therapeutic blood level is maintained for about 24 hr. One injection of 20,000 international units per kilogram bodyweight daily is sufficient. Benethamine penicillin will give therapeutic blood levels for 3 days whilst Benzathine penicillin will give a prophylactic blood level for 3 weeks. Penicillin is inactivated by the presence of metals so as far as possible all-glass syringes should be used. Penicillin is also destroyed by alcohol, phenol, formalin, hydrogen peroxide, tincture of iodine, etc., and so these substances should not be used for storage of syringes or for disinfection of the skin.

Streptomycin given by intramuscular injection acts rapidly and its action persists for 9 to 12 hr. For systemic effect it must be given parenterally as it is almost completely non-absorbed from the digestive tract and for this reason is used orally for enteric infections.

The Tetracyclines are a group of antibiotics with similar basic chemical struc- tures. Their antibiotic action extends over most of the important bacterial diseases and for this reason they are known as broad spectrum antibiotics. In our clinic we use "Tetracycline", "Chlortetracycline" and "Oxytetracycline". "Chlor- tetracycline" may be given intravenously or orally. When given orally there is good absorption of the drug and this produces an effective blood level lasting for 6 to 8 hr. When given intravenously the activity is approximately 8 times that of orally administered "Aureomycin". Solutions intended for intravenous admini- stration should be well diluted and this route should only be used when oral ad- ministration is not practicable. Once made up, the injection solution must be used at once as it deteriorates rapidly under normal conditions. The drug is never administered orally on an empty stomach but should always be given after food. The oral dosage is 12.5 to 25 mg per kg bodyweight twice daily for 3 to 5 days.

When given intravenously the dog receives 10 mg per kg bodyweight initially and half this dose on the following day. "Tetracycline" is given in the same dosage as "Chlortetracycline". With "Oxytetracycline" the blood levels and mode of administration are essentially the same as for "Chlortetracycline". With intravenous injection 10 mg per kg bodyweight are given initially and 5 mg per kg the following day. If "Oxytetracycline" is given intramuscularly or subcutaneously, the dose is 10 mg per kg bodyweight once daily and for oral administration 25 mg per kg bodyweight 3 times a day.

Chloramphenicol is rapidly absorbed following oral administration and is used at an average dose of 50 mg per kg bodyweight daily for 3–5 days. An injectable preparation is also available.

Combinations of different antibiotics or antibiotic/sulphonamide mixtures are possible and this is shown in Fig. 64, but combinations of "Chlortetracycline", "Oxytetracycline" and chloramphenicol with penicillin are not recommended because they may be antagonistic to each other.

Ampicillin is one of the group of synthetic penicillins which have a wide spectrum of activity against both Gram negative and Gram positive organisms. This antibiotic is used in canine medicine mainly in the treatment of respiratory, enteric and urinary infections in a dose of 5–10 mg per kg every 12 hr.

Neomycin is used by the oral route for the treatment of enteric infections and in ointments, creams and lotions for ear, eye and skin infections. This antibiotic is ototoxic and nephrotoxic when used systemically and should not be used by this route.

7. Bandaging techniques

It can be extremely difficult to fix a well fitting bandage to a temperamental dog, as animals usually try to get rid of dressings or bandaging by scratching, rubbing or biting. In many cases, therefore, it is necessary to protect the bandage by various means (collars, muzzle, leather boots, etc.). If the bandage is put on too tightly, e. g. on the limbs, it may lead to obstruction to the circulation, or if it is put on too loosely it is easily removed by the patient.

Some typical bandages used for the dog will now be described. A bandage for the head is sometimes necessary after ophthalmic operations. To cover one eye, one puts on a monoculus, but the binoculus (Fig. 65) constitutes a better protection. In brachycephalic types of dog, eye bandages are contra-indicated because of the short nose. We use bandages of medium width (3–6 cm) and figure of eight turns are applied in such a way that both the patient's ears help to retain the bandage. It may be necessary to make a longitudinal cut in the bandage through which the ear can be drawn (Fig. 66). In order to protect such an eye bandage from being clawed off by the patient, it is advisable to put an Elizabethan type collar on the dog (see Fig. 34), the radius of which should be as great as possible. In small breeds this collar should almost touch the ground when the animal is standing.

Following various operations on the ear, e. g. docking, opening of aural haematomas, aural resection, etc., it is necessary to apply a secure bandage. If the operation is unilateral, the unaffected ear can be used as a grip for the bandage as was described in the case of the eye (Fig. 67). Bandages for both ears can be made to lie correctly and securely if part of the neck is included in the bandage. The ears are laid together over the head and the bandage is then applied in figure of eight turns. When removing such a bandage it should only be cut along the ventral aspect of the throat and not over the top of the head. In the treatment of aural haematomas, it is often necessary to ensure that the ears are firmly immobilized on the top of the head. For this purpose a net shopping bag can be used to fix

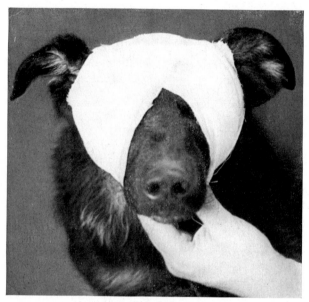

Fig. 65. Binocular bandage completed.

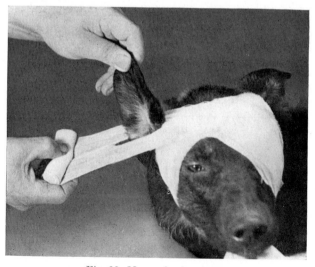

Fig. 66. Monocular bandage.

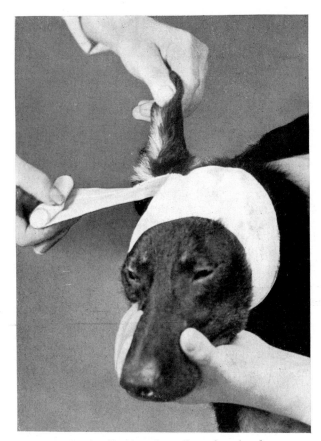

Fig. 67. Application of a unilateral ear bandage.

the ears firmly and this type of strapping also allows adequate ventilation of the enclosed ears.

In bandaging the neck the bandage is applied in spiral turns. Where the whole length of the neck is to be included, the bandage is applied over some turns of cellulose in order to give it a good hold. Where the area concerned is in the region of the throat, e. g. after operations on branchial cysts, the ears should be included in the bandage as described for bandaging the eyes. When bandaging the thorax a withers-saddle bandage is employed. This is applied by encircling the thorax behind the forelimbs, then taking the bandage over the neck of the animal and back between the two forelimbs, crossing over the thorax behind the forelimbs and then passing the bandage again forward between the forelimbs and returning over the withers. An abdominal bandage is difficult to fix on the dog because the abdomen in this species is rather conical in shape posteriorly (Figs. 68 and 69). The bandage which is most secure in this situation is one which is combined with the withers-saddle bandage described above (Fig. 70). To cover operation wounds in the abdominal region a strip bandage is often used. With this type of bandage,

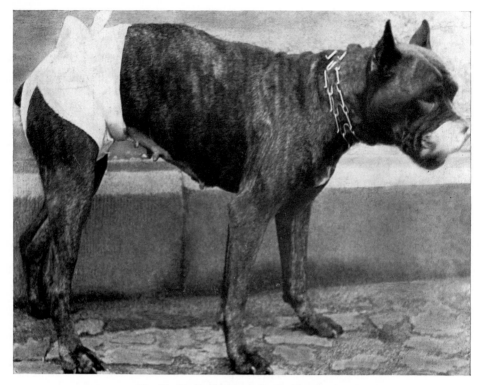

Fig. 68. Badly-fitting abdominal bandage.

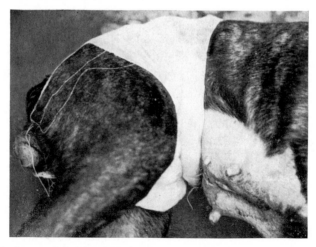

Fig. 69. A crumpled abdominal bandage will constrict the region of the wound.

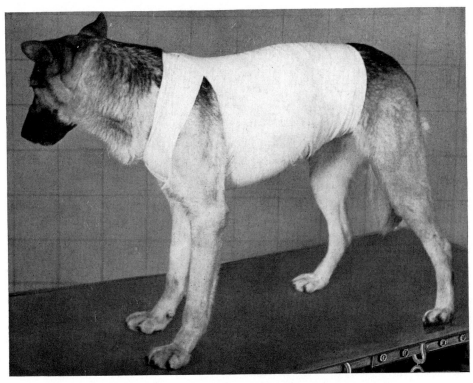

Fig. 70. Abdominal bandage combined with a withers-saddle bandage.

immediately following the operation the wound is dressed with a strip of gauze, which is fixed to the skin by continuous large sutures (Fig. 71).

The pelvic area is not often bandaged as the external genitalia render the application of a well-fitting bandage impracticable in this region.

Turning to bandaging techniques for the limbs, the paw bandage is of some importance, being indicated mainly in those conditions where there is inflammation between the toes, but also in wounds of the extremity. The toes are separated by inserting pledgelets of cotton wool between the toes and in the grooves between the pads (Fig. 72). Where there is a dewclaw, a small pad of cotton wool should be interposed between the claw and the skin. The foot bandage should be taken up to cover the carpus or the hock joint, otherwise it will tend to come off. Such bandages should be protected from damp and wear by some form of waterproof cover or "shoes" (Fig. 73). When a bandage is to be applied to the more proximal part of the forelimb, it should be combined with the withers-saddle type bandage for greater security. If the foot is to be left free the bandage must not be applied too tightly or there will be interference with the circulation and consequent swelling of the toes (Fig. 74). As the hindlimb of the dog is rather cone-shaped it is very difficult to apply a bandage which will remain in place.

Tail bandages usually require the use of adhesive plaster to keep them in position.

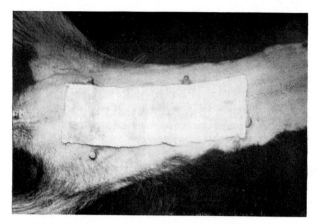

Fig. 71. Strip dressing.

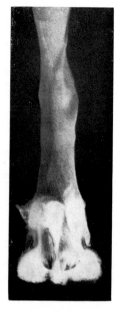

Fig. 72. Preparation of the foot for bandaging by insertion of cotton wool pads in the interdigital spaces.

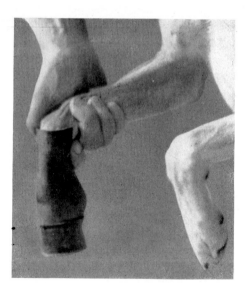

Fig. 73. Leather shoe to prevent wetting
of the bandaged foot.

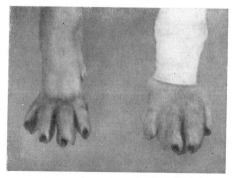

Fig. 74. Congestion of the toes due
to overtight bandaging.

8. Analgesia and anaesthesia

Local anaesthetics are substances which are capable of temporarily abolishing the passage of sensory impulses in nerves with which they are brought into contact. By this action they impart anaesthesia of the area of the body supplied by that nerve. In assessing the importance of local anaesthesia in canine surgery, one must remember that the patient needs to be adequately restrained, and this may necessitate the use of a tranquilliser or general anaesthesia. The oldest form of local anaesthesia is that produced by cold. From 1859 the cold produced by the evaporation of ether from the skin was used, this being replaced at the turn of the century by the use of ethyl chloride.

Ethyl chloride is marketed in glass tubes with a lever opening a narrow jet at one end. The tube is warmed in the hand for a few minutes which evaporates some of the fluid, thus increasing the pressure within the vial. When the lever is opened, the pressure expels a thin stream of ethyl chloride on to the site of operation which becomes white and hardened as it freezes. It is important not to freeze the tissues too severely or necrosis can result. The spray may also cause devitalisation of the tissues if the freezing is too prolonged. As ethyl chloride vapour is explosive, it should not be used in the proximity of a naked flame. Cold anaesthesia can only be used on the skin and is useful for minor superficial procedures such as opening of abscesses, etc.

When the anaesthetic activity of cocaine became appreciated, injection anaesthesia, which can be divided into infiltration anaesthesia and regional anaesthesia, was introduced into surgical practice. Later the dangers of addiction to cocaine were realised and various para-aminobenzoic acid esters were found to be safe, effective substitutes. A typical member of this group of substances is procaine. With local anaesthetics the lowest effective concentration should be used to avoid any risk of toxic side effects. Procaine used in high concentrations has occasionally caused toxic effects in the smaller breeds of dogs. The blood concentration necessary to paralyse the medullary centres is close to that producing convulsions; prior to and during these there is usually deep general anaesthesia. The toxicity risk can be minimised by using a low concentration of procaine and combining it with adrenaline to slow the rate of absorption. It must be remembered, however, that if large quantities of the combined solution are used, toxic effects of the adrenaline may arise. The lethal dose of procaine is extremely variable as the rate of absorption may vary considerably from different sites of injection and also with different concentrations of the solution used. The lethal dose thus varies between 40–400 mg per kg bodyweight, the average being about 150 mg per kg bodyweight. The lower limits of the lethal dose are approached if a 20 kg dog is given a total of 40 ml of a 2 % solution of procaine for infiltration anaesthesia. Concentrations of the agent greater than 2 % should not be used otherwise the vasoconstricting action of the adrenaline is counteracted by the vasodilator effect of the procaine, with consequent increased absorption of the adrenaline and the risk of toxicity.

Infiltration anaesthesia is performed by injecting small quantities of the solution fairly close together into the tissues. The sensory fibres are thus "chemically severed" by the procaine solution and the surrounding tissues together with

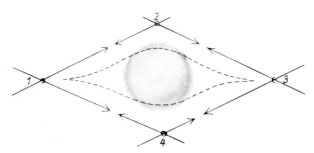

Fig. 75. Hackenbruch's anaesthetic infiltration. – – – – – – the probable incision.

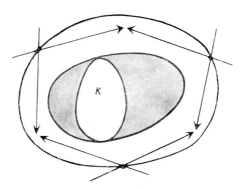

Fig. 76. Anaesthetic infiltration of a limb. K = bone.

their overlying skin or mucous membrane are rendered insensitive. For this purpose it is usual to employ a 2 % procaine solution, anaesthesia commencing in 7–8 min and lasting for about half an hour. Where the patient is a small or a young dog, it is advisable to dilute the solution of procaine to 1 % or even 0.5 % to lessen the risk of toxic reactions.

More rapid and extensive local anaesthesia can be obtained with the more recent agent, lignocaine, which is used in concentrations of 0.5–2 % for infiltration anaesthesia. It is somewhat more toxic than procaine.

Infiltration technique consists of inserting the needle subcutaneously as far as the hub in the direction of the part to be anaesthetised, and injecting the solution as the needle is withdrawn. In sensitive animals or especially painful areas, the injection can be made as the needle is inserted, allowing time for the anaesthetic effect before proceeding with the injection of the next area. If the infiltration is along the line of a proposed surgical incision, then the subcutis and the muscle layers should also be infiltrated once the skin has been anaesthetised. Where the area to be anaesthetised is extensive, the injections are made at two or more points in the form of Hackenbruch's quadrangle (Fig. 75). Where the surgical site is more than superficial, e. g. in some neoplasms, the area is injected in a triangular shape from four or more injection points, thus anaesthetising the whole field of operation. Pedunculated tumours can be adequately anaesthetised by injecting the anaesthetic solution into the stalk or its base. For anaesthetising a limb, infiltration is carried out by injecting around the limb at three or more points (Fig. 76).

Fig. 77. Dorsal view of the lumbosacral foramen. F. l. = the lumbosacral foramen; c. =
the iliac spine.

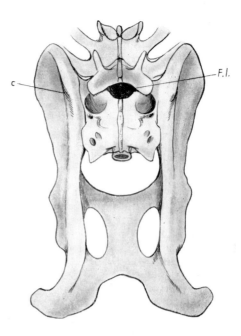

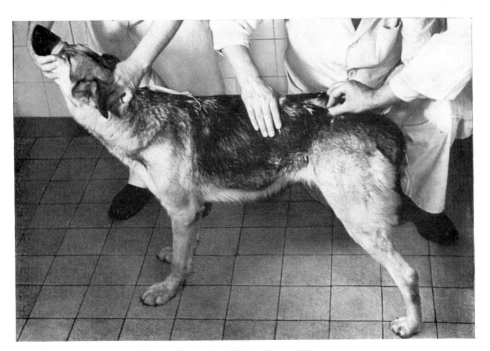

Fig. 78. Locating the lumbosacral foramen.

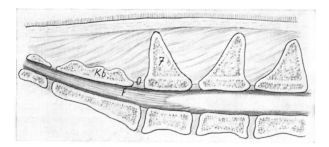

Fig. 79. Topography of epidural anaesthesia. 7 = the 7th lumbar vertebra; Kb = the sacrum.

Infiltration anaesthesia is contraindicated where there is any inflammatory condition of the subcutaneous connective tissues or if there is any risk of ischaemic necrosis, e. g. amputation flaps.

Regional anaesthesia is performed by injecting the anaesthetic solution around the nerves supplying the part. In canine surgery, the most important application of this technique is in the use of epidural anaesthesia. In our clinic, we do not employ regional anaesthesia of the head, as in surgery of this area we prefer the animal to be under the influence of a general anaesthetic.

Epidural anaesthesia is induced with the dog in the standing position, one assistant standing at the head to ensure that the latter is held higher than the lumbosacral area. A second assistant supports the pelvis with one hand and with the other presses down the spine at the thoraco-lumbar junction, thus fixing the animal for injection. The tail is left free, as in case of a faulty injection there may be reflex raising of the tail, a useful warning sign. The injection site (the lumbo-sacral foramen) lies at the point of intersection of a line joining the external angle of the ileum and the midline of the vertebral column (Fig. 77). The site can be determined by feeling for the iliac angles with the thumb and middle finger of one hand whilst the index finger locates the depression of the lumbo-sacral foramen (Fig. 78). The hair is clipped from the site, the skin defatted with ether and disinfected with iodine. A needle of suitable length is inserted through the skin and subcutaneous tissues slanting slightly forward. The foramen is covered by the interarcual ligament and this offers a slight resistance to the passage of the needle (Figs. 79, 80). If the needle has been correctly placed, the spinal cord cannot be damaged as it has become the filum terminale at the level of the 7th lumbar vertebra. If cerebro-spinal fluid escapes through the puncture site, the injection must not be made, as it is probable that the needle has passed between the 6th and the 7th lumbar vertebrae (Fig. 81). In older animals there may be ossification of the lumbo-sacral junction and in this case the injection must be made between the 6th and 7th lumbar vertebrae. This type of injection is called Peridural anaesthesia. A 2 % solution of procaine is employed, the amount of the injection varying from 2 ml in the case of a dachshund up to 7 ml for a Great Dane. The injection should be made over a period of about 30 sec, careful attention being paid to the animal's respiration and any tail movements as mentioned above. When the injection has been completed, the dog is held in a sitting position with the head held high. If the injection has been correctly made, the hindlimbs show signs of weakness after 5 min and this progresses into a state of flaccid paralysis (Fig. 82).

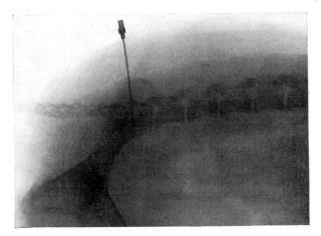

Fig. 80. Epidural anaesthesia. The needle lies in the lumbosacral foramen.

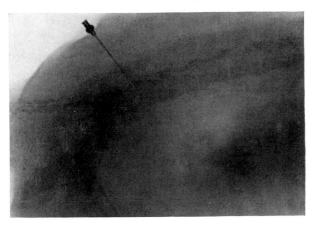

Fig. 81. Epidural anaesthesia. The needle lies between the 6th and 7th lumbar vertebrae.

Surgical anaesthesia, however, is not complete for about 10 min after completion of the injection. It is important not to restrain the dog on its side or back until this period has elapsed otherwise respiratory paralysis might ensue. In weak or debilitated animals, paralysis of the peripheral blood vessels may occur during epidural anaesthesia.

Epidural anaesthesia is indicated in all operative procedures in areas of the body caudal to the umbilicus, being particularly useful in laparotomies, e. g. hysterectomy, Caesarean section, etc. In Caesarean sections the puppies do not suffer from the effects of the anaesthetic and the bitch can care for them immediately the wound is closed.

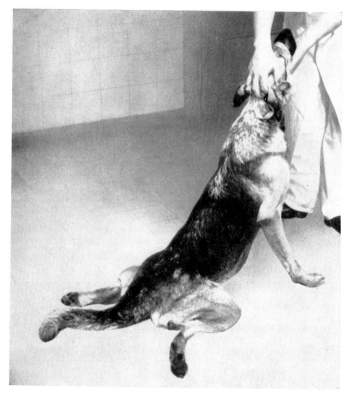

Fig. 82. Epidural anaesthesia is established. The patient assumes the attitude of a seal.

Topical anaesthesia (surface anaesthesia) induced by the application of cocaine to a mucous surface, was first introduced into surgery by the Vienna eye specialist, Koller. When applied to a mucous membrane, cocaine produces anaesthesia within 5–10 min and pallor due to its vasoconstrictor action. Unfortunately cocaine is an addictive drug so its use is strictly controlled and is now limited to certain ophthalmic operations. Amethocaine is a much more efficient surface anaesthetic, being 10 times more powerful than cocaine although somewhat more toxic. For this reason solutions more concentrated than 2 % should never be used. When instilled into the eyes amethocaine causes a chemosis (oedema of the bulbar conjunctiva), so its use in this field is contra-indicated. A 2 % solution of lignocaine may be used in the eye and a 1–4 % solution can be used for topical anaesthesia of other mucous membranes. The most powerful surface anaesthetic is cinchocaine. This is not an ester of benzoic acid, but a quinoline derivative, and is used as a ½–1 % solution.

It is important to remember that when the eye is anaesthetised by a topical anaesthetic, it should be protected from accidental trauma, as the protective corneal reflex has been abolished.

For the production of general anaesthesia in the dog two main groups of agents are used; those given parenterally and those given by inhalation. The anaesthetics given parenterally are injected at a computed dosage rate intravenously, subcutaneously, intraperitoneally or intramuscularly. To some extent these agents are uncontrollable in that once administered their action depends upon the metabolism of the body and their rate of excretion. Although the duration of an anaesthetic can be influenced by the administration of certain drugs, it is difficult to hasten recovery from an anaesthetic which is too deep. Amongst the anaesthetics used parenterally are the barbiturates, chloral hydrate and rarely, biomethol ("Avertin").

Premedication may be employed to lessen the stages of excitement, to make the patient more amenable to handling, and combined with local anaesthesia for minor surgical procedures. Where morphine is used as the premedicant, sedation is preceded by a stage of restlessness to a greater or lesser degree. The dog will walk about, raise its hackles, salivate, vomit, urinate and defaecate, and these signs may persist for up to half an hour before narcosis supervenes. It is therefore advisable to fast the patient before administering morphine. The dog becomes sleepy and comatose but can be readily awakened by touch or loud noises. Increasing the dose of morphine will not abolish reflexes; on the contrary, reflex excitability is increased and cramps may occur. By its action on the smooth muscle of the gut, morphine can produce relaxation and inhibition of peristalsis, which may lead to paralytic ileus. The dose of morphine when used as a narcotic is 5 mg per kg bodyweight of the hydrochloride threequarters of an hour before surgery. The action will persist for upwards of an hour.

Another narcotic in use is "Polamivet", which has two components, one with marked analgesic and spasmolytic powers and the other with an atropine-like action on the vagus nerve. The substance was introduced by BERGE and MULLER in 1949 (Tierärztl. Umschau, 4, 372). In debilitated or toxic patients the analgesic effect is usually attained, but local anaesthesia may be required. In young, healthy dogs it may be difficult to achieve a satisfactory state of narcosis with the drug. There appears to be an enhanced sensitivity to noise following the administration of "Polamivet". Fatalities have been recorded following the use of the drug in the brachycephalic breeds, e. g. Boxers, Pekingese, etc. The agent may be injected intramuscularly, subcutaneously, or intravenously. By the latter route the computed dose should be injected over a period of two minutes. The dose rate is 0.5 ml of the prepared solution per kg bodyweight with an absolute maximum dose of 15 ml in the heavy breeds, e. g. Great Danes, etc. When used for premedication, a dose rate of 0.05–0.1 ml is employed. Used in this manner post-anaesthetic excitement is lessened and induction is smoother and quieter.

Among the injectable anaesthetic agents, the two mainly used in our clinic are narcobarbital ("Eunarcon") and "Thiogenal". "Eunarcon" is a short-acting anaesthetic, surgical anaesthesia lasting for 10–35 min and with a short recovery period. The drug is contra-indicated in very old or young animals, debilitated animals and small dogs whose total weight is below 5 kg. The computed dose of 0.3 ml per kg is drawn into a 10 ml syringe and diluted to 10 ml with normal saline. Three ml of this solution are injected rapidly (20–30 sec) and the remainder slowly to effect, a close watch being maintained on the respiration and pulse rate. Where premedication with "Polamivet" has been used, the computed dose rate should be reduced to 0.1 m*l*. Anaesthesia is complete when there is abolition of the corneal reflex and relaxation of the masseter muscles.

Thiogenal is an ultra-short acting anaesthetic agent, the recovery period being very brief. Its use is contra-indicated in young or debilitated dogs. The dosage used is 35–40 mg per kg bodyweight, made up as a 10 % solution and injected intravenously. The first half of the computed dose is given fairly rapidly (20 sec) and the remainder more slowly to effect. In young dogs, the respiratory centre seems to be rather hypersensitive, so the injection should be made slowly in these patients.

So-called potentiated anaesthesia represents an advance in the use of the barbiturates described above. In this technique the effect of the barbiturate is increased by the use of an agent which has no inherent anaesthetic action. These agents act by interference with the metabolisation of the barbiturate. The phenothiazine derivatives produce a reduction in cell metabolism, which is especially marked in the central nervous system. In the brain, a phenothiazine derivative such as acepromazine will cause a greatly potentiated narcosis when administered in conjunction with "Polamivet" [BRASS, Dtsch. tierärztl. Wschr. (1954) **61**, 160, and KLUG, Mhefte Vet. med. (1957) **12**, 106]. A dose of 2–3 mg per kg bodyweight is injected intramuscularly or subcutaneously ½–¾ hr before giving "Polamivet". After a period of about one hour, narcosis and analgesia develop to a stage sufficient for most surgical procedures to be performed, although sensitivity to noise stimuli remains active. In very painful operations, such as aural resections, etc., the analgesia does not appear to be sufficient, so other methods of anaesthesia should be used in these cases. There is a fall in blood pressure and subsequent drop in body temperature when these agents are employed, so the dog should be kept warm during both the operation and recovery.

Chloral hydrate can be used in the dog as a narcotic, but it may produce a paralytic effect upon the vasomotor centre, and the dog is especially susceptible to its toxic effects on the heart and liver. The drug is best given as a rectal infusion at a dosage rate of 0.5 g per kg. The rectum must be emptied by an enema and then a 10 % solution of the drug in a mucilaginous medium is run into the rectum through a rubber canula. The animal's tail is then held pressed down for a while to discourage expulsion of the fluid. Narcosis begins in ½–¾ hr and may persist for about 4 hr.

Inhalation anaesthetics are given via the lungs and, being rapidly excreted by exhalation, are readily reversible and consequently more controllable. The blood level of the anaesthetic is directly dependent upon the concentration of the drug in the inspired air (vapour tension). The level of anaesthesia can thus be regulated by altering the vapour tension of the gas in the inspired air.

Formerly we used ether as our inhalation anaesthetic as it is very safe in the dog, there being no undue fall in blood pressure or observable toxic effects, even when the anaesthesia is prolonged. The anaesthetic grade of ether should be used and if there is any question as to its purity it should be tested by mixing with a little potassium iodide. If the ether turns brownish-yellow, then it is unsuitable for anaesthetic purposes as the toxic peroxide and aldehyde have been formed by oxidation. Ether may be used in a simple open mask after suitable premedication, or oxygen may be fed through an ether vaporizing chamber set in a waterbath and led into the trachea through an endotracheal tube (Fig. 83). To introduce

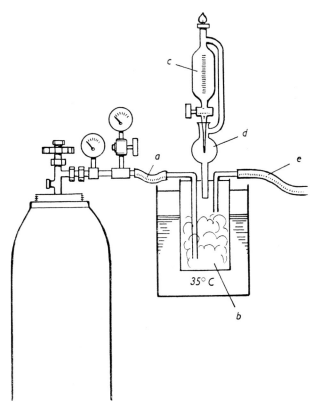

Fig. 83. Diagram of inhalation anaesthesia. (a) Oxygen supply; (b) vessel for evaporation of ether; (c) ether reservoir; (d) drip apparatus; (e) supply of the ether — oxygen mixture to the patient.

the tube, the dog is restrained on its back with head and neck extended, the mouth is opened and the tongue withdrawn with forceps. The tube is now passed along the soft palate (Fig. 84), the epiglottis is raised with the end of the tube which is then inserted into the glottis during an inspiration. The correct positioning of the tube can be checked by moving the tube slightly backwards and forwards; with the other hand on the trachea one can appreciate the feeling of the tube passing over the corrugations of the tracheal rings ("Washboard feeling"). The tube is fixed by a bandage round the jaws (Fig. 87). If too much oxygen is administered through the tube, hyperoxygenation may occur and the animal will stop breathing. If the oxygen supply is discontinued, the carbon dioxide building up in the tissues will usually stimulate respiration again in a short while; this process can usually be accelerated by administering a little carbon dioxide by blowing down the tube a few times. Both the foregoing methods of ether inhalation suffer from the disadvantage that quite a large amount of ether is liberated around the dog's head with unpleasant effects on the surgeon and his staff, but more important creating the danger of explosion. For this reason it is important that anti-static

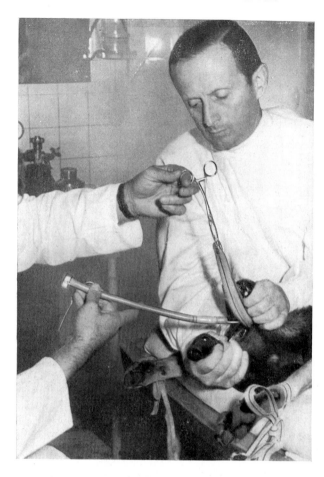

Fig. 84. Intubation anaesthesia.
With the tongue pulled out the
Rüsch catheter is introduced
into the trachea under usual
control.

Fig. 85. Mode of action of the
Rüsch catheter. The inflated
rubber collar clcses the glass
tube representing the trachea.

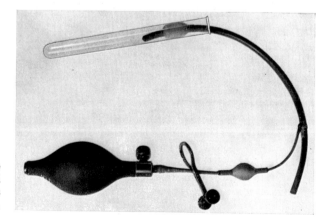

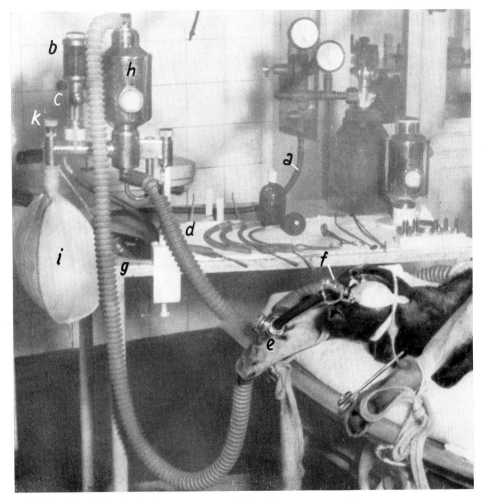

Fig. 86a. Intubation anaesthesia. (a) oxygen supply; (b) ether reservoir; (c) drip apparatus; (d) supply of the ether−oxygen mixture; (e) Y-valve piece; (f) attachment for the intubation tube; (g) outlet for expired air; (h) soda line canister; (i) rebreathing bag; (k) excess pressure valve.

precautions should be observed and no electrical equipment should be used during the operation.

For some years we have preferred halothane anaesthesia. Halothane is many times more active than ether. It causes little or no irritation of the respiratory tract and provokes little excitement. With rapid administration (2–5 min) it is almost completely excreted again through the lungs in 10–15 min. This, among other things, explains the fact that it is readily controllable. Its narcotic range is about equal to that of ether and the interval between respiratory stasis and cardiac

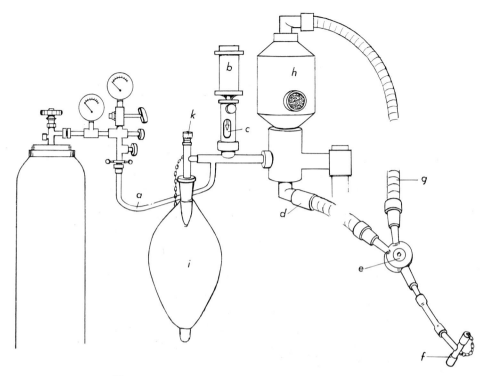

Fig. 86 b. Schema of intubation anaesthesia apparatus
(see Fig. 86 a).

arrest is very small. After inhalation of halothane, bradycardia and hypotonia
may occur. Damage to the liver and kidneys is very seldom seen. At present its
relatively high cost is a disadvantage. We therefore use halothane for the dog
almost exclusively in a closed system with endotracheal intubation.

In the hands of an experienced anaesthetist, this highly potent anaesthetic is
a considerable advance in the anaesthesiology of the dog. Halothane is not explosive
and therefore opens up many new fields in the surgery of small animals.

Closed circuit anaesthesia has recently been introduced into veterinary surgery.
In this technique the trachea is sealed off by an endotracheal tube fitted with an
inflatable rubber cuff (Fig. 85) so that the lungs can be mechanically expanded
even when the thorax has been opened. Oxygen is mixed with the anaesthetic gas
and passed into a reservoir rubber bag. Intermittent compression of this bag
allows mechanical expansion of the lungs, the bag serving to damp down the
pressure so that the lungs are not over-distended. It is usual to incorporate an
adjustable expiratory valve into the circuit as an added safeguard against over-
inflation. The anaesthetic mixture is then led into a Y-shaped valve (Fig. 86a and
b) containing two unidirectional valves. At inspiration the outlet valve closes
and the gases flow to the patient, at expiration the inlet valve closes and the

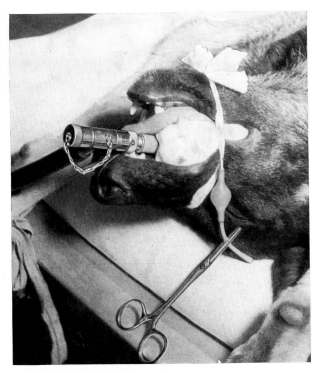

Fig. 87. Intubation anaesthesia. After the Rüsch catheter has been protected with cotton wool swabs and the jaws have been closed with a bandage, the patient can be connected to the ether—oxygen apparatus.

expired air passes into a soda lime container which absorbs the carbon dioxide content. This process can be represented in the form of a chemical equation:

$$CO_2 + Ca(OH)_2 = CaCO_3 + H_2O + Q$$

where Q is the amount of heat produced by the reaction. The heat produced can be used as an indication that carbon dioxide is being absorbed, but most soda limes contain an indicator which turns a light bluish-violet colour when their absorbent power is exhausted.

With these techniques balanced anaesthesia can be maintained for considerable periods of time, but even with these methods anaesthetic accidents may occur. Spasm of the glottis, evidenced by sudden cessation of respiration, may occur during induction with inhalation anaesthetics especially with refractory animals. In these cases, the spasm can only be overcome by forcibly opening the glottis, centrally acting analeptics being useless. Vomiting during anaesthesia is dangerous due to the risk of aspiration pneumonia, so animals must always be starved before operation. During induction at the stage of narcosis, the tongue may fall back into the pharynx and occlude the airway. This accident can be prevented by drawing the tongue forwards with forceps. During anaesthesia there is usually a marked fall in body temperature due to paralysis of the heat regulating centres, so that the operating theatre should be kept warm and the dog wrapped up during the recovery period.

Editor's note: It is unwise to apply direct heat to the patient as overheating may occur due to paralysis of the centres. Many leading surgeons prefer to keep the theatre cool as this tends to lessen surgical shock.

Respiratory or cardiac failure during anaesthesia may be caused by overdosage of the anaesthetic agent or individual idiosyncracy of the patient. In cardiac arrest, adrenaline should be given intravenously or intracardially, and may restart the heart beat. Where there is surgical shock, blood accumulates in the splanchnic area with a resultant diminution in the circulating blood volume. Countermeasures involve increasing blood volume by the use of whole blood transfusions, plasma, saline solutions (Ringer) or blood volume expanders such as dextran. The latter are preferable to saline solutions as the greater size of their molecules enables them to persist in the blood for a longer period.

In cases of central collapse, the centrally acting analeptics are indicated, the best known of these being leptazol. This drug is given intravenously until the respiration and circulation have become normal and the reflexes are again present. According to the size of the dog, the dose usually lies between 0.5 and 1 ml of the 10% solution. Certain anaesthetic agents will depress the respiratory centre, especially morphine and its derivatives. Increased frequency of respiration can be produced by decreased oxygen tension and a slight increase in carbon dioxide content of the inspired air. If the blood becomes saturated with carbon dioxide, the respiratory centre will be paralysed. If the oxygen and the carbon dioxide tension in the blood are reduced simultaneously, Cheyne—Stokes respiration will occur. In this phenomenon, periods of apnoea alternate with periods of slowly increasing and deepening respirations. The condition is usually seen in moribund subjects. An increase in the acidity of the blood (acidosis) produces stimulation of the respiratory centre with a consequent increase in the depth and to some extent the frequency of respiration. In this case the patient is unconscious and exhibits stertorous breathing (KUSSMAUL's respiration), the increased respirations sometimes producing an acid deficit (Hyperventilation alkalosis). Alkalosis may also be caused by loss of chloride (by persistent vomiting) or by failure of urinary excretion of alkalis. Because of the depressant effects of most anaesthetic agents on the respiratory centre, respiratory stimulants, e. g. leptazol, nikethamide, caffeine, camphor, etc., should always be to hand in the operating theatre.

Where respiratory failure occurs but the heart is still beating, forced oxygenation of the lungs should be carried out as soon as possible. It is advisable to incorporate about 5% carbon dioxide in the oxygen mixture to stimulate the respiratory centre. Sometimes the respiratory centre can also be stimulated by reflex stimulation of the skin, e. g. cold applications, light slapping, massage, etc. Ammonia and smelling salts stimulate respiration by their action on the trigeminal nerve. Despite the great advances which have taken place in veterinary anaesthesia, deaths continue to occur probably due to the fact that so little attention is paid to the pharmacological and physiological principles involved, and that the necessary facilities and drugs for dealing with anaesthetic emergencies are not immediately available. An anaesthetic tray should be laid out before the administration of any anaesthetic. On this tray should be set out respiratory and circulatory stimulants, specific antidotes if available, hypodermic syringes, scissors, tongue forceps, mouth gag, endotracheal tubes and oxygen apparatus.

9. Euthanasia

When euthanasia must be performed, obviously only the most painless and certain methods should be used. Many members of the general public believe that animals brought for euthanasia are subjected to experimentation, so the owner is always asked to be present when the dog is put to sleep.

The use of prussic acid, strychnine, etc., for euthanasia is to be condemned. "Pentobarbitone" is recommended at a dose rate of 200 mg per kg bodyweight given intravenously. The injection should be given slowly otherwise there may

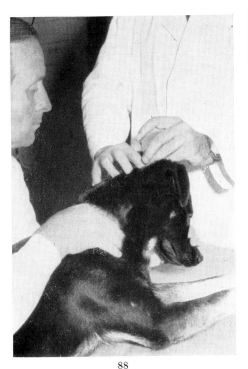 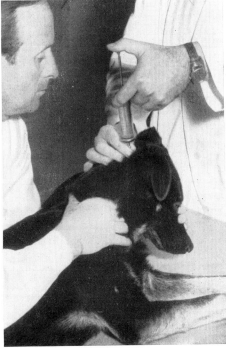

88   89

Fig. 88. Locating the occipito-atlantal foramen.

Fig. 89. Injection into the occipito-atlantal foramen.

be excitement, which may be interpreted as a pain reaction by the owner. Once the dog is anaesthetised the remainder of the dose may be given as rapidly as possible. This drug is rather expensive and the amount used can be reduced by inducing anaesthesia and then injecting 10–30 ml of a saturated solution of magnesium sulphate intravenously as rapidly as possible. Another method is to inject up to 20 ml of ether through the atlanto-occipital foramen. The technique is not too difficult in the anaesthetised animal. The head is strongly flexed towards the sternum and the depression of the atlanto-occipital foramen is located just posterior to the occipital protuberance. A strong needle is inserted through the depression (Fig. 88, 89) and if it has been positioned correctly, cerebrospinal fluid will emerge from the needle. Magnesium sulphate or ether can also be injected intra-cardially in the anaesthetised animal, using the 4th, 5th or 6th intercostal space on the left side where the apex beat is most easily appreciated. The needle should be sufficiently long to reach and enter the heart and should be thrust home decisively, otherwise the heart may be pushed away by the needle. Even if no blood enters the syringe, one can tell by the transmitted heart movements of the needle that the heart, in fact, has been entered. One can use other barbiturates to induce the initial anaesthesia.

Occipital puncture without prior anaesthetisation may be employed but there may be reactions from the dog to the pain of the actual puncture. Saturated solutions of magnesium sulphate injected rapidly intravenously will produce a painless death but there may be motor excitement and the dog may cry out. In newly-born or very young puppies, 5–10 ml of ether injected through the fontanelles into the brain produces sudden death.

10. X-ray technique

Revised by S. Schlaff

In his earliest work on the origin of X-rays Roentgen established that the rays are produced wherever cathode rays impinge upon matter. Cathode rays and X-rays have many properties in common, as for example, the production of fluorescence and absorption in every kind of material. However, in spite of this, they are not the same. Cathode rays are corpuscular radiations, while X-rays are electromagnetic oscillations. X-rays are, in fact, forms of radiant energy like other electromagnetic radiations such as light and heat rays. They are distinguished from the other radiations by the particularly short wavelength and the very high energy associated with this.

With X-rays, one is always dealing with a mixture of rays of different wavelengths between 0.016 and 60 mμ, i. e. from 0.16 to 600 Ångström units (1 Ångström unit, 1 Å $= \dfrac{1}{10}$ mμ).

X-rays are of varying wavelengths for the following reasons. The high tension on the X-ray tube usually does not have a constant unidirectional voltage. The highest voltage produces a radiation of short wavelength, while the lower voltages produce rays of longer wavelength. Quite apart from this the electrons penetrate to different depths in the focal spot. The electrons which are slowed up near the surface excite "hard" radiation of relatively short wavelength, while the electrons that have penetrated more deeply produce a "soft" radiation of longer wavelength. In radiology, the terms "hard" and "soft" mean greater or lesser capacity for penetration.

As with all waves the typical characteristics are reflexion, refraction, inter-ference, diffraction and polarisation. On the basis of the Law of Conservation of Energy, X-rays can arise by transformation of other types of radiation of similar high energy, e. g. in the spontaneous disintegration of uranium, in which fast electrons liberated produce X-rays by impinging upon matter. One applies this artificially in the electron tubes (see p. 84).

The typical elementary properties of X-rays are:

1. Capacity for penetration.

2. Excitation of fluorescence.

3. Photographic effect.

4. Formation of secondary and scattered radiations.

5. Ionisation of gases.

6. Biological action (Cell damage).

Only (1) and (4) will be discussed now; the other properties will be considered in later sections.

X-rays have the property of penetrating a body, but in doing so they are more or less absorbed. The thicker the body, the more it absorbs the X-rays. Moreover, the absorption is different in different materials; it depends on the chemical nature of the substance and on its density. For example, lead absorbs X-rays almost completely, while aluminium only does so partially. The individual constituent parts of the animal organism behave in an entirely similar way; bones absorb much more of the rays than soft parts.

Whenever X-rays penetrate into matter, there is absorption or weakening of the energy of the rays. The absorption is greater, the softer the X-rays. Hard rays are not absorbed so much but instead are more strongly scattered. In every process of absorption of radiation, including light, the radiant energy remaining behind in the absorbing material becomes transformed into other types of energy; the same happens with X-rays. The appearance of "secondary radiation" depends on different processes. A part of the absorbed X-ray energy is used for the produc-tion of "characteristic secondary radiation" which is characteristic of the absorb-ing material concerned and there is a transformation into X-rays of another wave-length. Moreover, during the absorption of X-rays, electrons are released, so that in this way X-rays are converted into corpuscular radiations. The "scattered radiation" is an important component, which is radiation deflected from its original direction.

The degree of scattering and absorption depends on:

1. The quality of the radiation.

2. The atomic weight of the matter, since substances composed of light atoms scatter relatively more and those composed of heavy atoms absorb to a re-latively greater extent.

3. The thickness of the layer, since every centimetre of the layer scatters and absorbs about the same percentage of the radiation coming through from the previous centimetre.

In the process of absorption, the energy is completely taken up and transformed by the atom involved, while in scattering, the X-ray gives up only a part of its energy and goes on in a different direction.

The X-ray equipment may be divided into:

1. The X-ray apparatus proper, which includes electrical installations such as the current generator, the control desk, the X-ray tube, etc.
2. The ancillary equipment:
   a) For the examination itself (couches, stands, etc.).
   b) Special appliances (aiming devices, diaphragms for excluding scattered radiation, etc.).
   c) Accessories (cones, grids, cassettes, etc.).

To generate X-rays, one needs high tension above 1000 V. In radiology a distinction is made between half-wave, 4-valve-, 6-valve- and condenser-discharge apparatus. The electrons produced in the X-ray tube by the cathode filament must traverse an electric field in order to reach the anode. For this purpose, a unidirectional voltage must be applied, if possible continuously across the X-ray tube. The alternating current (a. c.) of the mains supply changes its direction 50 times a second to the positive side and 50 to the negative; thus the periodicity is 50. Each cycle consists of two half-waves. Within each cycle, there is an increase of voltage from zero up to a maximum positive value and then a decrease to zero, with a subsequent further decrease to reach a maximum negative value followed by a return to zero. These voltage changes can be represented graphically as a sine wave (Fig. 90).

The simplest X-ray apparatus is the half-wave apparatus, in which the electrical connection is as follows:

Mains current-transformer-X-ray tube.

The two poles of the transformer are connected directly to the X-ray tube. If the negative pole is on the cathode the current flows (On-load phase), while if the positive pole is on the cathode, the passage of current through the tube is blocked (No-load phase). Only a half-wave of each cycle is utilised. The advantages of the

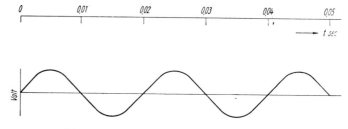

Fig. 90. Alternating current (mains voltage).

apparatus are cheapness, small space requirement and simplicity, while the main disadvantage is the low output. Moreover, the tube is easily destroyed by sparking back.

The a. c. is utilized better in the 4-valve apparatus. Here tubes similar to X-ray tubes – "valves" – function as valves for the alternating current. In these high-vacuum tubes, passage of the current is only possible if carriers of the electricity are available, as is the case with the filament as cathode; thus with negative polarity of the filament the electrons migrate to the anode. The passage of current is only possible in this one direction. The valves are connected up in a Graetz rectifying circuit (Fig. 91). In each half-wave, the two diagonally placed valves act as current transmitters or blocks, as the case may be. This circuit guarantees utilisation of both phases of the a. c. Some continuity of the voltage arises from the overlapping of the waves, though this is incomplete (Fig. 92). The sequence of the electrical connections is: mains current-transformer-rectifier-X-ray tube. In this apparatus, the X-ray tube does not have to function as a valve as well as in the half-wave equipment. The cycle-oscillation, which still persists with the 4-valve apparatus, is noticeable particularly with short switching-on times, since then a rapid fall in voltage occurs.

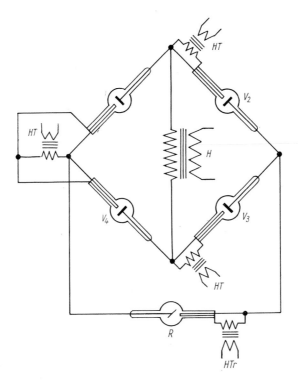

Fig. 91. Circuit diagram of Graetz's circuit. H = High tension transformer; V_1-V_4 = Valves; HT = Filament transformers for the valves; HTr = Filament transformer for the X-ray tube; R = X-ray tube.

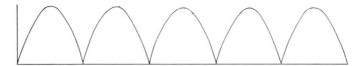

Fig. 92. Rectified alternating current (single phase current).

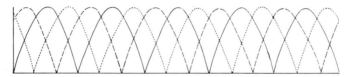

Fig. 93. Rectified three-phase alternating current.

In order to obtain a still higher output, one uses a 3-phase current with the 6-valve apparatus. This current is produced by the combination of 3 alternating currents with the same frequency and the same amplitude. In contrast to single phase a. c., the 3-phase current produces in each cycle 3 positive maxima, which follow one another in thirds of a cycle. With the additional rectification of the negative phases in the 6-valve equipment, six peaks occur in each cycle, so that there is an almost uniform flow of current (Fig. 93). Here the rectifying valves are also connected in a Graetz circuit. One can attain a further smoothing of the current variation by means of accessory condensers. The 6-valve equipment delivers a constant potential for the X-ray tube, with only slight pulsations and thus makes possible a uniform loading of the tube. This apparatus is suitable for high-output radiography, penetrating film techniques and all methods which demand the shortest possible exposure times.

In the condenser discharge apparatus, condensers are charged up with small current generators and then can be discharged at constant potential with very high currents in almost any short times as required.

The first type of X-ray tube, which was in use for a long time, was the gas tube (or ionization tube), which was characterized by three "poles" – the cathode, the anticathode and the supplementary anode – and in which a certain degree of vacuum had to be maintained. Besides other disadvantages this type of tube had the major defect that only a small part of the energy was converted into X-rays.

The usual type of X-ray tube today is the electron tube, or Coolidge tube, which has only two poles – the cathode and the anode. Inside there is a high vacuum at 10^{-7} mm Hg pressure (Fig. 95). The process of generation of X-rays takes place in the following way. If a metal is heated sufficiently by an electric current, it gives off electrons. The necessary electrons are obtained from a tungsten wire spiral brought to incandescence by means of electrical heating. They leave the cathode through the action of the high voltage applied across the tube and impinge with considerable velocity on the anode; here they produce the X-rays. The great advantage of the electron tube lies in the fact that the number of electrons

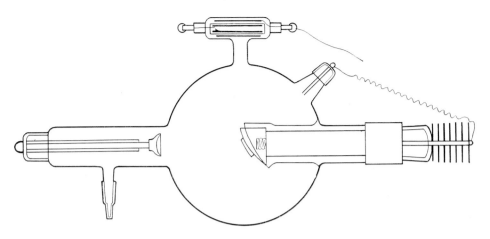

Fig. 94. Ion tube with concave cathode, tungsten anticathode and anode.

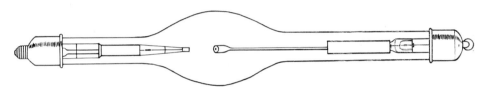

Fig. 95. Electron tube with massive tungsten anode.

can be controlled by means of the heating current. Independently of this, the quality of the radiation can be regulated by alteration of the tube voltage.

That part of the anode on which the electrons impinge with great velocity is described as the focal spot (or focus). It consists of tungsten, whose melting point is 3380 °C. The form and size of the focal spot depend on relative dimensions of the cathode. The ideal focal spot for diagnostic X-ray tubes should be as small as possible and in the form of a point, in order to guarantee sharp pictures. However, this is very difficult in practice, since the heat load would be too great. The focal spot can have the form of a circle, a rectangle or a band. This last form is the most ideal because of the relatively slight heating. The band form is attained by the so-called rotating anode. Here the anode has the form of a plate, which is set into very rapid rotation, so that in an exposure time of, for example, 0.1 sec the focal spot covers a distance of 63 cm. In this way we can keep the focal spot very small, because not only does it fall on one point but in practice many focal spots lie side by side. Thus the thermal loading of the anode is significantly less than with the fixed anodes.

The efficiency of an X-ray tube is only about 0.5 % under the usual working conditions. The whole of the remaining electrical energy is transformed into heat,

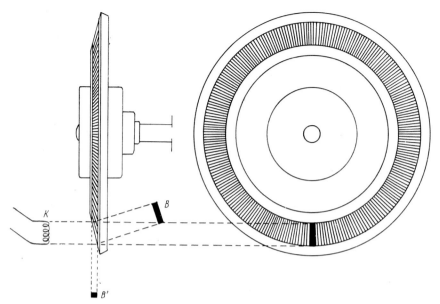

Fig. 96. Diagram of rotating anode plate. K = cathode; B = true focal spot; B′ = effective focal
spot; with rotation of the anode, the true focal spot moves on the plate.

which is developed at the focal spot and must be dispelled. The various possibilities
for cooling are:

1. Cooling by radiation. This depends on the fact that a system heated relatively
   to the environment gives off its heat to the environment. This process is usual
   only with a small electrical load or in combination with other types of cooling
   (Fig. 97).
2. Cooling by conduction, which is possible in three forms:
   a) As metallic conduction, e. g. when the shaft of the anode is of heavy copper.
   b) As fluid conduction with water or oil.
   c) As gaseous conduction, almost exclusively with air.

Besides the current generator and the X-ray tube, the X-ray apparatus includes
the control desk. In the usual model this contains the mains current inlet, the
leads to the primary of the transformer, the control transformer and the resistances,
the fuses, the measuring equipment, the dials for regulating voltage, current and
time and the switch gear. The high-voltage transformer, the heating transformer and
the rectifying valves are placed either in another part of the equipment or actually
in the control desk. A voltmeter on the desk measures the tension on the mains in
volts or the voltage of the transformer primary and can be adjusted to 200 V.
A second measuring instrument is the milliammeter, which measures the tube
current at the moment of taking the film or of the fluoroscopy. Besides these two
measuring instruments, we also have various regulating dials according to the
type of equipment, as, for example, for the tension on the X-ray tube in kV

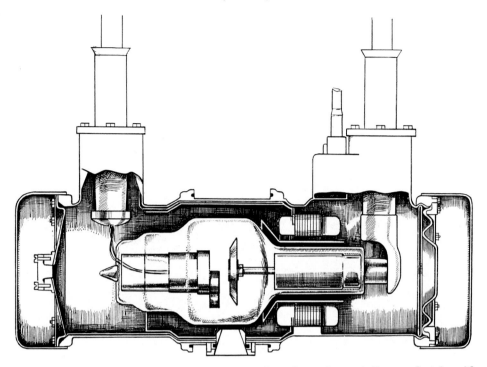

Fig. 97. Schematic cross-section through the oil jacket of a modern rotating anode tube with radiation cooling in oil.

(kilovolts), for the tube current in mA (milliamperes), etc. By milliampere seconds (mA sec) is meant the product of the current in milliampere and the time in seconds, e. g., 40 mA sec = 400 mA ×0.1 sec or 200 mA ×0.2 sec.

The X-ray tube is surrounded by a housing, which fulfils a double purpose; it serves for protection (1) against high tension, since it prevents the staff from getting close to the X-ray tube and (2) against radiation, since besides the useful beam, which emerges through the radiation window, no radiation worth mentioning can leave the housing. This is achieved by means of a lead casing and in addition by air or oil.

The ancillary X-ray equipment already mentioned includes, besides the stands, which serve for fixing or suspending the tubes, the appliances for making the examination, for which we distinguish equipment for taking films and for screening, though this equipment may be combined.

The equipment for radiography includes the stand and the table, which usually has a built-in grid, and accordingly is described as a grid table. As an accessory a chest stand with a built-in grid can be very useful for taking films of the patient in the standing position.

The equipment for fluoroscopy is either fixed (stationary apparatus) or mobile (tilting apparatus). Behind, or below, the supporting plate, which is transparent to X-rays, is the X-ray tube at a fixed distance. The fluorescent screen consists of

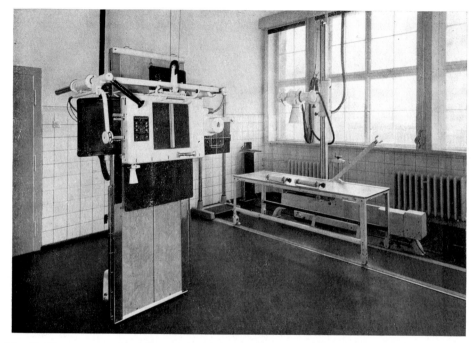

Fig. 98. X-ray room with tube stand with rotating anode tube. Flat grid table, chest X-ray stand, tomograph. Fluoroscopic equipment with rotating anode tube for tilting and for taking spot films. (High School Illustration Department.)

lead glass and in modern apparatus is coupled with the X-ray tube, however being adjustable to a certain extent in all directions (Fig. 98).

For certain examinations (e. g. of the gastro-intestinal tract), the spot film aiming device has proved to be a valuable accessory to screening equipment. By means of a special appliance on the fluorescent screen, one can take spot films in the course of screening.

Two advantages are to be gained by the application of a wide range of diaphragms and grids, viz. (1) the staff can be protected from unnecessary exposure to radiation by limitation of the primary beam to the dimensions required by the picture, and (2) scattered radiation is reduced and limited. One must distinguish (1) aperture diaphragms, which keep the useful beam of radiation as narrow as possible and (2) diaphragms and grids to eliminate scattered radiation.

1. Aperture diaphragms. The simplest form is the cone which consists of radio-opaque material. The radiographic cones have a fixed cross section but can easily be interchanged for other cones of different sizes (Fig. 99). By the application of the cone we give a certain amount of protection to the staff, and also to the animal, from unnecessary exposure to radiation, an improvement of the quality of the picture by narrowing of the beam of radiation to the necessary degree and facilitation of the set-up, since the cone indicates the direction and

Fig. 99. Different cones. In front are
two compression cones for fluoroscopy.
(High School Illustration Department.)

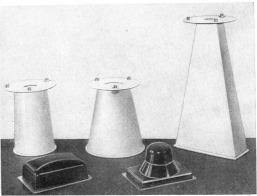

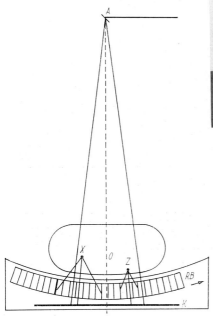

Fig. 100. Grid (diaphragm for eliminat-
ing scattered radiation). A = anode;
X and Z = scattering centres; K =
cassette; O = central ray; RB = grid.

form of the beam. In order to be able to alter the size of the image during the
course of the screening, fluoroscopic equipment is generally provided with a
double slit-diaphragm, which can be altered by hand levers.

With localising equipment and for screening, occasionally we also make use
of the compression cone (Fig. 99), with which we can compress or displace
interfering layers of tissue above the object to be examined, without having
to put the hand into the X-ray beam. In this way, we get a reduction of the
mass of scattering material and at the same time bring the object nearer to
the film or the screen.

2. Diaphragms to reduce scattered radiation. Today these are almost solely
used in the form of grids. In these, numerous strips, which are either parallel
or slightly inclined to the middle, are ranged side by side in such a way that
radio-translucent and radio-opaque material alternate with one another (Fig.
100). These grids certainly transmit the primary rays which travel in straight
lines and produce the image, but they keep back a considerable part of the
scattered radiation, which is ineffective for image production. A stationary
screen, of course, gives an image on the X-ray film (Fig. 101) and to prevent
this one uses moving grids. The running time of the grid must always be somewhat longer than the corresponding exposure time, in order not to give an

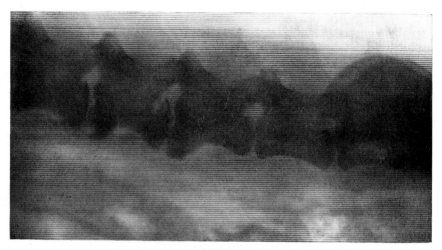

Fig. 101. Picture with a stationary grid.

image of the grid in its end position. If the grid is constructed of particularly thin elements, one speaks of fine grids. In the case of the so-called Bucky diaphragm, the screens are arranged in the form of a honey-comb.

As well as the scattered radiation which is intentionally eliminated, a small part of the radiation, which actually participates in the image formation, is also unfortunately removed. This loss varies according to the type of grid and can be compensated for by using a higher current or a longer exposure time. The so-called "grid factor" is the number by which the exposure intensity must be multiplied in order to get the right exposure when using a grid; it is 2.5 for the usual grids.

Among the most important points in working with X-rays is radiation protection. The 197 pioneers of radiology throughout the world, who up to the present have definitely lost their lives as a result of the effects of exposure to radium and X-rays acquired in the course of their professional work, should be an impressive warning of the dangers of these rays. Unfortunately, the rays produce no subjective or objective symptoms, but the steady accumulation of exposure over the years, often over decades, leads to severe injuries. Today we know enough about the biological action of X-rays to be able to protect ourselves against them.

X-rays always act upon living cells to produce an injury. It was thought at one time that small doses of X-rays exerted a stimulating effect but this is erroneous. If the amount of radiation is too small, there is no effect and then one speaks of a "tolerance dose". After the action of the rays, independently of the dose level, a certain time always elapses before the appearance of detectable sequelae, the so-called "latent period". As latent dangers arising from the continued summation of small and even very small individual doses, a number of late manifestations of radiation damage threaten the staff in the form of leukaemias and malignant tumours, premature ageing, shortening of life span and increase in the rate of hereditary changes.

The cell nucleus appears to be most susceptible to injury by radiation. According to its degree, the damage can occur as alterations of the hereditary properties of the cells, abnormal cell division and death of the cell nucleus with subsequent breakdown.

Among the detectable functional and morphological changes of individual organs and organ systems, one must distinguish between changes which are to be attributed to the local action of the rays on the organ itself (local effects) and those which are to be regarded as secondary manifestations of a general injury seen in the organ in question. Besides the local effects, there are also general effects which consist of weakness and lassitude, lethargy, loss of appetite, nausea and perhaps vomiting, colicky abdominal pains and diarrhoea. These phenomena as a whole are described as X-ray sickness. This lasts a few days but can drag on for up to two weeks. It is most pronounced after irradiation of the abdominal cavity with large doses. In this stage one finds a multiplicity of pathological changes in the soluble constituents of the blood and in the blood cells.

Of the local effects, radiation injury of the skin is the one most fully documented. After irradiation, reddening of the skin may appear, the so-called "X-ray erythema". This reddening is only the expression of an inflammation and does not represent radiation injury. This begins with blistering. A still more intense degree of X-ray burn is necrosis of the skin. In the most severe cases there is refractory ulceration, which can become malignant after persisting for many years. All these injuries are due to avoidable errors in technique, such as working with the unprotected hand or even with the hand protected with a lead glove in the primary beam.

Proceeding from the morphological signs of injury, organs and tissues can be arranged in the following series of decreasing radiosensitivity: lymphatic organs, such as lymph nodes, spleen, thymus and lymphatic tissue in other organs; bone marrow; testes; ovaries; mucous membranes of the gastro-intestinal tract; skin and its appendages; cartilage; growing bones; glandular organs such as the liver, adrenal, kidney, salivary gland; lungs, central nervous system, skeletal musculature; connective tissue; bones.

Diseased tissue has a particular sensitivity to X-rays, especially tissue involved in active cell division, such as tumour tissue. One takes advantage of this in X-ray therapy.

The tolerance dose of radiation, i. e. the maximal dose of X-rays that can be tolerated without injury, is established compulsorily at the present time by the Recommendations of the International Commission on Radiological Units, as revised at the 7th International Congress of Radiology in Copenhagen in 1953. This amounts to 0.3 r per week for exposure of the whole body or 1.5 r per week for exposure of the hands and feet only (see also Industrial Protection Regulation 950 Application of X-rays in Medical Establishments, of 25. 11. 1954). The unit of measurement of the quantity of X-rays is 1 r (Roentgen). This is the amount of X-rays which produces in 1 cm^3 of air at 760 mm mercury pressure and temperature of 0 °C, ionization corresponding to one electrostatic unit (e. s. u.) of ions of each sign.

It is important to know that for genetic effects in relation to radiation injury, no tolerance dose is discernible. All radiation exposures are cumulative, however low the dose-rate.

The best protection against X-rays is the avoidance of unnecessary proximity to the radiation source.

In the German Democratic Republic the health supervision of X-ray personnel has been controlled by an Implementing Regulation in the Statutory Notice No. 35 of 13. 5. 1957. According to this, every person who works with X-rays must undergo an examination every 6 months which comprises full blood count, urine testing, and thorough inspection of the skin, visible mucous membranes, hair and nails and also in the case of women, careful check on the calendar of the menstrual cycle. Moreover, once a year a chest X-ray should be taken and a general medical examination carried out.

Reference must be made here in detail to the most important measures for radiation protection, since there is still too much laxity in applying these precautions.

It is very important that all personnel concerned with X-rays should be thoroughly instructed. Systematic and thorough explanation can greatly reduce rashness and carelessness. By recognising sufficiently the dangers of being involved with X-rays, unnecessary close proximity to the source of the rays is largely avoided.

Accurate recording concerning the risk of exposure of the staff is an aid to careful control. A further reduction of the radiation exposure, above all of the animal attendants, can be attained by tying up the animal with the owner holding the head. This is possible with all dogs for up to a few films. For very restless animals, tranquillizers can be useful.

An essential aspect of the protective measures is the condition of the rooms in which the staff work. All these must be well ventilated, with the fresh air drawn immediately from the open air outside. The walls of the rooms in which people work, and also those in which they reside, should be painted with a bright colour. The X-ray rooms should be at least 3.30 m high, to reduce the effect of scattering of radiation from the roofs and walls as much as possible. Apart from small machines which are switched on and off by the person making the examination, all X-ray apparatus must have a separate control room, which must be in contact with the X-ray room by means of a grid for speaking through, or equipment for two-way speech, and approached through a door. An observation window must ensure a good overall view of the X-ray room. The control room must have a second access independent of the X-ray room. No-one should have to enter rooms with a risk of radiation, in order to reach his place of work.

All the arrangements and measures for protection are to be checked annually in the industrial safety inspection. However, the best test is always the measurement of the maximum amount of radiation in the X-ray rooms. By means of these measurements, it can be clearly established, what are the levels of scattered radiation and which place the worker must occupy, so that he is not exposed to more than the permissible dose. In any case, protective clothing must be worn in the X-ray room.

The protective clothing should reach high enough to cover the collar bone and should protect the body at least 30–40 cm below the waist-line. A thickness of lead rubber is recommended for the examination aprons corresponding to a lead equivalent of 0.25–0.5 mm. Protective gloves should have a lead equivalent of 0.25 mm. Protective clothing must be fully washable. The gloves and the aprons must be carefully looked after and checked since they become dangerous if they

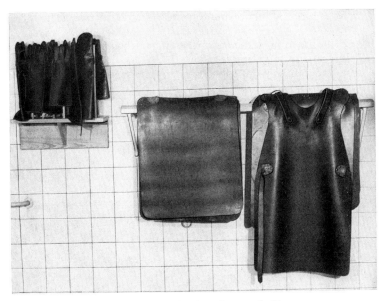

Fig. 102. Glove stands and apron holders.

are full of cracks. For this reason the aprons should never be left lying folded together, but must be hung on a rounded holder, perhaps 20 cm wide; also the gloves should be put on stands (Fig. 102).

In any application of X-rays, the amount of radiation is to be kept as small as possible. The useful core of radiation is rigorously cut down by the apertures to give a narrow beam. Insufficient closure of the diaphragms raises the degree of risk due to scattered radiation. The most certain shielding is obtained when all X-ray tube housings are fitted with diaphragms and collimators. However, the cone also produces a really good narrowing of the primary beam. A set of cones should always be kept in readiness, from which the smallest possible is fitted before taking the picture. The X-radiation must be filtered as strongly as the purpose of the particular use permits. In accordance with Para. 8, Section 5, of the Industrial Protection Regulation 950, the minimum filtration for tensions up to 60 kV is 1 mm aluminium equivalent and for tensions above this 2 mm aluminium equivalent. Diagnostic X-ray units with nominal voltages above 75 kV must be fitted with insertable supplementary filters, so that with tensions up to 125 kV total filtration of 3 to 4 mm Al or 0.2 mm Cu can be used, and over 125 kV 5 mm Al or 0.3 mm Cu.

The greatest dangers are with fluoroscopy. Since during the screening the dog must be placed in different positions, it must be held by the staff. Thus, the danger exists that even with the shortest possible exposure time, the person holding the dog, and also the person doing the examination, exceed the maximum permissible dose. For this reason it must be pointed out that fluoroscopy is to be reduced as far as possible. Instead of screening, insofar as this is not absolutely necessary, it is better that one or two more photographs should be taken. The fluoroscopic screens must always be linked to move with the X-ray tube. They should never be arranged to be movable independently, since otherwise there is a danger that the person doing the investigation is hit by the unshielded primary beam. Further, in fluoroscopy, the minimal amount of radiation possible should be employed. This means that it is necessary that the person doing the screening should be sufficiently dark-adapted. There must be a diaphragm for narrowing the useful beam to the smallest possible area, which is adjustable during the procedure. The use of viewing screens is only allowed if it is indispensable in the individual case from the point of view of veterinary medicine.

However useful, it is always very dangerous to put the hand into the direct beam between the X-ray tube and the screen for the purpose of palpitation of the patient. In such cases, one can use a compression cone fixed on the screen. Everyone present in the X-ray room during the screening must wear protective clothing.

By observing all radiation protection measures and with the necessary caution on the part of the staff, it is possible to keep the dose of radiation far below the prescribed maximum permissible level.

In the next section, the setting-up of an X-ray room with its control (and service) room is described briefly. The Clinic and Out-patient Department for Small Domestic Animals of the Karl Marx University, Leipzig has been used as an example.

The X-ray room should be as large as possible with an inside ceiling height of 3.30 m, in order to reduce the scattered radiation. In the Industrial Protection Regulation 950, Para. 6, Section 5 requires the fluoroscopy equipment to be set up so that in the examination of standing patients the distance to the nearest wall of the room is at least 2 m. In the X-ray apparatus to be seen in Fig. 98, the equipment concerned is the 6-valve-unit TuR D 1000 of the VEB (People's Own Undertaking) Transformer and X-ray Works, Dresden, provided with an Ultra-Kostix Stand, an Ultraskop-Z (fluoroscopy table tilting through 90°), a flat grid table, a chest X-ray stand, a supplementary tomograph and an Ultra spot-film device. The lighting of the X-ray room is controlled by switches from the two entrance doors and from the control desk and the red light from the control desk and from the position of the person making the examination. As legally required, both the X-ray room and the control room receive both daylight and fresh air through a window. Apart from the protective aprons and gloves, which are kept on a wall on special holders and stands, the accessories such as cones, syringes contrast media and also the films and cassettes are kept in the control room.

The X-ray room and the control (and service) rooms are provided with rubber floor-covering, as required by Para. 12, Section 4, of the Industrial Protection Regulation 950. Both rooms are ventilated after each photograph, and in the winter at least hourly.

We will now deal with the photographic material. It is well known that X-rays have the property of penetrating through matter. This occurs to a greater extent, the lower the specific gravity or the atomic number of the element. The X-rays are attenuated by the matter traversed. This attenuation is the more pronounced the larger the atomic number of the material and the greater the thickness of the layer. Lead has atomic number 82 and aluminium 13, and therefore aluminium

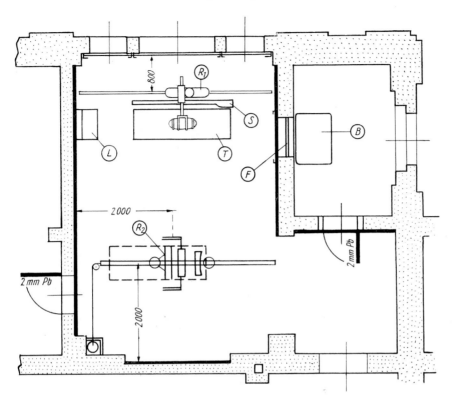

Fig. 103. Plan of X-ray room (as in Fig. 98). R_1 = radiography tube; R_2 = Fluoroscopy tube on; tilting equipment; T = flat grid table; S = tomograph; L = chest X-ray stand; F = lead—glass window; B = control desk.

is penetrated considerably more easily than lead. The bones of the animal body correspond to atomic number about 20 and soft tissue 7. Due to the differing density of the various parts of the object, which accordingly attenuate the X-rays more or less strongly and because of the property of X-rays of blackening X-ray film, it is possible for us to produce an X-ray picture of the organism. The final property of X-rays, which plays a part in X-ray photography, is the excitation of fluorescence by certain salts. The fluorescent screens in fluoroscopic apparatus are coated with a salt of this type, e. g. zinc cadmium sulphide.

However, the images on the fluorescent screen are only visible at the moment of fluoroscopy. In order to retain the image, one utilises the property of X-rays of blackening photographic films.

Through an exposure to radiant energy, which can be X-rays or even light rays, an invisible image is produced in the photographic emulsion, which is described as the "latent image". The actual light-sensitive substances are compounds of silver with halogens (generally bromide as silver bromide), which are present in the photographic emulsion in the form of minute crystalline bodies. If now in X-ray photography the rays penetrate through the tissues and act on the layer of light-sensitive emulsion, the silver bromide grains are excited by the splitting-off of small amounts of bromine to form what are called silver nuclei. This change, caused by the X-rays and remaining as the latent image, is made visible by the process of photographic development. In radio-opaque parts of the object no excitation of the silver bromide grains takes place, for here there is no exposure. Since no bromine is separated off, no blackening results. In the development process, the bromine is removed from the silver bromide grains by means of the reducing substances of the developer, so that in the exposed areas, black metallic silver remains behind, and from this the image is formed.

The unexposed silver bromide is washed out of the emulsion layer by the fixation. The unexposed areas thus appear transparent and clear, while the exposed portions appear grey to black, according to the degree of the exposure.

There is a fundamental difference between the action of X-rays and of light rays. The light acts only superficially, while the X-rays alter the layer in its whole depth. For this reason, the X-ray film is what is called a double film, i. e. it is coated on both sides. The X-ray film has a transparent base, generally of acetylcellulose, which may be coloured. Between the base and the photographic emulsion, which is prepared from a mixture of silver bromide and gelatin, there is an adhesive layer. The light-sensitive emulsions are provided with a skin to protect them against mechanical effects. The double-sided emulsion has the advantage that the contrast is doubled as a result of the blackening of the two layers.

The base is now coloured blue in many cases. This so-called blue film minimises dazzle when examined before a strong light and increases the contrast.

The special requirements of an X-ray film are sensitivity, contrast and clarity. Each X-ray is characterised by its gradation curve, from which one recognises the sensitivity and the contrast of the film material. By sensitivity in X-ray photography is meant the quantitative influence of the exposure on the light-sensitive layer; the smaller the dose of radiation required, the more sensitive is the X-ray film. Sensitivity depends in the first instance on the grain size; the larger and coarser the grain, the higher is the sensitivity. In the interest of the sharpness of the image, however, the grain size must be kept small.

By contrast is meant the difference between the deepest black and the clearest white of the negative. This contrast difference is also known as the image range.

The gradation curve mentioned may be determined by exposing a film stepwise to X-rays and then developing it. The density step wedge obtained in this way is evaluated with the aid of photo-electric equipment, and the magnitude of the blackening related to the exposure. The values determined in this way are drawn as a graph, in which the abscissa is the logarithm of the exposure and the ordinate is the photographic density. On the basis of such a gradation curve for any film, we can determine whether its curve is flat or steep and whether the film is sensitive or not very sensitive. A normal gradation shows harmonically graded density increases, while with the hard or steep gradation the steps of intense blackening and the white steps are extended far into the grey region in the middle. The steeper the slope of gradation curve, the greater are the contrast properties of the film. A soft or flat gradation shows quickly, on the contrary, grey tints in the white part of the density step wedge, while intense blackening is actually not reached.

What are the advantages and disadvantages of the different film gradations? X-ray film with a very steep gradation gives particularly striking contrast and for this reason gives the impression of good definition. Due to the relatively wide development tolerance of such a film, exposure errors can be compensated to a certain extreme in developing. However, no clearly recognisable reproduction of detail is present in the extremely black and extremely white parts of the negative on account of the marked differences of contrast.

A sensitive X-ray film of low gradation possesses only a small development tolerance. On account of the higher sensitivity, however, a shorter exposure time is possible; this limits the blurring due to movement – which is advantageous with animals. There are no extremely black and extremely white parts; more shades are present in the grey region, and the possibility of recognition of radiographic details is improved.

It is also possible to influence the contrast by the choice of kV and mA sec; this is applicable to all types of film. Lower kV and more mA sec always produce radiographs with greater contrast than higher kV and lower mA sec.

By the use of X-ray intensifying screens, it becomes possible to shorten the time of exposure of an X-ray film to 1/15th to 1/20th, according to the "intensifying factor" of the screen. Moreover, by this method the contrast is increased. It is an interesting fact that, for radiographs taken with screens, the X-rays themselves are only responsible for about 5 % of the image production, while the other 95 % is due to the light from the screens.

The intensifying screens consist essentially of calcium tungstate, which with various additives is spread as an emulsion on a base. On exposure to X-rays, the screens light up with blue fluorescence. To guarantee a uniform exposure, the X-ray film, which is always coated on both sides, requires the use of two screens, which are called a screen-combination or a screen-pair. Such a screen-combination consists of two different screens; the one on the tube side is called the front screen and the one on the side away from the tube the back screen. The arrangement of the screens and the film is basically as follows:

Tube – Patient – Front Screen – Film – Back Screen.

The front and back leaves of the screen must be well separated since the front leaf is thinner. The X-rays fall first on the front screen and excite it to fluoresce and then penetrate through the film on to the back screen. This receives the remainder of the rays, which have been partially attenuated in the front screen and in the film, but lights up more strongly on account of its greater thickness. In this way, both sides of the film receive about the same exposure. Only the special intensifying screens for hard radiation technique consist of two equal leaves, since for tensions over 100 kV the penetrating ability of the X-rays is so great, that for practical purposes there is no attenuation in the screen and film.

In radiological diagnosis, three different types of screen are used: the coarse-grained screen (the most highly intensifying screen) with very good intensification but only moderate image sharpness, the medium-grained screen (universal screen), with average image sharpness and good intensification, and the fine-grained screen with very good image sharpness and low intensification. Good amplification is always at the expense of image sharpness and vice versa.

In a possible interchange from one type of screen to another, it is best to alter only the mA secs and not the tension, in order to avoid gross errors of exposure.

The screens must be treated very carefully, since even very slight damage can lead to defects on the film. Screens should never be splashed with water or held with moist hands, since with moisture the film sticks firmly to the screen and on removing it, the protective skin is torn off the screen. It is advantageous to join the screen combination with adhesive strips on one long edge like the covers of a book, or to stick it carefully into the cassette.

The cassette provides a light-tight container for the film and presses the film and the screens firmly together. Cassettes are made almost invariably of metal and should be as flat as possible, so that the film can be brought as close as possible to the patient. The cassette base, which is on the tube side, must be transparent to the rays and usually consists of a thin layer of light metal. The cassette cover, which faces away from the tube, is appreciably thicker and opaque to the rays, so that the back-scattered radiation does not fog the film.

With time, the effects of wear become apparent, as shown by bulging of the base plate of the cassette in the middle, leading to a lack of definition on the X-ray film, especially in the centre of the image. If the fasteners on the cassette are worn or damaged, there may be imperfect closure of the cassette with light entering from the sides and fogging the film.

By far the best sharpness of the image is produced by X-ray exposure without screens on "individual pack" films. These radiographs, however, require a high exposure and for this reason can only be applied in thin parts of the body, such as the extremities.

From what has been said it is obvious that it is not easy to select the right film and the right screens for the particular case. It is therefore advantageous to select from the vast number of types of film and screens available one film and set of screens and accustom oneself to these. Special films or screens are then only used for special radiographs – with hard radiation technique, for extremities, etc. Thus for a long time we have used almost exclusively the most highly sensitive film (Agfa-Rapid, Kodak-Supervidox) and the universal screen. In this way, the continual changes to different exposure conditions were eliminated and relatively short exposure times were attained. This limited the lack of definition due to movement to a minimum, a point of particular importance with animal patients.

There are three basic requirements for a dark room:

1. The dark room should occupy as central a position as possible in relation to the X-ray rooms as a whole, to save unnecessary journeys in the course of work.
2. The size should correspond approximately to the work load, i. e., a dark room should be neither too large nor too small.
3. The dark room must be able to be well ventilated, in the simplest way by a window, which can be reliably blacked out.

The entrance to the dark room should be built in such a way that at entry no light can come in from the outside. In smaller departments, in which only one person deals with the dark-room work, it is often sufficient to put up a sign "No Entry", which lights up in front of the dark room during working. However, whenever several people go in and out in the course of their work, such an expedient no longer suffices.

The most ideal entrance without doors, or any possibility of an accidental light leak, is the labyrinth entrance which, however, has the disadvantage that it needs a lot of space. A light lock with two doors is serviceable in a similar way but there is no completely unobjectionable method of closing off both doors, so that light leaks easily occur. One door with a round curtain fixed in the dark room can act as a simple light lock.

Cleanliness is a basic principle for work in the dark room. It is absolutely necessary to have a "dry" side and a "wet" side, and this arrangement must be observed consistently. By the "dry" side is meant the section in which the films are stored, put into the cassette, stretched in the frame and labelled. The hands must be really dry.

On the "wet" side stand the tanks for development, intermediate washing, fixing and final washing. The floor of the dark room should be kept dry. It is better if the floor is slightly inclined, has a drain and is covered with a wooden grid.

X-ray films ought to be processed only with proper dark-room illumination; the provision of dark-room lighting is very important. One needs bright general space lighting and special illumination for the working area. A prerequisite for good lighting is a suitable ceiling and wall-paint, which should be chosen to be as bright as possible. The ceiling light for general space lighting should shine first on to the ceiling, to give indirect illumination. For the illumination of the working area there are many filters, of which colours from reddish-brown to yellowish-green can be selected. The best shade of colour for the lighting is the green. It is advantageous to fix a working light over the dry side and another over the wet side. With the use of 15 watt bulbs the dark-room lamps must be placed at least 75 cm above the working area, while for 25 watt bulbs the distance should be one metre. Moreover, the lamps should be fixed so that no direct illumination of the photographic films is possible. The film should be exposed to the dark-room lighting for only a short time, while it is being put into the cassette and during labelling. In doing this, bright and reflecting bases are to be avoided. The tank must be closed with a lid during the development. As far as possible, the development should only be checked by inspection at a distance of about 1 metre away from the light source.

Since light filters age with time and then partially transmit unfiltered light, the safety of the lighting system should be checked once a year. This test can easily be carried out in the following way. A film is cut into two parts in the completely darkened room. One strip is covered with black paper. The other strip is illuminated with the dark-room lamp after switching on the light in a series of steps, of duration 30 seconds, 60 seconds, 90 seconds and 120 seconds, respectively, for each quarter of the area. After completely blacking-out, the two strips of film are stretched in one frame and developed. An exposure of less than 120 seconds ought to be imperceptible, otherwise the filter must be changed. For testing the safety of the dark-room lighting, test patterns are supplied free of charge on request by various firms.

X-ray films are developed almost exclusively in a tank. Tank development has a numer of advantages, among which may be mentioned better control of the process, reduction of the number of film defects, better and more uniform treatment of the film, more thorough utilisation of the baths and negligible

7*

oxidation by the air. Film holders are necessary; these are made of stainless steel (V2A or V4A) or plastic. The V4A-holders are best, since they are least corroded by chemicals. Plastic holders which are resistant to the photographic chemicals are also very practicable in use, but they have the disadvantage that they hold the large sizes of film badly and easily become distorted by the heat in the drying cabinet.

For drying films it is advisable to acquire a drying cabinet. By this means one gets rapid drying and a great economy of space.

The next matter for discussion is the film-processing in the dark room. It is well known that up to the moment when the film goes into the fixing bath, one can work only with the dark-room lamp. After taking the film out of the cassette only a preliminary marking is put on the exposed but still undeveloped film. This is best done with a pencil. The final identification label is put on after drying.

The film is then stretched in the holder and dipped into the tank of developer. The X-ray developer contains Metol, hydroquinone, sodium sulphite, soda and potassium bromide. The developing agents proper (the reducing substances) are the Metol and the hydroquinone. Metol is a "surface developer" which acts quickly, while the hydroquinone is a slowly acting "depth developer". It is very important for the work in the dark room that the films are fully developed since otherwise the hydroquinone is not completely effective and the negatives are not sufficiently secure. The sodium sulphite is intended to bind the oxygen from the air and the water, since the developers Metol and hydroquinone have a great affinity for oxygen and deteriorate very quickly as a result of the combination with it.

The developers require the presence of alkali for their activity, and this alkaline reaction is guaranteed by the soda. The potassium bromide serves as a regulating substance; it prevents a too rapid and uncontrolled tempo in the reduction process.

The chemical process of development is in short and simple terms as follows. The X-rays and light rays loosen the chemical union of the silver halide. Accordingly, by means of the developer, the exposed silver can be reduced easily to metallic silver. With an appropriately long action of the developer, the non-exposed silver is also reduced.

The duration of development is determined by the age of the solution and the temperature and also to a certain extent by the type of exposure. For an unused developer, one can lay down approximately the following optimal times of development:

	Duration of development	
Temperature	Normal	Maximal
	minutes	minutes
16 °C	7	9
18 °C	6	8
20 °C	5.5	6
22 °C	4.5	5
24 °C	3.5	4
26 °C	3	3.5

The normal temperature of the developer should be if possible 18 °C. As a rule of thumb, one can remember that for a temperature increase or decrease of 2 °C, about 1 min is subtracted from or added to the time of development.

In urgent cases, where minutes matter, as in the X-ray control of surgical measures, a rapid developer can be used. Either one warms the usual developer to 26 °C or one works with a catechol developer, for which the development time at a temperature of 26 °C is only about 10–20 sec. However, the method of rapid development is not ideal, since the films developed in this way are far inferior in contrast and durability to films developed in the normal way.

During the chemical process of development, the bromine of the silver bromide of the emulsion layer combines with the alkali of the developer. In this way potassium bromide is formed and this delays the development. Moreover, the strength of the Metol and hydroquinone decreases and the developer is used up. Every film takes several drops of developer solution with it on removal from the tank, so that from time to time the tank must be filled up. Topping up with "replenisher solution" is best. The "replenisher" is devised to correct the alteration of the developer with use. In this way the developer can be kept constant for quite a long time, so that the time of development remains the same.

The tank for development must always be closed with a cover and moreover the fluid level should reach to the edge of the tank, to keep the layer of air between the cover and the developer as thin as possible. In this way, premature oxidation of the developer by the air is prevented.

After the development of the film comes the intermediate washing. The alkaline developer can be largely removed from the surface layer, if the film is washed in running water, while the developer continues to work in the depth of the emulsion. The intermediate washing in running water ought to last at least 20 sec. It is better, however, to bring the alkaline process to an end by means of a stop bath. For this purpose a 1 % acetic acid solution is used with about $\frac{1}{2}$ min washing. Since alkaline developer gets continually into the stop bath with the film, the acid reaction of course decreases, so that the bath must be tested now and then with litmus paper for its acid content.

After the intermediate washing the film goes into the X-ray fixing bath. This is a 20–40 % solution of sodium thiosulphate ("hypo"), which has an acid reaction because it also contains potassium metabisulphite or sodium bisulphite. In the fixing bath, the unexposed silver, which is of course not reduced, is dissolved out of the emulsion. The alkaline developer still present in the emulsion is neutralised by the acidity. In a fresh fixing bath the films clear after 3 to 4 min and can be examined briefly with the light. They must then still be fixed for about three times as long, since insufficiently fixed films show brown spots after a time. On the average, one reckons with a fixation time of 20 min. The fixing bath deteriorates after some time. To test the fixing solution, a layer of 4 % potassium iodide solution about one finger's breadth is poured onto a half test-tube full of the solution. The solution remains clear if the fixing bath is still usable, but it becomes cloudy when it is exhausted. One must also take care that the solution in the fixing bath does not become too warm, since otherwise the emulsion softens.

When the film is fully fixed, it is placed for about half an hour into running water for the final washing. The chemicals of the fixing bath ought to be fully washed out of the film. With an insufficiently long final wash, traces of the fixing solution still remain in the emulsion and produce browning. In the washing, it is important that the films should not come in contact with one another but are rinsed round with water from all sides.

The drying of the X-ray films takes place either in a dust-free space at room temperature or in an electrical drying cabinet. The temperature in the drying cabinet should not exceed 40–45 °C, otherwise the emulsion is easily damaged.

After drying, the corners by which the film was fixed in the holder are cut off, since they look untidy and remain for a long time.

After this, there is the final labelling of the film, which is best done with white Indian ink. It is useful to put the films immediately into paper envelopes, in order to avoid damage.

Subsequently, the film goes into the X-ray record office, in which it must be kept for a least 6 years, since it is to be considered as a document. The film belongs to the producer of the radiograph and can be loaned to a court or to the veterinary surgeon treating the case. The owner of the animal has no claim to the film, even on loan.

As a result of faulty treatment of the film, during exposure and during the process of development, there are now and then film defects. These must be considered in some detail, since they can make radiological diagnosis very difficult.

Thin pictures with little contrast are generally produced by the application of kV levels which are too high, in other words by radiations which are too hard. This occurs particularly with low output machines with short exposure times and high kV values. Pictures of this sort may also arise by taking X-rays of thick patients without grids. These errors are best avoided by using soft radiation, more mA and rather longer exposure time.

A thin picture can also arise from under-development, e. g., as a result of too short development, or too cold or exhausted developer. This error can be recognised best by examining the blackening of edge of the film where there are no intervening tissues. If the film is held against a source of light, one can see a finger held behind the film. The fault can only be avoided in development by correcting the time and the temperature of the developer.

Overblackened films can be caused by over-exposure, as is often seen with thin parts of the body. The product mA sec is too large. The image emerges too rapidly during development. Overblackened films also arise from over-development, particularly with developer which is too warm or fresh. In general, on these films development fogging occurs in association with the intense blackening.

Under the influence of a strong source of light (daylight or light from a lamp) upon the film before or during development, a reversal of the light and dark areas takes place as a result of the characteristic behaviour of the photoemulsion. This is described as the solarisation effect (Fig. 104).

Circumscribed areas of blackening of the film in the form of minute points or tree and lightning figures arise as a result of electrical discharges (Fig. 105), when the film becomes electrostatically charged by friction in unpacking from the wrapping or removal from the cassette too rapidly. Films must be taken out in such a way that all friction is avoided.

Very intense blackening of the edges of the films is usually caused by faulty cassettes, which let in the daylight. The blackening is always more pronounced on one edge of the film, where the cassette fastener does not close tightly.

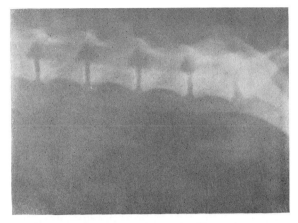

Fig. 104. Solarisation effect.

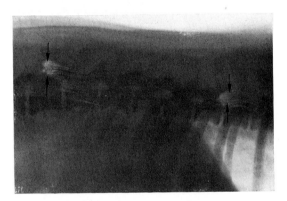

Fig. 105. Electrical discharges.

Fogging (Fig. 106) occurs on films from a number of causes. It can arise as a result of too fresh or too warm developer, previous exposure of the cassette to X-rays, radiations which are too hard or intense, scattered radiation during radiography, too frequent inspection of the film during development – from oxidation – and old films. X-ray films should, if possible, not be stored for longer than six months.

Yellow fogging appears as greyish-yellow dirty fogging after excessively long development and also with developer which is too warm or fresh or exhausted.

If developer is carried into the fixing bath during the brief intermediate washing, the fixing bath shows an insufficiently acid reaction. In this way, dichroic fogging is produced; this is an iridescent, reddish-green coloured haze.

Large, bright patches with indefinite edges resembling zones are observed, when the films hang too closely together in the developing tank and stick to one another or on to the wall of the tank (Fig. 107). Similar but dark patches arise from the

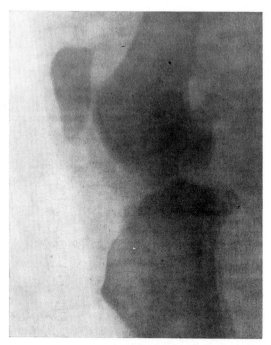

Fig. 106. Fogging.

films sticking together in the fixing bath, since the fixing solution cannot then act and the developer goes on working (Fig. 108). Accordingly, in all tanks it is important to leave sufficient distance between the films.

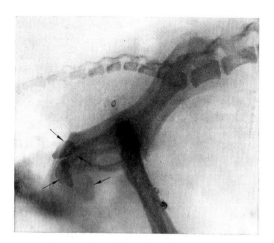

Fig. 107. Films stuck together in the developer.

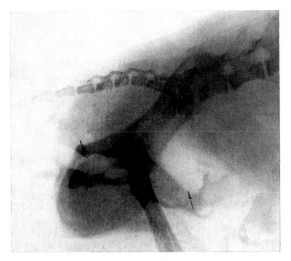

Fig. 108. Films stuck together in the fixative.

If the work in the dark room is dirty and the film gets splashed with water, developer or fixing fluid before development, spots arise at these places. Moderately dark patches on the negative are seen after spotting with water (Fig. 109), dark patches after developer and bright patches after fixative (Fig. 110).

The screenless single envelope-packed film is very sensitive to pressure. A slight pressure on the unexposed emulsion makes it insensitive, and strong pressure more sensitive. Therefore the pressure points are lighter or darker than their surroundings (Fig. 111). This is why the single film should only be held at the corners and should be handled with care.

If the hands of the dark-room staff are moist or greasy, the fingers leave impressions behind on the film, upon which the developer cannot act. This gives rise to fine, bright lines in the form of finger prints.

Damaged places on the screens, which of course produce less light, give sharply defined light patches, which always lie in one and the same place and only on one side of the film (Fig. 112). These defects can only be avoided by proper treatment and care of the screens.

Occasionally, one sees on films numerous, closely packed, point-like transparencies with a thin, dark edge, which arise from bacterial erosion (Fig. 113). These points are best recognised in oblique incident light. The bacterial erosion is due to colonies of bacteria growing on the gelatine of the emulsion, aided by warm and moist storage.

In the following paragraph radiographic technique and the measures to be observed in connection with it will be discussed. Basically there are two possibilities for X-ray examination, fluoroscopy and radiography.

In fluoroscopy almost the whole of the energy of the X-rays is transformed into the fluorescent light of the screen. In contrast to the radiograph, which is, of

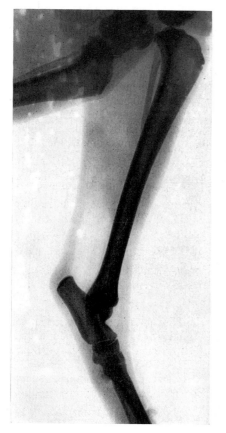

Fig. 109. Spotting with water.

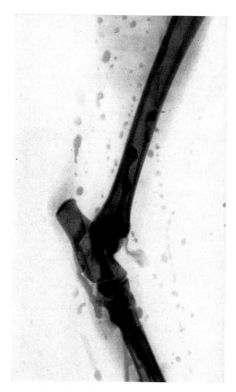

Fig. 110. Spotting with fixative.

course, a negative, on screening, an object which is penetrated by the rays only with difficulty, e. g. bone, appears as a dark area, like a shadow, while an object which transmits the rays easily, e. g. lung, appears bright. For this reason one also speaks of shadows in radiographs although in these cases, instead of shadows, light areas are to be seen. Fluoroscopy has a number of advantages. The animal can be held in any position, its body can be rotated and turned during the screening and the movement of individual organs can be observed and assessed. One disadvantage is that there is no permanent picture, but the greatest disadvantage of fluoroscopy is the dose of radiation to the person doing the examination and to the staff holding the animal.

In the case of the radiograph, a permanent picture is obtained but this only puts on record the state at the time of exposure. Further, only one plane of the object is represented in the image. Yet, in the radiograph, we have a negative which can be considered carefully and assessed and can be called upon for comparison even after a considerable time.

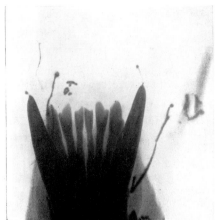

Fig. 111. Pressure site due to bite.

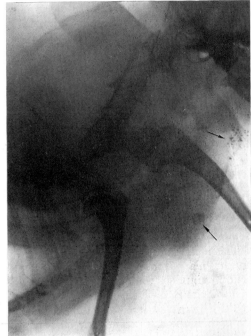

Fig. 112. Screen marks.

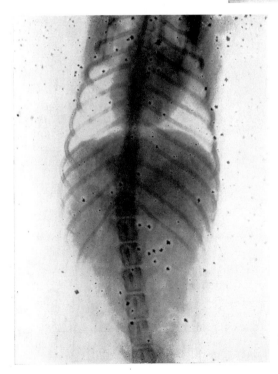

Fig. 113. Bacterial erosion.

The X-ray image shows a projection rather like a silhouette and this applies both for screening and radiography. It is well-known that, on account of their parallelism, the sun's rays lead to a projection which is correct in size and shape, as appears in silhouettes. On the contrary, the X-rays arise from a very small source, the focal spot of the anode, and are accordingly divergent. This fact leads to definite laws for image formation, termed the laws of the central projection:

1. The image is always larger than the object (Fig. 114).
2. The larger the distance of the object from the focal spot, the smaller is the enlargement (Fig. 115). The same result is obtained with reduction of the distance from the object to the film (Fig. 116).
3. The farther the film is removed from the X-ray tube, the greater is the surface hit by the rays. The surface area involved is increased four times by doubling the distance and nine times by trebling the distance. Since the X-rays are now distributed over a larger area, the region of the surface originally considered receives only a quarter or a ninth, as the case may be, of the quantity of radiation, i. e. the intensity of the X-rays decreases with the square of the distance.

This means that those parts of the body which lie furthest away from the film appear enlarged and distorted, while the parts close to the film give an image which is approximately the correct size. Therefore one must bring the parts of the body of particular interest into as close proximity to the film as possible. The enlargement is also eliminated by means of long distance radiography. For this, a focus-film distance of about 2 m is chosen, but the distance is limited by the reduction of the intensity of the X-rays. Further, in order to get an approximate spatial impression of the object, two radiographs can be taken in different planes. Since the X-rays diverge, one must take care that the central ray falls as closely as possible in the middle of the picture.

Every straight radiograph represents all the layers of tissue through which the rays have penetrated. It is termed a summation image. If a part of the body near the edge is to be displayed preferentially, contact radiography is used. The part of the body concerned is brought as close as possible to the film, while the window of the tube for the exit of radiation is brought close to the opposite point on the body. By this means, there is a blurred enlargement of the parts distant from the film, while the layers near the film give a sharp image of the correct size. On account of the short focus-object distance, however, the radiation dose to the skin is much greater than in a normal radiograph.

The following factors are of particular importance for the quality of an X-ray image:

1. The photographic material.
2. The contrast.
3. The sharpness.

The photographic material has already been discussed in detail.

By contrast is meant the difference in the blackening of adjacent parts of the image. The greater this difference, the greater is the contrast. The contrast, of course, depends on the kind of organ and the thickness of the object. If dense parts of organs lie next to less dense parts, as for example, bones beside air-containing organs, there are good contrasts. Very thick layers strongly reduce the

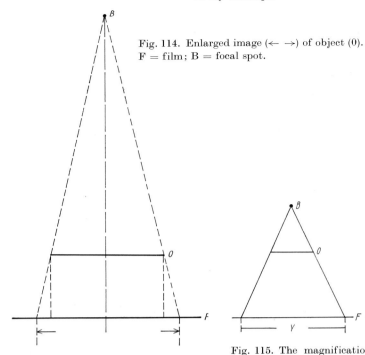

Fig. 114. Enlarged image (← →) of object (0).
F = film; B = focal spot.

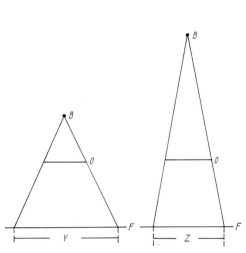

Fig. 115. The magnification (Y, Z) decreases with increase of the focus-object
distance (B).

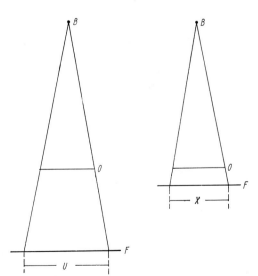

Fig. 116. The magnification (U, X) becomes less with decrease of the object-
film distance (0–F).

contrast on account of the unavoidable scattered radiation; for this reason the use of grids is indicated for all large patients or bulky layers of tissue.

In addition, the quality of the radiation has a great influence upon the contrast. The tension is primarily responsible for this. Hard rays (high voltage) result in poor contrasts, while soft rays give intense contrasts. Within limits the pictures obtained with both methods are very satisfactory for use. With too great a degree of hardness, the contrasts are so slight that the discrimination of the structure and of the fine details of the picture suffers. At the other extreme, with low voltage, the rays can no longer penetrate through the more strongly absorbing sections. Apart from the voltage, the exposure time influences the contrast, though in practice this is not of much importance. The development process influences the contrast, as we have already seen.

By sharpness of the image is meant the nature of the boundary of the individual parts of the picture, e. g., at bone. For a high degree of sharpness, the edges of the elements of the image must be smooth and sharp.

Blurring, which may appear in some circumstances, is due to a number of causes:

1. Geometrical blurring. This is conditioned by a large focal spot, each point of which for practical purposes produces its own image. The impression of blurring due to geometrical factors is strengthened further if the distance between the focus and the object is too short, since for short distances those parts of the object most distant from the film give a particularly blurred image. There is an inverse relation for the distance between the object and the film; a large object-film distance results in marked enlargement and distortion. Taking into account these three factors, the following formula is obtained for the geometrical blurring:

$$\text{Blurring} = \text{focal size} \times \frac{\text{object-film distance}}{\text{focus-object distance}}.$$

2. Kinetic blurring. This is due to movement of the whole of a restless patient or to the movement of individual organs during the exposure, e. g. the movements of the lung during respiration. To obtain a good degree of sharpness of the image, every effort must be made to keep the patient as quiet as possible during the time of the exposure. This is the reason why so much importance should be laid on the positioning of the animal. Even a shift of $1/10$ mm is clearly recognisable in the X-ray image as blurring. Therefore, radiographs of organs subject to movements as, e. g., the heart and the lung, require short exposure times.

3. Material blurring (blurring due to the film and screens). The most important cause of this is the coarse grain of the film and above all of the screen, particularly with highly sensitive films or with coarse-grained screens. In addition, the developer can increase or reduce the blurring of the image, according to whether it is a coarse working or fine working developer.

To combat blurring, all three factors must be improved. The sharpest radiographs are obtained by the use of a small focal spot, and a fine-grained film without a screen and with the patient in a position of complete rest. As kinetic blurring is greater than the other two factors, it appears e. g. to be advantageous to increase the geometrical blurring by having a rather larger focal spot and offsetting this, to reduce the kinetic blurring by means of shorter exposure time.

Before positioning the animal for the radiograph, one must be quite clear about the path of the rays with which the picture should be taken, in order to show the presumed pathological state to best advantage.

The path of the rays which is most commonly used in dogs is the frontal, which is always designated as latero-lateral. It can come in from the right or left. It has become standard practice with us, to lay the patient on the left side, except for special pictures. This has above all the advantage of better representation of the heart. In preparing for a radiograph with the rays in the latero-lateral direction, the dog must be restrained lying on the left side (Fig. 117). We are of the opinion that binding down the "patients" is neither more complicated and time-consuming than holding nor more painful for the animal. With calmness in the X-ray room and in the presence of the owners, the dogs can be bound down for positioning in nearly all cases without any resistance. Radiation exposure of the staff can thus be reduced to a minimum.

The second most important direction of the beam for the thorax or abdomen is the sagittal. For a ventro-dorsal radiograph, the dog is bound down on its back lying on all four extremities (Fig. 118). For a dorso-ventral radiograph, the patient lies on the abdomen (Fig. 119). For chest radiographs, the owner keeps the dog's mouth closed for the moment of the picture, to avoid blurring due to breathing.

These three directions of the beam (latero-lateral, ventro-dorsal and dorso-ventral) and the corresponding measures for fixing the animal are suitable for all radiographs of the abdomen, chest, neck, head and vertebral column.

For the extremities, the designation of the positions for radiography is somewhat different. With the medio-lateral view, the rays pass through the extremity from the inside to the outside and the film lies on the outer surface. If the extremity is X-rayed from the front to the back or from above to below, this is designated for the front leg as dorso-volar and for the back leg as dorso-plantar and the reversed position (from the back to the front) as volo-dorsal or planto-dorsal respectively. With these radiographs also, the patients can usually be restrained with bands on the table, so obviating the need for staff to hold the patient in the majority of cases. For radiographs of the extremities particularly in the medio-lateral view, the extremities must be fixed as far as possible from one another, in order to avoid overlapping by the image of the limb in which one is not interested and which is at some distance from the film. With the anterior extremities, the one to be photographed is brought near to the film and stretched far forward, while the other one is stretched far back. In this way, the very frequent overlap of the images of the shoulder blades is also avoided. With the posterior extremities, one stretches the one to be X-rayed far back, while the other one is angled sharply sideways and to the front.

With the skull, one designates the frontal direction of the beam as latero-lateral while the axial is called submento-vertical or vertico-mental (from the region below the chin to the crown of the head and vice versa).

In order to press the patient as closely as possible on to the cassette or grid table, we use a compression band which can be fitted on to the table on both sides and shifted in an adjustable manner. It is laid over the patient and drawn tight (Fig. 117).

In particular cases, radiographs of the patient standing or sitting are necessary, e. g. for showing a fluid level in hydrothorax. The chest X-ray table is well suited

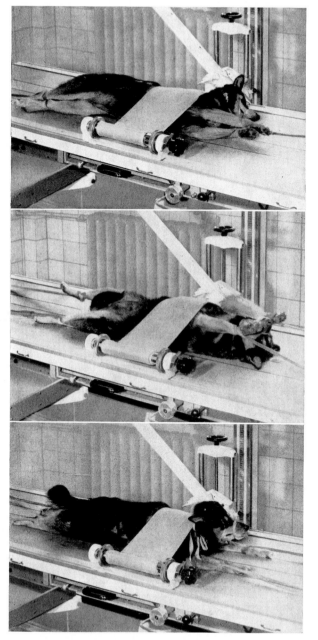

Fig. 117. Positioning of the dog for radiography in the latero-lateral ray direction. For better immobilisation a compression bandage was placed on the thorax. (University Department of Illustration).

Fig. 118. Positioning of the dog for radiography in the ventrodorsal ray direction. (University Department of Illustration.)

Fig. 119. Positioning of the dog for radiography in the dorsoventral ray direction. (University Department of Illustration.)

for this and has the advantage of a vertical grid, thus allowing pictures to be taken with a grid with the patient standing (Figs. 120, 121).

After the animal has been positioned for the photograph, the X-ray tube is brought into position. In addition to the centering of the tube, the choice of the distance is a very important point. For one thing, the enlargement of the object changes with the distance and for another, the intensity of the X-rays decreases with the square of the distance (see page 108). For this reason it is expedient, if possible, always to keep the distance from the focus to the film the same, e. g.

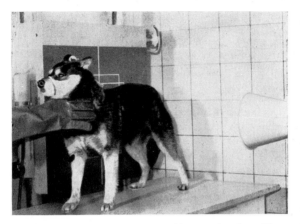

Fig. 120. Lateral radiography with the patient standing on the chest X-ray stand. (University Department of Illustration.)

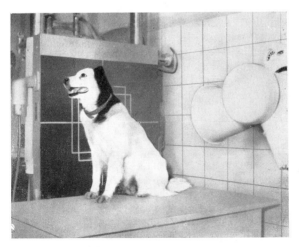

Fig. 121. Lateral radiography with the dog sitting on the chest X-ray stand. (University Department of Illustration.)

8   Christoph, Diseases of Dogs

always 100 cm. Shortening the distance implies an essential reduction of the exposure time, for 70 cm one half of the time necessary at 100 cm. Increasing the focus-film distance leads to a considerable increase of exposure time; for 140 cm, the exposure time must be double that which is used for 100 cm. A departure from 100 cm is only undertaken for contact radiographs and with the hard radiation technique (see page 126).

For what is called the centering of the X-ray tube, i. e., the focusing, the most important concept is the central ray. By this is meant the axis of the cone of radiation. For most radiographs, the central ray should be at right angles to the mid-point of the film, where the organ to be photographed lies as centrally as possible.

All the staff, except the one holding the head of the animal, now leave the X-ray room. In the control room, everything is set ready and at the moment when the patient is lying most quietly, the radiograph is "shot". The best time for this is when the dog has breathed out, since then the respiratory movements stop for a fraction of a second. With restless dogs, it is better to keep the mouth and nose closed for the moment of the picture.

What exposure conditions are to be used for the radiography required? It is very difficult to give exact instructions but tables of exposure valves and other aids are available. These values are altered by the use of a different film (e. g. with the most highly sensitive X-ray film), a different screen, single pack film, etc. Moreover the exposure times for the same picture are different for every apparatus. For this reason, it is recommended that as far as possible one should always work with the same kind of screen (e. g. with the universal screen) and use the same film. In our hands, the universal screen and the most highly sensitive film (e. g. Agfa-Rapid) have stood the test of time. For specially positioned cases, one must now and then of course fall back an another screen. For photographs of the lower sections of the extremities, the screenless single pack film is worth recommending.

To avoid errors of exposure, we have drawn up an Exposure Table, which contains all the standard radiographs and in which for each radiograph the values for small, medium and large dogs are set out. This table refers only to the most highly sensitive film with the universal screen or to the screenless film with the use of 6-valve apparatus. We are of the opinion that errors of exposure are more easily avoided with the help of the table than with any other aid. Accordingly, it is reproduced here. Attention must be drawn to the fact that it cannot be applied uncritically to every other machine but will give some guide.

At this point something must be said briefly about the restriction of scattered radiation. One must always avoid having the beam of radiation unnecessarily large; that would mean a substantial increase of the scattered rays and accordingly a deterioration in the quality of the image. A simple means of reducing the size of the beam is the cone, which is interchangeable and limits the beam all round. If one combines the cone required with a light projector, the choice of the most favourable field and the centering are greatly facilitated, since the field is made visible on the skin of the patient with the light beam.

The scattered rays which are still present must be prevented from affecting the film. This can be achieved with the grid, which is placed between the object and the film. The grid is only of benefit if a great deal of scattered radiation arises from large masses of body tissue. With the use of grids, the exposure time is, of course, increased, since the lead lamellae also remove part of the primary radiation.

Something must now be said about the choice of film size. It is to be borne in mind that the objects always form images which are somewhat enlarged; this is particularly noticeable with short distances between the focus and object and long distances between the object and the film. It should also be remembered that the films are about 1 cm smaller than the cassettes on each side. The following sizes are in general available:

$$9 \times 12 \text{ cm}$$
$$13 \times 18 \text{ cm}$$
$$18 \times 24 \text{ cm}$$
$$24 \times 30 \text{ cm}$$
$$30 \times 40 \text{ cm}$$
$$15 \times 40 \text{ cm}$$
$$35.6 \times 35.6 \text{ cm}$$

The table gives the usual sizes for the various radiographs.

For radiography of the extremities, the long and narrow film sizes are the most suitable. If they are not available, two pictures can be taken on one film, since as a rule, it is necessary to have two pictures in planes at right angles to one another, e. g. medio-lateral and dorso-volar. For the first picture, half the film, or cassette, is covered with a radio-opaque plate; then this plate is laid on the previously exposed part and the second picture taken on the other half. Obviously the pictures should correspond at the top and the bottom on the two halves.

In the following section, the technique of contrast methods and some special radiographic procedures will be summarised briefly. It is well known that a picture with plenty of contrast is necessary for diagnosis. If, however, adjacent tissues show no very great differences in absorption, they will not stand out sufficiently from one another. In the application of artificial contrast media, it depends less on reproducing the organ in question directly in the picture than in attempting a cast, with filling or covering from within with substances whose X-ray absorption is greater or smaller than the adjacent parts of the body.

The positive contrast media are substances whose atomic weight is greater than that of the tissue, so that they give a more intense shadow density than the organs. Preparations of iodine, barium, bismuth and bromine are mainly used as positive contrast media. For increasing the density of the shadows, a tri-iodination of the molecule has been carried out in modern contrast media.

The negative contrast media have a lighter atomic weight and their X-ray shadow is of lower density than that of the body tissues. The most important negative contrast media are air, oxygen and nitrous oxide.

We have two different possibilities for the incorporation and excretion of the contrast medium. First there is the normal physiological route, with the direction either normal or reversed, as with contrast filling of the gastro-intestinal tract per os or rectally. Secondly, the excretion of the contrast medium, which has been incorporated into the body by some method, is left to the body itself with the help of the blood stream, as in the filling of the renal pelvis after intravenous injection of contrast medium.

Data for radiographic examinations with a 6-valve unit (rotating anode tube) and the most highly sensitive film (Agfa-Rapid) with universal screen or single pack film (Agfa-Sino) and a focus-film distance of 1 metre

Region	Direction of the X-ray beam and positioning of the dog	Cassettes (C) or Single pack film (S)	Film size cms	Grid	kV	mA. Secs	Remarks
1. Skull, frontal	Latero-lateral, dog lies on the side, the head to be fixed against the back of the neck	C	18/24 to 24/30	— +	50 54 56 52 55 60	28 32 45 45 47 50	
2. Skull, axial	Submento-vertical or vertico-submental, lying on belly or back	C	18/24 24/30	— +	50 54 56 52 55 60	28 32 45 45 47 50	
3. Lower jaw	Vertico-submental, back position, film is pressed in below the teeth	S	13/18	—	60 64 67	62 68 75	
4. Teeth	As in 3 or latero-lateral with dental film	S	13/18 or dental film	—	As in 3 or 45 48 52	As in 3 or 20 25 30	Focus-object distance 40 cm
5. Cervical spine	Latero-lateral or ventro-dorsal, side or back position, head to be well fixed	C	18/24 24/30	+	50 56 60	30 45 55	
6. Thoracic spine	Latero-lateral or ventro-dorsal, side or back position	C	24/30 30/40 15/40	+	55 58 65	35 45 65	

7. Lumbar spine	As 6.	C	13/18 to 30/40 15/40	+	55 60 65	35 55 65
8. Pelvis	Latero-lateral, side position	C	18/24 24/30	+	52 60 65	35 50 65
9. Pelvis and hip joint	Ventro-dorsal, back position, hind legs to be stretched far behind, patella must point upwards	C	18/24 24/30	+	50 55 60	35 40 60
10. Scapula and shoulder joint	Latero-lateral, side position	C	18/24 24/30	+	56 58 60	35 47 55
11. Humerus	Latero-lateral, side position	C	13/18 24/30	+	52 56	35 40
	Dorso-volar, belly position, foreleg to be drawn far forward	S	13/18 18/24	−	62 65 70 60	65 75 90 50
12. Elbow joint	Latero-lateral, side-position	S	13/18	−	60 62 65	60 70 80
	Dorso-volar, belly position, limb to be drawn forward	S	13/18	−	60 62 65	65 75 85
13. Radius and ulna	Latero-lateral, side position or dorso-volar, belly position as 12	S	13/18 to 24/30 15/40	−	60 63 66	65 75 85
14. Carpal joint and carpus	Latero-lateral and dorso-volar, as 12	S	13/18 18/24	−	60 62 64	60 65 70

Region	Direction of the X-ray beam and positioning of the dog	Cassettes (C) or Single pack film (S)	Film size cms	Grid	kV	mA. Secs	Remarks
15. Toes	Latero-lateral, side position	S	13/18	—	58 60 62	60 65 70	
	Dorso-volar, belly position	S	9/12 13/18	—	60 62 64	62 67 72	
16. Femur	Latero-lateral, side position, or perhaps dorso-plantar, back position, limb to be fully stretched	C	13/18 to 30/40	—	47 48 50	15 20 25	
17. Knee joint	Latero-lateral and dorso-plantar, as 16	S	9/12 13/18	—	60 64 68	60 75 85	
	Planto-dorsal, belly position, limb fully stretched and to be drawn backwards	S	13/18	—	60 64 68	65 80 90	
18. Tibia and fibula	Latero-lateral, side position	S	13/18 to 24/30	—	58 60 62	60 65 70	
	Dorso-plantar, belly position, limb extended and to be pulled forward and laterally	S	13/18 to 24/30	—	60 62 64	60 65 70	
19. Ankle joint	Latero-lateral, side position	S	13/18	—	60 64 68	60 75 90	
	Dorso-plantar, as 18	S	13/18	—	58 62 65	60 70 80	

20. Tarsus	Latero-lateral, as 18	S	13/18	—	60 64 68	60 75 90	
	Dorso-plantar, as 18	S	13/18	—	58 62 65	60 70 80	
21. Whole limb	Latero-lateral, side position	C	15/40	—	45 47 50	15 18 22	
22. Thorax (lungs)	Latero-lateral, side position	C	18/24 to 30/40	+	54 57 60	30 40 60	
	Ventro-dorsal, back position	C	18/24 to 30/40	+	56 58 65	35 45 55	
	Hard ray technique, latero-lateral	C	18/24 to 30/40	—	95 100 105	10 12 14	Focus-object distance: 170 cm. Object-film distance: 20 cm
23. Abdomen	Latero-lateral, side position	C	13/18 to 30/40	+	52 56 60	35 45 60	
	Ventro-dorsal, back position and dorso-ventral, belly position	C	13/18 to 30/40	+	54 58 65	35 45 65	

For each group there are always three values, of which the first is for small dogs, the second for medium-sized dogs and the third for large dogs.

Radiographs with contrast media should usually be taken in two planes and certainly if one wants to determine the accurate localisation of a foreign body or a pathological state.

There are numerous forms of application of contrast media in radiology but only a relatively small number of these have found a place in the routine investigations of veterinary medicine.

Examination of the stomach. This is often associated with the study of the intestinal tract (Fig. 300). This method is the one most frequently applied in veterinary medicine. The aim of the examination of the stomach is to render visible the mucosal relief and the form and position of the stomach, or the possible presence of an invisible foreign body, as well as the detection of an enlargement of the liver. As contrast medium an aqueous barium sulphate suspension in the ratio of one part contrast medium to two parts water, or one to one is administered by mouth. One mouthful is sufficient for relief presentation, but for complete filling of the stomach with passage through the intestine about 50 to 250 ml of the suspension are used. The radiographs are taken immediately after administration as well as after about 30 min and 1, 2 and 4 hr. The latero-lateral view has proved to be the most advantageous and may be combined with ventro-dorsal photographs and similar pictures in the standing position.

Examination of the intestine. Barium examination of the intestine is carried out in the same way as the examination of the stomach (Figs. 300 and 301).

Examination of the colon with a radio-opaque enema. Barium sulphate is also used for barium enemas, though the consistency is considerably thinner and more fluid; the mixture used for the stomach can be diluted with 5–10 times its volume of water. This contrast mixture is run into the rectum as an enema at body temperature, in order to demonstrate the rectum and the colon (Fig. 302). Recently, to improve the demonstration of the mucosal pattern and to study the movements of the colon, a contact laxative has been added to the contrast medium so that a more rapid evacuation is obtained. Despite this, some of the contrast medium remains adherent to the mucosa producing a good visualisation of the mucosal pattern. The radiographs should be taken immediately after the enema and after the evacuation.

Urography. The aim of urography is the demonstration of the position, size and form of the kidneys, ureters and bladder as well as the presence of urinary calculi. The functional efficiency of the kidneys can be assessed fairly accurately with the help of urography.

Cystography is most useful. For this purpose a positive contrast medium (potassium iodide, etc.) or a negative one (air) is introduced into the bladder by means of a catheter. Potassium iodide in 10% solution is considerably cheaper than the contrast media available commercially and is quite adequate for our purposes. The radiographs are taken immediately after filling the bladder with 10 to 30 ml of contrast medium and using the latero-lateral and ventro-dorsal views. The use of a negative contrast medium is particularly valuable for the detection of stones in the bladder.

For the demonstration of the kidneys and the ureters, only intravenous pyelography is suitable for use in the dog, since retrograde filling meets with considerable difficulties. In contrast to retrograde urography, in which the contrast medium is introduced into the kidney with the aid of a ureteric catheter, in intravenous urography the contrast medium is injected into the blood stream. After a certain time it is excreted through the kidneys (Excretion urography). The injection of 5–20 ml of the contrast medium can be made quickly or slowly, intravenously into the saphenous vein, but with rapid injection of the tri-iodinated contrast medium; a careful watch must be kept on the pulse and respiration. The radiographs are taken 5–30 min after the beginning of the injection. In our experience radiographs at 7, 14 and 21 min after the injection are most useful. If excretion is not completed after 21 min, further X-rays are taken every 20–30 min.

One gets the best pictures with the ventro-dorsal direction of the rays. An increased filling of the renal pelvis is obtained by compression of the ureters just in front of the pelvic brim with the help of a football bladder or a rubber ball, which is pressed tight with the compression band. This compression should be started only after the first X-ray picture, i. e. after 7 min, so that an unambiguous assessment of the renal function is guaranteed. Further, the combination of intravenous urography with a retropneumoperitoneum is advantageous.

Fistulography. In order to ascertain the form and extension of a fistula, the contrast medium in an amount of 5 to 30 ml – according to the size of the track and of the base of the fistula – is injected under pressure into the track. The opening of the fistula must then be closed as firmly as possible. As contrast medium one generally uses viscous media. The radiographs are taken a few minutes after the injection and always in two planes at right angles to one another.

Sialography. By sialography is meant the demonstration of the otherwise unrecognisable salivary glands and their ducts with the aid of a contrast medium. By this means obstructions of the ducts and salivary calculi which may be present can be rendered clearly visible. For filling the salivary ducts the contrast medium is injected into the parotid duct for the parotid gland, through the salivary papilla or into Bartholin's duct on the sublingual caruncle for the monostomatic sublingual gland, into Rivini's duct in the sublingual pad for the polystomatic sublingual gland, or into Wharton's duct for the mandibular gland. The pictures are taken in two planes as soon as possible after filling with the contrast medium.

Pneumoperitoneum. For this a negative contrast medium, as e. g. atmospheric air or oxygen, is insufflated into the peritoneal cavity. The aim of the pneumoperitoneum is the presentation of an image of the diaphragm, spleen or liver edge and with tumours, the recording of the size and the limits of the tumours. For this purpose, a canula is inserted into the peritoneal cavity laterally to the linea alba between the umbilicus and the symphysis pubis and filtered air insufflated in an amount of about 700–2000 ml. If the canula is not introduced sufficiently deeply but lies only in the subcutaneous fatty tissue, subcutaneous emphysema develops (Fig. 122). In general, the appearance of a tympanitic percussion note is sufficient to establish whether the abdomen is satisfactorily filled with air. The X-ray photographs are made according to the condition under investigation in the latero-lateral, ventro-dorsal or dorso-ventral view and these positions may be combined with elevation of the head or pelvis (Figs. 372 and 373). Untoward reactions have not been observed so far.

Pneumoretroperitoneum. The insufflation of air into the retroperitoneal connective tissue space is intended to give a good radiological presentation of the kidneys, especially their outer contours, form and position and of the rest of the urinary tract. After the introduction of a vaginal speculum of the right size into the rectum,

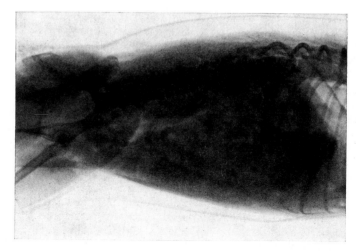

Fig. 122. Extensive subcutaneous emphysema after error in the induction of a pneumoperitoneum.
(Spitz.)

a canula about 10 cm long is inserted between the anus and the base of the tail and
under fluoroscopic control the canula is pushed forward into the connective tissue
space between the rectum and the vertebral column. Air is then insufflated in
amounts varying between 300 and 700 m*l*. For the radiographs the same positions
are used as for a pneumoperitoneum, though the ventro-dorsal view with elevation
of the pelvis is the most suitable (Fig. 381).

Radiographs with enlargement. If the distance of the object from the film is
increased and at the same time the distance of the focus from the object is decreased
(see Figs. 115 and 116), the result is an enlarged image of the object (Figs. 123 and
124). This can be utilised to obtain radiographs with enlargement, e. g. in the
case of intervertebral discs. We use the ancillary enlargement equipment "TuR"
DZ 103 made by the VEB Transformer and X-ray Works, Dresden, which is
capable of enlargements of 1.5 : 1 to 2 : 2 (Fig. 125). For increasing the distance
of the film from the object to be photographed, the cassette carrier is arranged
to be movable vertically and linked with the cross arm of the stand by means of
a parallel motion guide rod. The guide rod has a centimetre scale, with which the
enlargement factor (V) can be determined as follows from the ratio of the distance
from the focus to the film (FF) to the distance from the focus to the object (FO):

$$V = \frac{FF}{FO}.$$

With a large focus-film distance, the use of a grid is superfluous.

Tomography. On ordinary X-ray photographs there is the risk that different
objects are projected on top of one another, since there is certainly a summation
image, thus individual parts may escape assessment. With the help of tomography,
any required section through the body can be studied and only the objects which
lie at the level of this section give a sharp image, while all the parts which lie higher

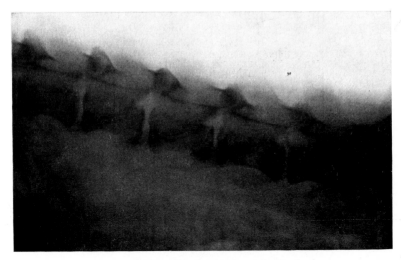

Fig. 123. Radiograph of normal vertebral column.

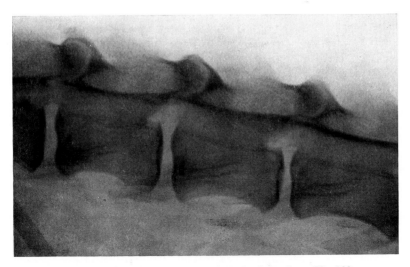

Fig. 124. Enlargement of the vertebral column from Fig. 123.

or lower appear blurred (Fig. 126). If, during the exposure, the tube is moved to one side and the film to the other side, only the layer which lies in the place of the axis of rotation gives a sharp image. The other layers are, of course, represented but are so blurred that they give no definite image. Figure 127 shows the principle of tomography. The X-ray tube and the cassette (K) are linked in such a way that they both oscillate about the axis of rotation (D). The cassette is always kept parallel to the positioning plane in the patient. During the movement, all the

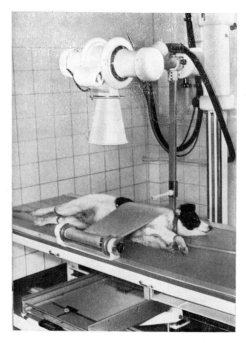

Fig. 125. Enlargement attachment. (University Department of Illustration.)

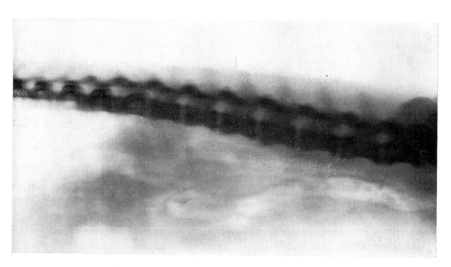

Fig. 126. Tomogram of the vertebral column.

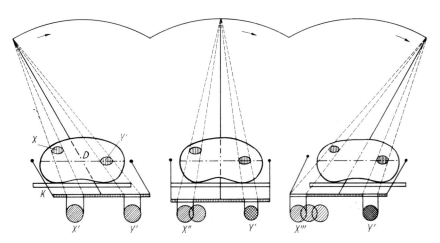

Fig. 127. The principle of tomography. K = cassette; D = centre of rotation.

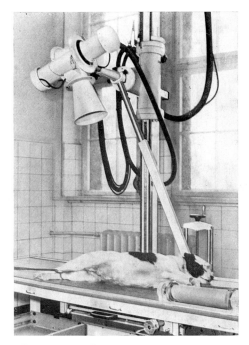

Fig. 128. Tomograph. (University Department of Illustration.)

structures in the plane of the section through D are represented as a sharp image
– e. g. Y gives the image Y' – while the parts lying outside the plane of the section
are blurred, as e. g. X'–X''' corresponding to X. The height of the plane of the
section can be adjusted as required by altering the axis of rotation (Fig. 128).
It is important to have the patient in a position of absolute rest for tomography,
since relatively long exposure times, of about 2 seconds, must be used. It is, therefore, advantageous to keep the patient quiet by means of a sedative.

The procedure has been improved on the technical side by the development of
simultaneous multisection laminography, in which with a single tube movement up
to 7 films arranged above one another at selectable distances are exposed at the
same time.

Hard ray technique. With this method certain structures, which in normal
radiography swamp other details, are penetrated by the hard rays excited at
high tension. This is utilised particularly in chest X-rays, since the parts which were
previously covered by the ribs and heart shadow, are then reproduced clearly.
With the hard ray technique one gets pictures which are not quite so rich in contrast
as the usual X-rays, but there is the advantage of better recognition of detail and
the possibility of rendering visible organs and parts of organs which had previously
been obscured. Moreover, the patients receive smaller doses of radiation with the
high tensions and the tube is subject to a lesser load. The disadvantage of the scattered radiations produced by the hard rays can be compensated for by various
means. For one thing, there is the possibility of using special grids and for another,
use can be made of Groedel's distance technique. For this, the distance of the film
from the object is chosen to be more than 15 cm. As a result of this space intervening, the greater part of the scattered radiations does not reach the film. The
focus-film distance must be increased above 150 cm, in order to overcome the lack
of sharpness arising as a result of the relatively large object-film distance.

We work with a focus-film distance of 170 cm and an object-film distance of
20 cm with 95–105 kV and 10–14 mA sec (see Table on p. 119).

II. Special Part

1. Diseases of the skin

The functions of the skin are well-known and will not be discussed here. The skin of the dog is only moderately supplied with sweat glands, these being mainly concentrated in the pads, the skin between the pads, and the external auditory canal. The skin itself is more sensitive to agents applied externally than that of man, the thicker and heavier the coat, the more sensitive the skin.

The patient suffering from skin disease should first be observed as a whole in order to gain a general impression of the extent of the disease and the distribution of the lesions. A closer examination of the individual lesions should then be made under a good light. In certain conditions, the use of a hand lens may yield valuable information, e. g. fungus infections, ectoparasites, etc. Microscopical examination of skin scrapings should be undertaken as a matter of routine in all skin diseases in the dog. The scraping is made with a sharp scalpel blade scraped at right angles to the skin at the edge of the lesion until it bleeds slightly. It may be necessary to take several scrapings from different lesions before a firm diagnosis can be made. The scraping is mixed with a little liquor potassium, a coverslip applied, and the slide examined under the low power objective of the microscope. In long-haired breeds it may be necessary to clip the dog short before the extent of the skin lesions can be ascertained. Effective treatment will usually necessitate close clipping of the patient so one should not hesitate to get the owner's permission at the outset.

In non-parasitic diseases of the skin, the cause may lie in disease of other internal organs, the skin lesions being a reflection of a more general condition, e. g. nephritis, hormonal dysfunctions, etc. It is advisable, therefore, to carry out a complete physical examination of the patient as recommended in Part I. According to KRAL (1959) Kleintier. Prax. **4**, 48–54, 12 % of all canine skin disease is of external origin, 10 % is due to infection and 72 % due to disease or dysfunction of the internal organs.

Pruritus (Itching of the skin). Pruritus indicates an itching of the skin with no observable associated skin lesion or parasites. The itching may be confined to certain areas of the body or may be generalised. The cause of the condition may be difficult, if not impossible, to determine, but known aetiological agents include allergic reactions, nervous conditions, nephritis, alimentary disorders, etc. There may be considerable differences in the degree of pruritus between individuals and between breeds, e. g. rough-haired breeds show pruritus more frequently than do the short-haired dogs. The initial pruritus may be complicated or perpetuated by traumatic damage to the skin which is self-inflicted by the biting and scratching of the patient.

Treatment of pruritus is, of necessity, largely symptomatic. Where the cause can be determined, specific treatment should, of course, be applied, but where the aetiology is unknown, an effort should be made to break the vicious circle of itch-scratch-itch. This may be accomplished by diverting the animal's attention by work in the case of working dogs and increased exercise in pet animals. A spell in the open air may help by renewing the blanket of air retained in the coat. A rub down with acidified water (1 cup of vinegar to 1 litre of water), weak salt solution or camomile tea will often diminish a general pruritus. Scratching may sometimes be prevented by binding the paws or application of an Elizabethan collar. Application of a 1–5 % solution of salicylic acid in surgical spirit may bring relief. Internally sedative drugs may be given, e. g. barbiturates.

Editor's note. The phenothiazine-derived tranquillisers are very useful in this condition, as some also possess an antihistamine action.

Doses of brewers' yeast (up to a fingertip daily), or tablets of vitamin B complex may be given as supportive treatment. Without doubt the antihistamines constituted an important advance in the treatment of pruritus but they have been largely superseded by the corticosteroids. In every case of pruritus, it is advisable to alter the diet of the patient, and in this connection the slightly laxative action of a milk diet may be beneficial. Artificial Karlsbad salts may also be used as a mild laxative, giving 1–5 knife points (as much as lies on the point of a knife) daily in the drinking water.

Alopecia. Alopecia is a falling out of the hair which is apparently not preceded by skin disease or infection with ecto parasites.

Alopecia congenita (Congenital loss of hair). Complete loss of hair is not often seen in practice because affected animals are usually destroyed by the breeder. Congenital alopecia is seen as a breed characteristic in various African, Chinese, Mexican and Patagonian dogs, such dogs usually being called "hairless". Except for a few hairy places at the tip of the tail and on the upper part of the head, these animals are usually completely devoid of hair. A slight degree of congenital alopecia, which is localised in a few areas of the body, is sometimes found in miniature pinschers, and this kind of alopecia may also be seen in whippets on the underside of the thorax.

Alopecia acquisita. This is considered to be a disturbance of the nutrition of the skin and the hair and is often seen in association with organic or infectious diseases. Hormonal imbalance may lead to alopecia, especially in the older dog, and it may also be seen during the puerperium. Some poisons may produce severe loss of hair, e. g. the rodenticide, thallium. Sometimes in the rough-haired breeds, alopecia may be seen immediately following stripping, the condition usually resolving itself without therapeutic measure.

The clinical picture of alopecia consists of a falling out of the hair, but no alteration in the actual structure of the affected hairs can be seen by careful examination with a hand lens. The normal and bald patches may be distributed quite irregularly over the body. Where the bald patches are circular in outline the condition is known as alopecia areata. Where the loss of hair is only slight it may only be perceived when one brushes against the run of the hair and with a lateral source of light. Usually, in alopecia there is no evidence of disease or inflammatory change in the skin. Treatment is mainly directed to improving the blood supply of the part.

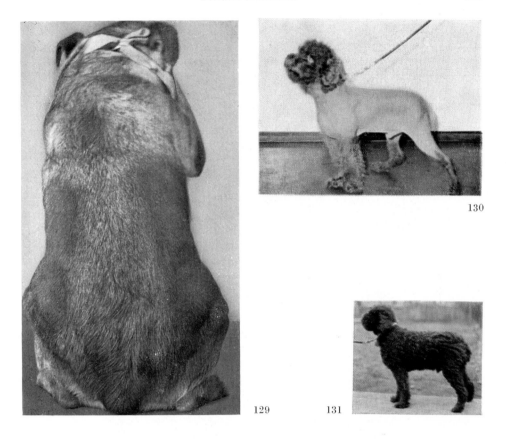

Fig. 129. Hormonal alopecia in a mongrel bitch, which resolved after castration. The symmetry of the alopecia in the lumbar region is characteristic.

Fig. 130. Hormonal alopecia (in a poodle) which responded at first to injections of testosterone, but castration ultimately brought about a cure. (Pathological examination of the testes: in the first testis there was fibrosis, in the second normal testicular tissue with slight increase of connective tissue.)

Fig. 131. The poodle shown in Fig. 130, ten weeks after castration.

In mild cases of alopecia, rubbing the affected areas with tincture of iodine may be effective. Often arsenic is prescribed as an alternative in the form of Liquor arsenicalis. The dose of arsenic is gradually increased during the course of treatment because its absorption after oral administration is slowly inhibited in the gut (arsenic resistance of the intestine). One or two drops more of the preparation are given on each succeeding day and the treatment is stopped when a dose of 15 to 20 drops a day is reached. With parenteral arsenical preparations the dose should not be increased as resistance of the intestine does not occur by this route. Where

9   Christoph, Diseases of Dogs

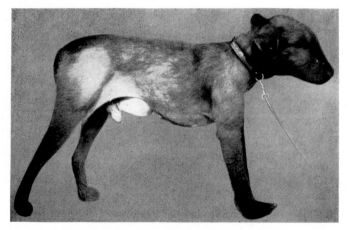

Fig. 132. Hormonal alopecia (Welsh terrier).

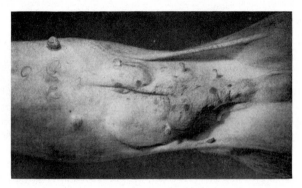

Fig. 133. Hormonal alopecia (Welsh terrier). Gynaecomastia and pachydermia of the prepuce
(see also Fig. 132).

hormonal imbalance is suspected to be the cause of the alopecia, hormone replacement therapy must be given (oestrogens or androgens).

The course of alopecia is not regular or uniform as it may appear rapidly and pass
into remission, or appear slowly and persist for a long period of time, resisting all
treatment. Hormonal alopecia would seem to have become more frequent recently.
It is difficult to ascertain whether it is due to dysfunction of the gonads or of the
thyroid. Good results have been obtained by castration in hormonal alopecias.
In most of such cases new hair growth is usually seen within about 6 or 7 weeks
of operation and the coat is completely restored 4–6 months post-operation.
Hypothyroid alopecia has been treated successfully with dry thyroid extract.
In these cases the clinical picture usually shows a symmetrical trichorrhexis,
usually in the lumbar region, which then develops into an alopecia, there being
no signs of inflammatory change in the skin. In a minority of cases there may be

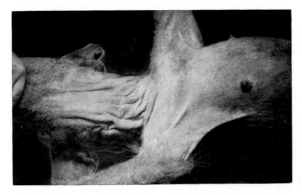

Fig. 134. Hormonal alopecia (Welsh terrier). Pachydermia of the neck.

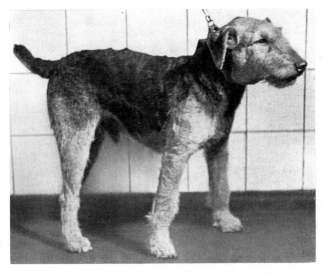

Fig. 135. The same terrier as in Fig. 132, 14 weeks after castration. The coat has grown again perfectly. The skin changes shown in Figs. 133 and 134 have completely disappeared.

signs of pruritus. The loss of hair finally affects the whole body, but the head, tip of the tail and the extremities of the limbs are not usually affected (Fig. 130). Male dogs with alopecia due to changes in the testes also show gynaecomastia, pachydermia of the prepuce and of the soft skin under the neck (Figs. 132, 133, 134). The general bodily condition of the dog is usually not affected although there may be some loss of vitality. In hypothyroid alopecias some cases are seen in which the hairless areas feel dry, rough and thickened, these areas being more strongly pigmented. The longer the alopecia had been in existence, the deeper the pigmentation. Well-developed formation of coarse adherent scales of the skin

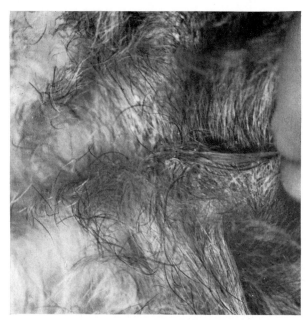

Fig. 136. Seborrhoea (Fox terrier).

may be noted and in more advanced cases still, closely placed, fine, blackish swellings may be seen projecting from the hair follicles. Marked gynaecomastia and enlargement of the prepuce may be present but these disappear after castration. Growth of hair commences within eight weeks after the operation. In long standing cases of alopecia, the affected areas are well demarcated and here and there outgrowths resembling warts may be seen. In these chronic cases also, the remaining hair shows increased scaliness and dryness, is finer and thicker than normal, and inclined to become matted. The treatment of hormonal alopecia is castration, or the administration of dried thyroid preparation in doses of between 100–400 mg daily, for a considerable period of time. After castration new growth of the hair occurs in 8–10 weeks after the operation (Figs. 131 and 135). In hypothyroid alopecia a sparse growth of hair can be seen after 3–4 weeks of treatment.

Seborrhoea. In this condition, which is rarely seen in the dog, there is excessive secretion of sebum of the sebaceous glands. The animal looks rather as if it has been dipped in fat, there being masses of fat droplets on the tips of the hair (Fig. 136). Treatment of this disease is extremely difficult, because after bathing the animal with fat emulsifiers, the seborrhoea only returns in a more severe form. Successful results may be obtained by rubbing in a 5% spirit of salicylic acid.

Trichoma (Hair villi). This occurs in long haired dogs and is formed by the matting of individual hairs. In many breeds, e. g. Komondor, this condition is acceptable to the breed standard. Where grooming has been neglected, matting of the hair can be so close (especially around the ears or on the neck) that it can be mistaken for a tumour.

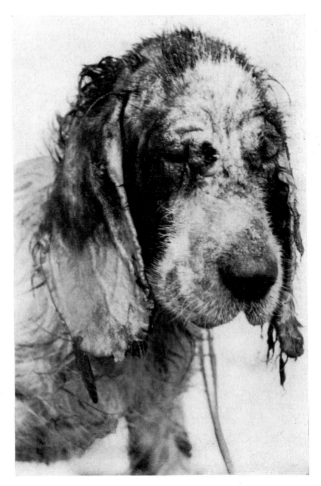

Fig. 137. Chronic eczema with marked corrugation of the skin due to pachydermia (Spaniel).

Trichorrhexis (Brittleness of the hair). This condition occurs quite commonly in sheepdogs in the withers region, and is popularly but erroneously thought to be associated with worm infestation. Individual hairs show a brushlike fraying, develop club-shaped thickening and finally break off. Short stumps of the outer hairs remain but the undercoat is fairly normal.

Treatment consists of clipping the affected area and rubbing with balsam of Peru.

Loss of pigment. Loss of pigment may occur either in the skin or the hairs. In the Chow there may be lightening of the blue tongue and some breeds show a variable loss of pigment in the normally black nose (Dudley nose). A pale nose may regain its former colour after a major operation. It is frequently reported that increased depth of nasal pigmentation is seen in dogs following a stay at the seaside. It has been suggested that this may be due to ingestion of seaweed. In older dogs pigment changes may occur as a result of endocrine disturbance, e. g. greying of age, etc.

Loss of hair pigment may occur following the injection of local anaesthetics containing adrenaline, following traumatic damage to the skin, or irradiation of the skin.

Albinism (Congenital lack of pigmentation). This condition in which there is a total absence of melanin from the body has not been observed in dogs.

Treatment. No effective method of treatment for lack of pigmentation is known. Tattooing of the light areas may be performed where there is evidence that photo-sensitisation may otherwise occur.

Eczema. There are many types of eczema and a similar number of recognised causes. The term implies an inflammatory process of the skin involving all the various layers and accompanied by pruritus. Causes of eczema can be divided into internal and external. Amongst the internal causes may be listed nephritis, consti-pation, pregnancy, the puerperium, cachexia, adiposity, diabetes mellitus, severe infections and allergies. External causes comprise mechanical, chemical and thermal injury to the skin. Under this heading must be included neglected grooming leading to soiling of the hair and skin and pruritus. Anal irritation, external otitis, ecto-parasites, inexpert trimming, chafing of the collar, discharges from wounds, etc., may all trigger off an eczema in a dog which is predisposed to the condition by one of the internal causes mentioned above.

Acute eczema is characterised by the rapid development of signs of inflammation of the skin, viz. reddening, swelling, exudation, etc.

Chronic eczema has a slow course with marked swelling or thickening of the skin, inflammatory signs being subdued (Fig. 137).

Clinically the skin changes commence with an inflammatory reddening and increased heat (Erythema), passing into nodular eczema, vesicular eczema, wet eczema, pustular eczema and finally scaly eczema. Some cases show all these stages in the development of the lesions whilst others commence with one of the stages remaining unchanged until the desquamation, which precedes resolution, occurs.

Different parts of the skin may be affected with different stages of eczema at the same time and so recovery occurs at different times.

Predilection sites are recognised for many forms of eczema. Intertriginous eczema is found where there is frictional contact between the skin of adjacent areas, e. g. scrotum, axilla, between the toes, etc. (Figs. 138, 139). In the latter site, intertriginous eczema must be distinguished from the swelling and inflamma-tory changes associated with entry of a foreign body, e. g. barley awn, etc. Such swellings should be incised under local anaesthesia and thoroughly explored. If this is not done, an abscess forms and bursts, leaving a discharging fistula necessitat-ing more radical surgery. Where the foreign body cannot be located, a bandage with 40 % ichthyol ointment is applied and renewed every two days. Eczema of the back is often seen, appearing first in the region of the crupper and extending forward to the withers. The condition often becomes chronic with connective tissue thickening (pachyderma, scleroderma).

The course of the condition is not always uniform. With proper treatment it may be expected that an acute type of eczema may be resolved in about two

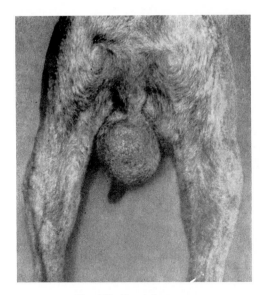

Fig. 138. Scrotal eczema.

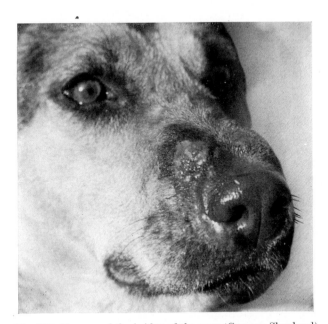

Fig. 139. Eczema of the bridge of the nose (German Shepherd).

weeks, but relapses are frequent. With a chronic eczema it is unwise to prognosticate about the duration as the condition often proves to be completely refractory to treatment. Cases which are apparently cured may relapse at any time. The general condition of the patient is usually not affected and even in severe eczemas regional lymphadenitis rarely occurs, unless there is secondary bacterial infection.

Parasitic skin disease must be excluded by thorough clinical examination and skin scrapings. The identification of the original cause of the condition may be almost impossible and treatment must often be empirical.

Treatment is mainly applied externally and locally. If an endogenous cause is suspected the necessary systemic treatment must be given. Any mechanical cause must be eliminated (ectoparasites, badly fitting collar, continual scratching, etc.) and some cases will resolve spontaneously once this has been done. It is always advisable to clip the hair from a wide area around the lesions and if the condition is generalised the whole body area should be clipped. The clipping is beneficial in that it allows light and sun to act on the skin surface and also removes matted and discharge-caked hair. The affected areas should then be thoroughly but gently cleansed with surgical spirit or, where the lesions are crusty, by the use of liquid paraffin or olive oil.

Drugs used in treatment may be applied in the form of ointments, creams, lotions, liniments or aqueous solutions. Powders should only be prescribed in cases of dry eczema as otherwise they tend to cake, allowing the inflammatory process to continue unchecked beneath. As eczema manifests itself in many different forms, we depend more on specific prescriptions rather than on ready made preparations. If the eczema is acute, medicaments must be applied care fully and gently, as too vigorous rubbing may exacerbate the condition.

Acute moist eczema is quite a common condition, often appearing very suddenly (overnight), the predilection sites being the base of the tail, the outer side of the upper thigh or the head, particularly below the ears. In these cases preparations are prescribed which have an anti-inflammatory and a drying, astringent action. The following prescriptions have been found useful:

R.   Linseed oil   } āā
      Calcium hydroxide soln   }
      Shake well before use

R.   Tannic acid   } āā   5 parts
      Linseed oil   }
      Calcium hydroxide solution ad 100 parts

R.   Tannic acid   10 parts
      Isopropyl alcohol   ad 100 parts

R.   Zinc oxide   20 parts
      Liquid paraffin   30 parts

In the prescriptions containing tannic acid, care must be exercised as liver damage may result from too prolonged application of this substance.

For the removal of scales and crust we use preparations containing salicylic acid:

R. Salicylic acid   2 parts
    Olive oil   ad 100 parts

R. Salicylic acid   6 parts
    Linseed oil   20 parts
    Isopropyl alcohol   ad 200 parts

If the eczema is of the encrusted squamous type the following prescription is useful:

R. Resorcinol   } āā   20 parts
    Sulphur
    Petroleum jelly   ad 100 parts

or

R. Icthyol   } āā   1 part
    Salicylic acid
    Zinc oxide ointment   ad   30 parts

To encourage desquamation the following can be recommended:

R. Salicylic acid   2 parts
    Zinc oxide   } āā   24 parts
    Starch
    Petroleum jelly   50 parts

R. Salicylic acid   2 parts
    Balsam of Peru   } āā   10 parts
    Potash soap
    Isopropyl alcohol   ad 100 parts

For long-standing eczemas which have become chronic, tar-containing preparations are especially valuable.

R. Coal tar solution
    Sulphur   } āā   25 parts
    Potash soap
    Alcohol   ad   50 parts

R. Coal tar solution   2 parts
    Liquid paraffin   ad   20 parts

R. Tannic acid   10 parts
    Coal tar solution   20 parts
    Petroleum jelly   ad 100 parts

In this group Lassar's Paste should also be mentioned. This is a zinc paste augmented by the addition of salicylic acid:

R. Salicylic acid   2 parts
    Zinc oxide   } āā   16 parts
    Liquid paraffin
    Lanoline   ad 100 parts

In the very chronic types of eczemas it may be necessary to cauterise the affected areas to stimulate healing. This can be done by painting the parts with 5–10% silver nitrate solution, ½–1% picric acid or ½–2% formalin. Ultraviolet radiation applied 2–3 times daily for 4–8 min at a distance of 80–100 cm is a very useful adjunct to the treatment of chronic eczema. In Vienna good results are claimed for radiotherapy in chronic eczema, but we have no personal experience of its use.

It is important to pay special attention to the diet of dogs suffering from eczema and the history should always include details of the feeding of the patient. Quite minor errors of nutrition can produce eczema in the dog. All spices, artificial flavourings, roasts and sauces should not be allowed in the diet. This does not mean that the dog should have a completely salt-free diet, as the importance of the sodium chloride blood level is well recognised. A fall in blood chloride results in outflow of chlorine ions from the tissues with eventual resultant dehydration. In any skin condition, optimum nutrition will always prove beneficial. Any tendency towards constipation should be corrected by the use of a mild saline aperient. The addition of a small quantity of brewers' yeast or the vitamin B complex to the diet is also recommended.

In very stubborn cases the use of non-specific protein therapy may be effective. Non-specific vaccines are available for this purpose. The mode of action of this type of therapy is not yet clear, but quite a number of individual effects can be detected and have been explained. The most important of these is an increase in cell function, accompanied by increased metabolism, increased activity of the reticulo-endo-thelial system and increased enzyme formation. Changes in the level of the blood serum proteins have also been detected. Frequently there is an increase in the globulin fraction and a decrease in the albumins. Hyperaemia and increased leucocyte counts have also been noted. Dosage of the various preparations varies but normally lies between 0.5–4 ml, depending upon the size of the dog, and is given by deep intramuscular injection three times a week. The course of injections should continue until 6–8 injections have been given; breaking off the course prematurely may lead to a relapse. One often gets the clinical impression that smaller doses produce a better response than larger ones, possibly the massive doses inhibit the regulatory effect of the central nervous system.

Autogenous blood therapy may also prove effective. Between 2–5 ml of venous blood, depending on the size of the dog, is withdrawn and immediately injected intramuscularly without any further preparation. Transient reactions in the form of inappetence, listlessness, etc., may appear but are usually mild. The injections may be repeated every 2–3 days but the course should not be protracted otherwise anaphylactic reactions may occur.

Vitamin H (Biotin) has been reported as beneficial; possibly its effect is due more to the fact that it improves the appetite and thus the nutrition than to any specific activity.

In resistant eczema ACTH in a dose of about 10 IU may be used (see p. 445) but has been largely superseded by the corticosteroids. Where hormonal dysfunction is the cause of the dermatosis (Fig. 140), hormone therapy should be instituted. In the bitch "oestrogens" are used and in the dog "androgens". In the bitch too high or prolonged dosage with these hormones may produce endometrial hyperplasia and pyometra.

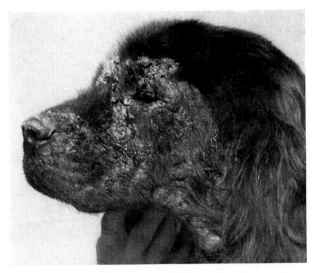

Fig. 140. Puerperal eczema of the head (Newfoundland).

Dermatoses can be divided into those which are exogenous and those which are endogenous in nature. Exogenous dermatoses may be caused by either mechanical or chemical agents.

Frictional callosities are caused by pressure and friction on the skin when the dog lies on a hard surface, bald patches appearing on the outside of the elbow or hock joint. The skin is thickened (scleroderma) and there is considerable des- quamation of scales from the affected area. No effective treatment is known.

Hyperkeratosis may be seen on the feet of dogs which have been prevented from using the pads for some time, due to illness or lamenesses, etc. Treatment is usually not required because this condition rapidly disappears once the pads are subjected to wear once more. In all old dogs hyperkeratoses appear lateral to the pads. These animals may be slightly lame because the elastic mechanism of the pads is impeded by these new growths. Treatment consists in removing the excess tissue first with scissors and later with a scalpel, after the horny portion of the pad has been softened by the use of warm baths. In this way the horny layer can be thinned down so that the elasticity of the pad is once more restored. The owner should be instructed to promote this result by the use of baths or ointment. In the latter, the keratolytic action of camomile can be used. After some serious systemic diseases hyperkeratoses may appear on the muzzle of the dog (Fig. 141). These may originate as a result of a drying up of the secretory glands of the muzzle, so that the normal moist nose is no longer present. As a result of this drying up, the muzzle is hard and rough and becomes rather horny. In these cases the owner should be advised to rub a little bland ointment into the muzzle several times a day in order to keep it flexible. In this respect it should also be noted that hyper- keratoses may also result from poisoning with the chlorinated naphthalenes (the

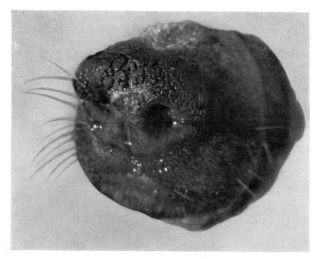

Fig. 141. Hyperkeratosis. Fissures on the end of the nose.

active components of wood preservatives). This results in a patchy falling out of hair, pachyderma, and the formation of scurf or scales on the upper and lower lips, the muzzle and the eyelids. Treatment in these cases is mainly symptomatic, but possibly the use of high doses of Vitamin A may be effective.

Another form of dermatosis which is caused mechanically is decubitus, and this is found chiefly in patients that are severely ill or cachectic. The lesions occur on the pelvis (tuber coxae), the elbow joint and sometimes on the head (on the zygomatic ridge). The essential measure in treatment of this condition is the provision of a soft bed. Frequent changes of bedding are also to be recommended in order to avoid any extension of the affected areas. The lesions should be treated with protective ointments or paste, e. g. Lassar's paste:

London paste is also to be recommended and is very useful for eczema caused by "scalding" with faeces, urine and wound exudates:

R.	Menthol	0.1 part
	Salicylic acid	0.3 part
	Zinc oxide	6.0 parts
	Starch	6.0 parts
	Lanoline	15.0 parts
	Petroleum jelly	15.0 parts

Where there is a condition of chronic thickening of the skin we use the term scleroderma. In most cases the underlying connective tissue is also affected. Alternative terms for the condition are sclerosis of the skin, pachyderma or elephantiasis. Scleroderma is caused by a recurrent irritation of the skin which is never very severe in degree. The skin is rough, inelastic and grossly thickened, in some cases coarse clefts appearing in the skin. The treatment of scleroderma is very unsatisfactory and in advanced cases the condition is usually completely refractory to all treatment. The application of hot, wet compresses combined with intensive massage of the affected area may produce a limited absorption of the thickened skin. The effect of such massage may be enhanced by the use of iodine ointments. Where there are superficial proliferations of the skin these can be removed under local anaesthesia, the wound surface being gently cauterised with silver nitrate.

Amongst the thermal causes of dermatoses are freezing, burning and erythema solar (sunburn). We have not seen freezing or sunburn in the dog in our area.

Chronic solar dermatitis has been described as a congenital abnormal reaction to solar radiation occurring in Collies and related breeds. The condition commences with a loss of hair on the bridge of the nose and gradually assumes an ulcerative character sometimes extending as far as the eyelids. The general condition of affected animals is not upset in any way. Attempts at treatment have been made in these cases with ACTH and corticosteroid but with variable results.

Burns may be seen quite often in the dog, three degrees of skin damage having been observed. So far we have not seen the fourth degree of burning which has been designated as frank carbonisation. It is mainly the small breeds which suffer from burns. With 1st degree burns, signs of acute inflammation appear with erection of the hair and severe reddening and possibly exudation from the skin. This degree of damage usually heals completely without appreciable scar formation, but with a certain amount of hair loss. Second degree burns show the formation of typical vesicles leaving no resultant scar formation, but considerable loss of hair which may persist for some years. Second degree burns are the type most frequently seen in practice, 3rd degree burns being comparatively rare (Fig. 142).

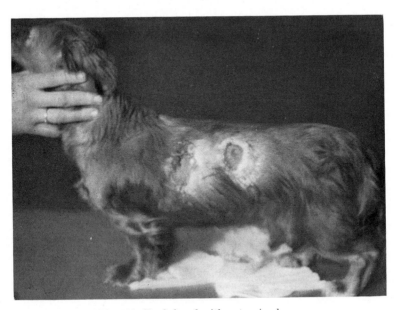

Fig. 142. Dachshund with extensive burn.

Treatment is mainly directed towards the prevention of toxaemia by absorption of breakdown products from the lesions. As well as local treatment the action of the liver should be bolstered by the administration of glucose, methionine, etc. Where there is a risk of toxaemia, corticosteroids may be used. In addition, the burnt areas are treated topically with liniments, ointments, etc. In order to stimulate granulation and at the same time achieve some astringent effect, tannic acid preparations may be used. The tannin tans the exposed corium and its nerve endings and so achieves an analgesic effect. The tannic acid may be incorporated in Ringer's solution, the burnt area being carefully dabbed every half hour with this fluid.

R.   Tannic acid   5 parts
       Ringer's solution   ad 100.0

The chemical causes of dermatoses are many and of a varied nature. The use of a sand/salt mixture on iced-up roads in winter can lead to interdigital eczema in the feet of dogs walking on the roads. The same effect may arise from walking on tarred roads in summer, from lime on building sites, or oil, etc. in garages.

Parasitic Skin Disease

Ticks. The tick found on dogs in Europe is *Ixodes ricinus*. The larvae, nymphs and adult ticks attach themselves to the tips of grasses or leaves and fasten on to any passing animal. The tick is most prevalent during the late summer months, dogs which have access to long grass or bushes being mainly affected. The tick sucks the blood of the host through its mouth-parts which are firmly buried in the animal's skin. If the tick is carelessly removed, the head is usually left in the skin of the host where it may give rise to suppuration. Application of a little ether or chloroform to the tick will relax the mouth-parts and the tick can then be removed quite easily.

Lice. Dog lice are of two varieties, the sucking louse, *Linognathus setosus*, and the biting louse, *Trichodectes canis*. Sucking lice tend to remain in one spot for some time and their bodies are set at right angles to the skin surface, whereas biting lice move around more freely with their bodies in the same plane as the skin surface. Lice are mainly found on the dog in late summer or autumn. Their eggs (nits) are laid attached to the hairs of the host and nests of such nits may be found on the head, especially the forehead or cheek. The movements and bites of the sucking lice lead to pruritus with resultant loss of hair and eczematous areas. The hair loss tends to be irregular with ill-defined margins. The remainder of the coat appears dull, lifeless and rough and areas of brittle hairs may appear. In the very young animal or one weakened by intercurrent disease, emaciation and anaemia may occur. For *treatment* any suitable contact insecticide may be used. In severe cases it may be necessary to clip the dog out before applying the powder or bathing the animal. It is advisable to withhold fats on the day of treatment, as fat may facilitate toxic absorption of the insecticide if the dog licks an appreciable quantity from the skin. The treatment should be repeated in 10–14 days' time to catch the larvae hatching from the eggs.

Fleas. The dog flea, *Ctenocephalides canis*, is a blood-sucking insect and may infest the dog in large numbers, particularly during the summer and autumn. Fleas breed away from the dog, depositing their eggs in corners and crevices in the animal's bed, or on the ground. Larvae hatch from the eggs and after several moults enter a cocoon stage, from which the adult flea emerges after a time varying from one week up to as much as ten months. The fleas may give rise to intense pruritus, some dogs being actually allergic to flea-bites, and the resultant scratching causes loss of hair and severe eczematous reactions. The pruritus may be severe enough to lead to inanition or even cachexia. *Ctenocephalides canis* is the inter-mediate host of the tapeworm *Dipylidium caninum*. It may be difficult to spot the fleas in a long-coated dog but indications are the presence of small red spots in the unpigmented skin, a brown scaly deposit on the skin and small, granular, brown specks amongst the hair, which are actually the faeces of the flea. Treatment is the same as for lice infestation. It is important to treat the animal's bed and kennel to destroy the eggs, otherwise re-infestation will soon occur. This is best accom-plished by scrubbing with boiling solutions of washing soda, and destroying any bedding and replacing it with newspaper, which should be removed and burned regularly. The usual disinfectants are no use even in very high concentrations. Kennels and outside runs, etc. can be briefly flamed with a blow lamp.

Harvest mite. The larval stage of the harvest mite, *Trombicula autumnale*, attacks the dog especially in the soft-skinned areas, e. g. between the toes, the lips, around the eyes, the ear, etc. Infection may be so heavy that the affected area assumes a yellowish-red colour. There is a marked pruritus with resultant loss of hair and eczema. Treatment is similar to that used for lice and fleas.

Sarcoptic mange. This is another parasitic disease and is caused by the burrowing mite *Sarcoptes scabei var. canis*. More rarely one finds Otodectic mange which is mainly in the ear and on the pinnae, and even more rarely Notoedric mange. Sarcoptic mange is usually transmitted by direct contact between one dog and another, but infection may also occur indirectly through the medium of clothing, blankets, bed boxes, etc. There can be said to be a variable incubation period in mange, dependent upon various factors. As regards the duration of this incubation period, the actual number of mites on the host body may determine the onset of clinical disease, so that with a small number the incubation period may extend to three weeks. In this respect climatic conditions exert quite an important in-fluence, so that in warm, damp weather there is a shortening of the incubation period, whilst cold, dry weather tends to prolong it. The incubation period may also be affected by the hygienic conditions under which the dog is kept, e. g. the standard of grooming may influence the time. Taking all these factors into account the incubation period may vary between a few days and three to four weeks.

The disease commences mainly on the hairless places of the body and because these areas are often unpigmented the small vesicles or nodules can be easily seen. The predilection sites are the abdomen, the flexures of the joints, the axillae and the head. As the disease progresses there is a marked desquamation of the skin and falling out of the hair which extends peripherally until the entire body is affected. Characteristic of sarcoptic mange, and a valuable differential diagnostic pointer, is the appearance of thickening of the margins of the ears.

When the infection is a mild one it may be difficult to make a positive identifica-tion of the mite by examination of a single skin scraping, so several scrapings should be taken in each case. The most suitable site for scraping is the area on the edge of a lesion where transition from diseased to healthy skin occurs. The clinical picture is seen as the type of eczema already described. In addition there is extreme pruritus as the activity of the mites stimulates the end plates of the cutaneous nerves. The itching is especially severe in a warm room or when the patient is lying in its bed, the warmth making the mites more active. If the patient is in the open air and is also distracted by exercise or work, the itching may disappear completely. Where the condition is extensive, there may be emaciation proceeding to a state of cachexia. With a severely weakened patient treatment may cause death, as the animal is unable to withstand the stress of treatment with specific parasiticides.

Notoedric mange ("Cat head mange"). This is caused by the mite *Notoedres cati* and is mainly transmitted by diseased cats to suckling puppies or young dogs. In the cat it occurs chiefly on the head, hence the name, but may appear elsewhere on the body. The infection is especially well marked on the outer surface of the ears and the edges of the pinnae. There is desquamation of the skin and the formation of grey, dry scabs, accompanied by marked pruritus.

Treatment of both sarcoptic and notoedric mange usually necessitates treatment of the whole body surface, and for this it is necessary that the whole body should be clipped out. In order to avoid large-scale absorption of the medicaments applied to the body, only one third of the body area is treated each day. Benzyl benzoate, sulphur preparations and gamma benzene hexachloride (BHC) are effective. When treatment with the contact insecticides is prescribed the directions for feeding given on page 142 must be observed. Application of the medicaments should be repeated after eight days. It is advisable to provide an adequate or even rich diet during treatment. In large animals fumigation with sulphur dioxide produces good results, but it is difficult to apply in the dog because of the different sizes of the various breeds, and also due to the different temperament of individual dogs. Sarcoptic and notoedric mange may be transmitted to the owner so the danger should be pointed out, and if infection is present the owner should be recommended to seek medical advice.

Another skin condition which has a course similar to that of mange, but is not a mange in this sense, is Demodicosis or hair follicle rash. This is caused by the demodex mite (*Demodex folliculorum* or *Demodex canis*). The mites, which are cigar shaped, travel along the shaft of the hair down to its root, causing an inflammation of the hair follicle. The mites multiply in the follicles and sebaceous glands producing a dilatation rather like the finger of a glove. Secondary bacterial infection, usually with staphylococci, causes the characteristic acne-like and purulent inflammation of the hair follicles and the sebaceous glands. Clinical disease only occurs when certain conditions of the skin favour the multiplication of the mite. Predisposing factors are: poor care of the hair, frequent washing with strong skin stimulants, faulty nutrition, or severe systemic diseases, e. g. distemper. During the post-war period we often saw the disease appear during teething. Direct infection of one animal from another does not occur, transmission experiments having proved negative. Demodex has been found in the blood, lymph glands and spleen of dogs which are clinically normal. The mites are even encountered in the organs and skin of aborted puppies, and thus it can be presumed that the mites have migrated through the placenta to infect foetuses in utero.

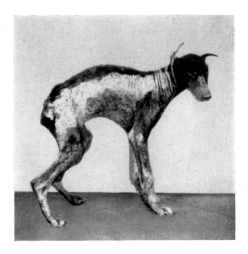

Fig. 143. Demodicosis with marked pachyderma of the skin of the neck.

Demodicosis affects mainly young dogs under 1 year old. Although apparently new infections appear in older dogs, these are mainly relapses from a previous infection. The following breeds show a special predisposition to the condition: Dachshund (especially the short-haired type), Short-haired Setter, Doberman, Boxer, German Shepherd, Fox and Scottish Terrier.

The clinical picture can be divided into two main types, squamous and pustular eczema, and according to the distribution of the lesions one can distinguish the localised form and the generalised form.

The squamous type is shown by increasing desquamation of the skin, combined with a moderate loss of hair. Usually no inflammatory change in the skin can be perceived. The colour of the skin may be light and pinkish, but in most cases it assumes a greyish-blue hue. Normally no pruritus is apparent.

The pustular type, in most cases, develops from the squamous type of lesion, although where the lesions are widespread the pustular form may be primary. In this form the skin may become quite swollen, hyperaemic and is sometimes called "red mange". The condition is called pustular due to the formation of nodules or pustules in the skin, about the size of a millet seed. The pustules are usually darkish or blueish-grey in colour but may be yellowish-grey. In chronic cases pachyderma develops, the skin increases in thickness and loses its elasticity, becoming corrugated (Fig. 143). Very often the skin surface is scaly. Again pruritus is usually absent.

In the early stages demodicosis is usually restricted to the head, the first lesions appearing mainly on the upper jaw below the eyes. The owner attributes little significance to these round, hairless patches, as they show no signs of inflammation and there is no obvious irritation. From the head the disease extends to the neck and the front of the chest, and later to the palmar surface of the front limbs as far down as the toes. It may extend further to the flanks and finally the whole body may be affected (Fig. 144). In atypical cases the disease may be closely localised, e. g. on the palmar surface of the hind legs. In each case the regional lymph glands

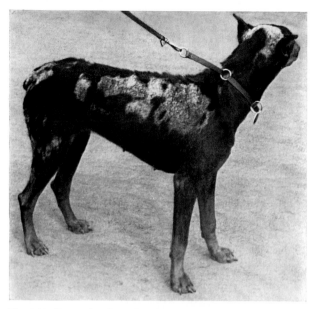

Fig. 144. Extensive demodicosis, squamous form (Doberman).

are always enlarged. Diagnosis is made by demonstration of the Demodex mite in a skin scraping or in the contents of a ruptured pustule.

Demodicosis can be a very protracted condition, although if there are only small foci of the disease it can usually be cleared in about two to three weeks. Spontaneous remissions are seen but they are very rare. In most cases the disease spreads at a variable rate over the whole body if treatment is neglected. In these cases treatment must be continued for several weeks or even months if a cure is to be effected, and many cases prove resistant to all therapy.

The prognosis of the condition should always be guarded, except where there are only a few foci of infection. Before treatment is commenced the case should be discussed with the owner as to whether he is willing to undertake the protracted course of treatment which is usually necessary. Where large areas are affected the whole body should be treated, but because of the risk of absorption of medicaments only one third of the body should be treated at one time. The recommended agent is best rubbed thoroughly into the skin with an old toothbrush in order to ensure optimal penetration. Occasionally signs of skin sensitivity appear in the form of oozing areas and in these cases the drugs should not be applied to these places, protective sedative skin preparations being used instead. Supportive treatment in the form of improved nutrition and the elimination of worms, etc., should be carried out. There is still no specific treatment for demodicosis. Contact insecticides are useful, Rotenone, the active principle of derris, being especially valuable.

In the pustular form of the disease the secondary staphylococcal infection may be checked with staphylococcal vaccine, or with an autogenous vaccine and non-specific protein therapy. In recent years the systemic insecticide Ronnel has been widely used for treatment of demodicosis.

The differential diagnosis of demodicosis from sarcoptic mange is relatively easy. The following typical signs of the two diseases are compared:

Sarcoptic mange	Demodicosis
Marked itching	No itching
Distribution on the head, eyes, median surfaces of the forelimbs and later of the hindlimbs and the feet, tail and abdomen	Distribution on the head, the area under the eyes, front of the chest, palmar surface of the forelimb, the lateral wall of the hindlimbs and feet
Tips of the ears thickened	Tips of the ears not thickened
Diffuse fall out of hair	Circumscribed bald areas
No enlargement of lymph glands	Enlarged lymph glands
Direct or indirect transmission possible	For clinical disease a special predisposition of the dog is probably necessary
Age of the dog of no significance. Re-infection in an infected environment is always possible	Primary infection only in young dogs. Relapse is possible in older dogs
Occurs in all breeds, especially long-haired breeds and the German Shepherd	Attacks short-haired breeds such as the Doberman, Boxer, Dachshund, Pointer, etc., but also the Fox terrier, Scottish terrier and Sheepdog
Microscopic identification of the mites difficult	Microscopic identification of the mite easy
Prognosis always favourable (except in debilitated dogs)	Prognosis doubtful or unfavourable
Spontaneous cure not yet observed	Spontaneous cure can occur now and again
Effective drugs available, therefore rapid cure possible	No specific drugs known, therefore therapy protracted
Cure has commenced when the itching ceases	Cure may be expected when hair recommences growth on the previously bald areas

Dermatomycoses are skin infections caused by fungal parasites. In these infections we include Yeasts, Hyphomycetes and Actinomycetes, but clinically the term dermatomycoses should be reserved for the skin conditions caused by hyphomycetes. The common characteristic of the pathogenic fungi of the skin is that their multiplication is asexual and accordingly these fungi are classified as fungi imperfecti. We use the classification given in the Manual of Clinical Mycology (PEZENBURG) (Kleintier Praxis. **5**, 81, 1960) and this divides the dermophytes into the genera, *Microsporon* (GRUBY, 1843), *Trichophyton* (MALMSTEIN, 1845)

10*

and *Epidermophyton*. The latter genus is of no veterinary concern as it has only been encountered as a cause of disease in man. The following pathogenic fungi are of importance:

Trichophyton mentagrophytes
Trichophyton rubrum
Trichophyton schonleini (Syn. *Achorion schonleini*)
Trichophyton verrucosum
Trichophyton megnini
Trichophyton gallinae
Microsporon audouini
Microsporon canis
Microsporon gypseum (Syn. *Favus*)
Microsporon distortum

In the dog the important pathogens are *Microsporon canis* and *gypseum*, and *Trichophyton mentagrophytes*.

Trichophytosis or Microsporosis is caused by various species of moulds of the genera *Trichophyton* and *Microsporon*. Predilection sites of the fungus are the hair follicle, the hair itself and the epidermis, and so one can distinguish endothrix (growing in the hair) forms and ectothrix (growing outside the hair) forms. Infection may be direct or indirect through the agencies of cleaning utensils, bedding, etc. Infection of man from dogs is also recognised and this may take a very virulent form.

There is usually an incubation period of one to four weeks and during this time the fungal spores enter the hair follicles and begin to multiply with resultant inflammation. In the less severe cases there is a marked scale formation with hair loss, or crusts or vesicles are formed and there is some suppuration of the hair follicles. The affected areas extend in a circular manner, due to the fact that infection spreads peripherally from a central point.

Trichophytia tonsurans maculosa is the most common form. In this condition circular, hairless patches appear on the body without any special predilection area. No inflammatory change is seen, but there is an increased desquamation of the skin resulting in scales of an asbestos-like appearance. These diseases are often first noticed when the coat is brushed or combed against the lie of the hair, and the dog is viewed in a lateral light. The hairs are bunched together and with a hand lens one can often see the fungal threads on the roots or the basal parts of the hair shafts. The circular areas may become confluent, in which case the circular outline may be obscured or lost. If hair growth recommences in these areas it can be assumed that a cure can be expected. Diagnosis is based on the clinical picture (circular lesions, bald patches and slight pruritus) but the diagnosis should always be confirmed by microscopic identification of the fungus. Skin scrapings should be taken from the margin of the diseased areas and into healthy skin. The fungal hyphae grow down from the surface of the skin into the keratinised part of the hair. The hyphae grow as the hair grows, showing a predilection for the newly keratinised part. The youngest part of the fungus is thus the deepest in the hair shaft. The older fungal hyphae reach the surface with the growing hair, break up into spores and this leads to a breaking off of the hair, giving rise to the characteristic bald patches. *Microsporon* gives a yellowish-green fluorescence with

Wood's lamp, but no fluorescence occurs with *Trichophyton*. Scales on the skin have a whitish fluorescence under the Wood's lamp. When using this test it should be remembered that some topically applied drugs may give a yellowish-green fluorescence. Certain identification of the fungus necessitates its cultivation on special media.

Where the infection is light and treatment is applied, the condition should be cleared in about three weeks. In severe infections, even with intensive treatment, the disease may drag on for months. Spontaneous remissions sometimes occur.

Treatment. With isolated foci of infection, the hair should be clipped, the skin defatted with ether, and then painted with tincture of iodine. A useful application is:

R. Chrysarobin   } āā   20 parts
    Birch tar oil
    Salicylic acid   10 parts
    Potash soap   } āā   25 parts
    Lanoline

This treatment must be continued for 8–10 days and, if necessary, repeated after a week's interval.

Where the infection is extensive then the whole of the body should be short clipped and washed in 7 % chloramine solution. This solution must be freshly prepared before use if it is to be effective. These baths should be given once daily for 4–5 days and then repeated after an interval of 2 days. The treatment cycle is repeated 3–4 times. Occasionally signs of sensitivity, in the form of erythema, appear, and in these cases the washes should be discontinued and bland soothing dressings applied. Oral treatment of ringworm with the antibiotic, Griseofulvin, has given good results in a dose of about 10 mg per kg bodyweight, continuing the treatment for 3–4 weeks. It has been shown, however, that treatment with Griseofulvin alone, whilst producing a clinical cure, may leave the affected animal in an infective condition. It is better to combine systemic Griseofulvin therapy with local antimycotic treatment. All objects in contact with affected animals must be thoroughly disinfected.

It would seem that there is a local immunity produced to reinfection with *Trichophyton*, as previously infected areas cannot be reinfected, even though other areas of the body become infected.

Favus is caused by the fungus *Microsporon gypseum* and is relatively rare in the dog, the short-haired breeds being most susceptible to the infection. Scabs form on the individual hair shafts and ultimately form concave plates or cups. If removed, a raw, moist area is left on the skin. Pruritus is rare with Favus. The disease often appears first on the head, especially the ears and then the legs. Frequently the condition is confined to the nail bed (onychomycosis) producing brittleness of the horn and subsequent deformation of the claw.

Treatment is similar to that used in other dermatomycoses. If the disease is generalised then an unfavourable outcome can be expected. The scabs should first be softened with 2–5 % salicylic acid, the lesions washed with ether and then painted with tincture of iodine.

Pyoderma is due to the entry of the organism *Staphylococcus pyogenes* into the hair follicles. This is usually secondary to traumatic damage to the skin, e. g. a

badly fitting muzzle, chemicals, eczema, etc. One has to distinguish between acne
and furunculosis, in which the inflammation of the tissues around the hair follicles
spreads peripherally.

In acne, the clinical picture is one of eruption of small pustules. If these pustules
are squeezed out they leave cavities which tend to bleed easily. Pus formation is
not invariable and frequently there is just a watery exudate from the pustules.
In many cases there are nodules without any fluid content, and these usually
heal with shedding of the affected hairs. The number of nodules is very variable,
at first only a few develop and these usually heal up after their contents are
expressed. When the infection is more chronic it may show a diffuse distribution,
so that the whole body might be affected. If the bacteria enter the blood stream,
the resultant bacteraemia may produce sudden outbreaks on any part of the body.
Where a long-standing acne heals up, a deformed area of skin may remain (acne
indurata). In this case the hair has fallen out, the hair follicles and the sweat
glands no longer produce their secretions and the skin is thickened by scar tissue
formation (sclerosis, pachyderma). The predilection sites for acne are the bridge
of the nose, the upper and lower lips, the angle of the lower jaw, the distal extremities of the limbs and the skin between the toes.

A furunculosis in which isolated lesions appear is seldom encountered in the dog.
The most characteristic type of furunculosis appears to be acute juvenile pyoderma
(lymphadenitis apostematosa), appearing in dogs about 4 to 10 weeks old, usually
on the upper and lower lips. These areas become very swollen and painful, and
purulent nodules appear which reach the size of a pea before breaking down and
exuding a brownish-yellow secretion. There is always an associated lymphadenitis
and there may be pus formation in these glands. The course of the bacterial
infections described above varies according to the case. A mild acne infection may
be cured in about two weeks, but if it is extensive, treatment must be very intensive
and even then the condition may last for weeks or even months. In acute juvenile
pyoderma there may be a rapid deterioration in the puppy's general condition and
death may even occur following general emaciation. Prognosis must be cautious
in acne, but in acute juvenile pyoderma it is always grave. Effective treatment
is initiated by removing the primary exciting causes. Individual nodules are
regularly expressed and then painted with iodine. Where the acne is more generalised
it is best treated with 40% ichthyol ointment rubbed in several times a day,
and this is supplemented by a course of treatment with sulphur ointment. Daily
irradiations of the diseased areas under the quartz lamp, for three to four minutes
at a distance of 80 centimetres may be useful. This local treatment should be
supplemented also by internal treatment as outlined on page 129. In this respect
the most useful measures are autohaemotherapy and an autogenous vaccine.
The autogenous vaccine is prepared from the organism grown from the contents
of the pustules. Usually 2–4 ml of the vaccine are injected every 2–3 days. If an
autogenous vaccine is not readily available, non-specific protein therapy, e. g.
boiled milk, may be used at a dosage of 1–5 ml. Arsenical treatment is also used
to increase the metabolism of the skin and thus aid recovery. Antibiotic treatment
in high dosage both systemically and injected locally, directly under the lesions,
is worth trying.

Skin tuberculosis must be mentioned among the bacterial dermatoses. This
usually occurs after trauma, large flat ulcers appearing on the wound surface and

the wound itself shows little tendency to heal. In spite of the most intensive treatment of the wound, a flat ulcer with a rolled edge persists. After suitable internal treatment (see page 473) the ulcer remnants must be surgically removed.

Streptotrichosis may show very similar skin lesions. These lesions appear initially in various parts of the body as circumscribed nodular thickenings. These break down releasing a thin brownish-red fluid. Larger or smaller abscesses may also occur with a tendency to produce fistulae and ulcers. All these lesions are fairly resistant to the usual therapeutic measures, but may respond to combined penicillin and streptomycin treatment given in high dosage for a long period (see page 473).

Dermatoses may also be caused by many internal diseases (endogenous dermatoses), e. g. nephritis, diabetes mellitus and insipidus, leucosis, advanced age, etc., may all produce dermatoses. These conditions will be described in more detail in the chapters dealing with the respective diseases. Dermatoses due to poisons and those appearing in infectious diseases will be discussed in the relevant chapters.

Urticaria (Nettle rash) is due to a serous infiltration of the papillary body, usually involving the vaso-motor nerves. External causes may be mechanical, chemical or thermal, but the possibility of internal factors must be borne in mind. In this connection, the predisposing cause may be a hypersensitivity to the condition amongst individuals or in certain breeds, e. g. the Boxer, short-haired Dachshund, Doberman, etc. The onset and course of the disease are very rapid and may only last a matter of hours. The prognosis is favourable and resolution often occurs spontaneously. The clinical picture is characterised by the sudden appearance of round, flat wheals, either over the whole body, or in certain areas, within the

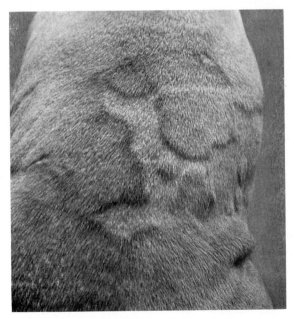

Fig. 145. Urticaria in a Boxer. Only a few parts of the skin are unaffected.

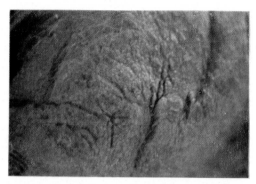

Fig. 146. Acanthosis nigricans in a Dachshund. The pigmentation, folding of the skin and the
pachyderma are characteristic.

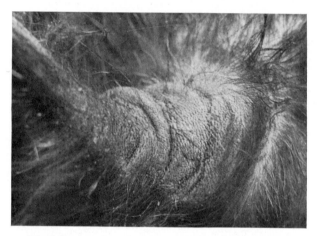

Fig. 147. Acanthosis nigricans at the root of the tail.

space of a few minutes. The first symptom seen by the owner is that the hair tends
to stand on end over the lesions (Fig. 145). Usually the urticaria commences on
the head, causing the so-called hippopotamus head. Good results are claimed
following the injection of 10 % calcium thio-sulphate in a dose of 2–8 m*l* given
slowly intravenously. Extravascular injection produces great pain and often
sloughing of the overlying skin. Vitamin C (ascorbic acid) in high dosage of up to
500 mg is indicated and possibly the anti-histamines may be added to the treatment
(see page 128). A mild laxative such as Carlsbad salts is advisable for several
days after the acute stage has subsided. Where possible the exciting cause should
be discovered and removed.

Acanthosis nigricans (Keratosis) is a skin condition due to a proliferation of the
stratum spinosum and papillary body, which later shows dark pigmentation and
cornification of the skin surface. The aetiology of this is unknown, but its course is

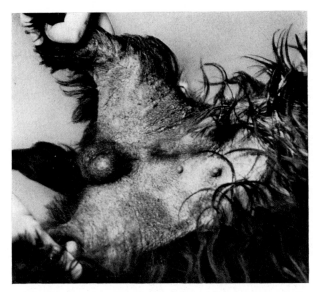

Fig. 148. Acanthosis nigricans symmetrically distributed on the inner surfaces of the thighs.

very protracted and may last for months or even years. Cures are rare, but there may be remissions in the course of the disease from time to time. Prognosis must be very cautious because of the prolonged nature of the disease and the fact that no effective treatment is known to date. Clinically the disease is characterised by the absence of any sign of inflammation. The affected areas of skin show abnormal pigmentation and roughness (Fig. 146), the grooves in the skin protruding like a grater or rasp (Fig. 147). Characteristic of the disease is the symmetrical distribution of the lesions, thus we find the skin of the folds of the carpus, the internal surfaces of the thigh and of axillae symmetrically affected (Fig. 148). Other areas affected are the scrotum and the under surface of the tail (Fig. 149). The disease can also appear at the transition from skin to mucous membrane (anus, vulva, lips and eyelids). Itching is variable. In most cases it is not seen but in a few cases it may be so intense that the healthy transition areas are reddened and swollen. If the disease becomes chronic the elasticity of the skin is markedly lost. The skin is rough and dry.

Treatment is begun with sulphur ointment or sulphur tar liniment. Satisfactory results are obtained with Chrysarobin in various prescriptions, e. g.

R.	Chrysarobin	1–5 parts
	Icthyol	5 parts
	Salicylic acid	2 parts
	Petroleum jelly	ad 100.0

Hot, wet compresses applied to the affected areas daily form a useful supportive treatment. Systemic therapy is as indicated for chronic eczema (see p. 138). Adrenal cortical hormones and the hormones of the anterior lobe of the pituitary

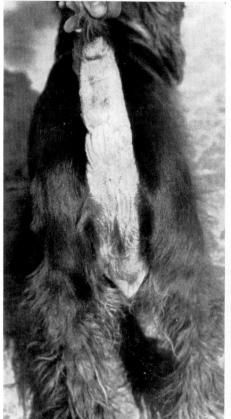

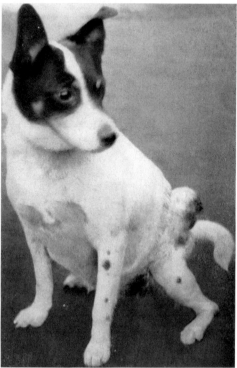

Fig. 149. Acanthosis nigricans on the tail.   Fig. 150. Skin tumour on the left flank.

gland are now being tried in the treatment of acanthosis nigricans. Successes in the treatment of this condition by castration, or adrenalectomy, or both have been claimed. As high doses of ACTH also produced improvement, it is supposed that the condition may be due to a partial insufficiency of the adrenal cortex. Some workers believe that a thyroid dysfunction is the basic cause of this condition and some cases respond to Thyroid Stimulating Hormone or thyroid extract.

Neoplasms. Amongst the tumours occurring in the skin and subcutaneous tissues are Fibromas, Lipomas, Sarcomas, Carcinomas and mixed growths. Adenomas arise in the glands of the skin and papillomas may be generalised over the whole of the body surface, especially in the older dog (Papillomatosis). The clinician must often decide whether a tumour is likely to be malignant or benign. As a general rule it may be said that a benign tumour grows slowly over a period of months, whilst the malignant type may reach a considerable size within a matter of weeks. Metastasis is an important feature of some malignant growths. Usually rapidly

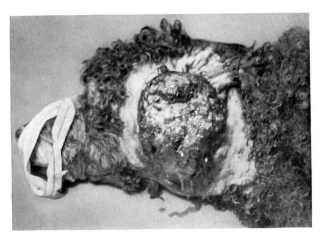

Fig. 151. Tumour on the head of a 10-year-old poodle.

growing tumours which tend to produce metastasis, or in which metastases have already occurred, are inoperable. In the examination of a tumour-bearing animal therefore, special attention must be given to the thorax (radiography) and the abdomen (radiography and careful palpation).

Skin tumours (Figs. 150, 151) are encountered most frequently in the older dog. There is no sex predisposition, but there is an increased susceptibility in the Boxer, Elkhound and Airedale, a moderate predisposition in the German Shepherd and the Rottweiler, and some degree of resistance in the Collie and the Fox Terrier.

The best treatment, where applicable, is the complete surgical removal of the neoplasm. Smaller tumours of the skin surface, especially if they are pedunculated, may be removed by ligature. In this procedure a loop of suture material is made around a pair of forceps, the tumour is seized with the forceps and raised, when the loop can be slipped around the base and drawn tight. Where the tumours are raised above their base and are still quite small, the bases are pricked with a needle in a cruciform manner to control the bleeding and they are then tied off. The neoplasm can then be removed by scissors.

Larger tumours can also be removed. An old method was to remove them by actual cautery, but this tends to leave a permanent scar which is unacceptable to some owners. The direction of the incision must be carefully assessed, so as to obviate any tension on the sutures tending to cause dehiscence of the wound. It is often necessary to do a plastic operation on the wound to ensure coaptation of the margins.

Technique. The operation area should be shaved, defatted with ether, thoroughly cleansed and painted with tincture of iodine. Tumours which lie within the skin are excised by incisions which are made with due regard to the skin tensions of the site. Tumours lying under the skin may be removed by a longitudinal incision over the tumour and careful dissection of the latter from its bed. It is important that haemostasis should be as complete as possible, otherwise slow haemorrhage will almost certainly result in further intervention becoming necessary some hours later. In such an eventuality, the whole of the wound must be opened up under a surface anaesthetic and all bleeding points effectively sealed off. Capillary haemorrhage can be arrested at operation by the use of gelatine sponge. The wound surface must be as dry as possible otherwise the sponge will not adhere. The haemostatic effect of the sponge may be increased by treating it with Thrombin to accelerate coagulation. As the gelatin is a good medium for bacterial growth it is advisable to drip 10,000 units of penicillin on to the dressing, before it becomes attached to the wound surface.

Formerly incisions were made so that, with the animal in the standing position, the wound was as vertical as possible. This ensured adequate drainage if necessary. In the present day of antibiotics and sulphonamides, incisions are made so that the least tension will result on the wound, especially in those areas where movement occurs.

The edges of the wound are closed with mattress sutures, any extra tension being taken up by deep interrupted sutures. If possible the incision should be oval rather than circular in outline, otherwise folding of the skin may result. A little antibiotic or sulphonamide suspension may be introduced under the sutured area. The deep sutures are removed on the 3rd post-operative day and the skin sutures about 8 days later. To produce increased blood supply to the healing wound, a 20% camphor ointment may be applied to the area daily. The usual counter measures to stop the dog biting or licking the wound should be taken, e. g. Elizabethan collars, etc. Healing may be accelerated in some cases by irradiation with red light.

Cysts are quite common in the skin and subcutis of the dog, their origin being rather varied. True cysts arise from transposition of foetal remnants of tissues or organs. There is no continuity with the epithelium, as the cyst develops independently under the skin and increases in size by growth of the cyst wall.

The cysts develop slowly and are round or oval in shape. Their surface is always smooth and they are sharply demarcated from the surrounding tissues. They are freely mobile under the skin and the overlying skin is not altered in appearance. The cysts are usually distended with contents which are of a fluid, pulpy or doughy consistency. Diagnosis is confirmed by exploratory puncture. The commonest type of cyst in the dog is the Dermoid (epithelial cyst). These occur beneath the skin. Simple dermoids are covered with smooth epithelium and contain a watery mucous fluid. In more complex dermoids there often appear trabeculae, so that the cysts appear to be divided into chambers. The cyst wall has the same structure as that of the outer skin – i. e. epidermis, papillary bodies, hairs and sebaceous glands. The contents of the cysts are doughy or pulpy, with a high fat content and of a greyish-white colour. Predilection sites for these dermoids vary with the individual breeds, e. g. in the German Shepherd, the back (withers) and the head (between the ears and on the bridge of the nose), in the Boxer, the bridge of the nose and on the brow. Treatment is by surgical removal.

Technique. As the dermoids are under the skin they can be extirpated after making a longitudinal incision through the overlying skin. In some sites, e. g. on the bridge of the nose, too much skin must not be removed, otherwise coaptation of the wound margins will be difficult.

Retention cysts are caused by a congenital or acquired obstruction of the ducts of the glands or glandular organs. If the ducts of the sebaceous glands of the skin are blocked, atheromas (sebaceous cysts) are formed. These can be palpated as globular structures, about the size of a pea or a cherry, bulging out on the surface of the skin and fairly mobile on their beds. The contents in this case are paste-like. As the cyst wall is rather fibrous and strong and lies in the dermis, it is fairly easy to enucleate the whole cyst. Treatment is by surgical removal by an elliptical incision.

Injuries of the skin are usually caused by accidents, bites, etc. In some cases the skin is actually detached from the body by the opponent seizing the dog by a fold of skin and worrying it. Small particles of dirt may be sucked under the skin by negative pressure, through the relatively small openings caused by the canine teeth and thus infection readily occurs. It is essential to search for the sites of these bite wounds and if they have closed up they must be opened and the extent of the skin detachment ascertained with a sterile probe. An instillation of a suitable sulphonamide or antibiotic solution can then be made into the affected area. If in spite of this treatment infection results, an incision must be made in the dependent parts of the wound and if necessary drainage tubes inserted. Tearing of the skin is repaired by suture following surgical cleansing and debridement if necessary. Injuries to the extremities of the limbs are often seen, caused by walking or jumping on broken bottles, etc. On the foreleg especially, these may be proximal to the carpal joint and in this site they often injure the ulnar artery. Copious arterial bleeding results which sometimes the owner controls by binding the limb above the elbow joint. For repair of this injury, the patient is restrained on its side (see Fig. 30), and local anaesthetic is injected proximal to the injury. Anaesthesia of the wound can be attained by painting the raw surfaces with 2 % lignocaine in addition to the regional anaesthesia. Any tourniquet or tight bandaging is then released, so that the renewed bleeding from the arteries concerned can be controlled with artery forceps and then ligatured. Finally the wound is closed with mattress

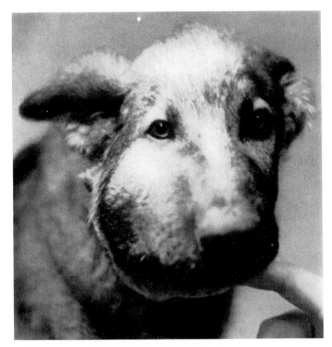

Fig. 152. Phlegmon with associated abscess formation on the head after an insect bite.

sutures, sulphonamide or antibiotic solution is instilled, and a firm bandage applied. Where there has been penetration of a joint, systemic antibiotics should be given for several days and a splint applied.

Phlegmon is an extensive inflammation of the connective tissue of the skin caused by the entry of pyogenic bacteria. It occurs quite frequently in the cheek, as it may be caused by the bite of an insect the dog has caught in its mouth (Fig. 152). This is an extremely painful condition, there is a general malaise and may be pyrexia. Treatment is chiefly by warmth (see physical therapy) and may be by the application of wet compresses, or the various kinds of irradiation. If there is pyrexia, systemic antibiotic treatment should be initiated. Abscess formation may result if the pyogenic process is not curtailed.

Abscesses of various kinds are quite frequent in the dog. Abscesses due to faulty injections are not very common and when they do occur are usually due to a reaction to the injected substance. Treatment is governed by ripening of the abscess and this can be brought about by drugs producing hyperaemia, e. g. camphor ointment (see page 47), wet, hot compresses and irradiation (see page 49). When the abscess is pointed, it is opened with the usual surgical precautions and routine antiseptic measures applied until healing occurs.

Docking of the tail. While it remains fashionable for dogs to have a short tail and ears in certain breeds, it is essential that the veterinary surgeon should master the technique of these operations. The tail is usually docked when puppies are

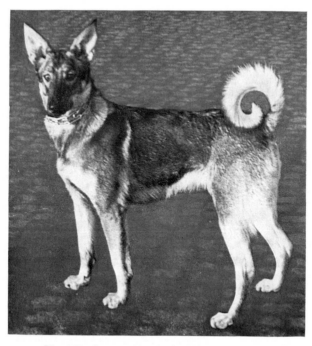

Fig. 153. German Shepherd with a curled tail.

Breeds in which the tail is docked.

Rottweiler Schipperke Breton Spaniel Entlebucher Sennenhund	Born with a stumpy tail, otherwise dock extremely short.
Bobtail	
Schnauzer (various sizes)	Shorten the tail if it is longer than 5 cm.
Pinscher Doberman Boxer Belgian Brussels } Griffons Brabant	Tail short, leaving about 3–4 tail vertebrae, the anus must be covered.
Airedale Fox Terrier Irish Terrier Welsh Terrier Yorkshire Terrier Lakeland Terrier Hunt Terrier	A third is amputated. In adult animals the end of the tail when held in the normal position should be on a level with the occiput, but the tail must not be curled.
Kerry Blue Terrier	Shorter than the other terriers, i. e. a full half.
Sealyham Terrier	Shorter still, about $^2/_3$rds being amputated.
Weimaraner Griffons Poodle-Pointer	Cut $^1/_3$rd to $^1/_2$, the length of the tail must be about half the interval between the beginning of the tail and the hock joint.
Cocker Spaniel Springer Spaniel	About $^1/_2$ to $^2/_3$rds amputated.
German Spaniel	Remove half the tail.
Poodle	Remove half the tail. In the Karakul clip the tail is usually docked rather shorter than in the standard clip.
Blenheim Ruby } Spaniels King Charles	Tail should be docked only as far as one joint.
Munster Lander (large & small)	The end of the tail should only be shortened if it is carried crooked.
Mongrels	Never dock the tails of puppies, only those of adults if they can be assigned by their appearance to a corresponding breed.

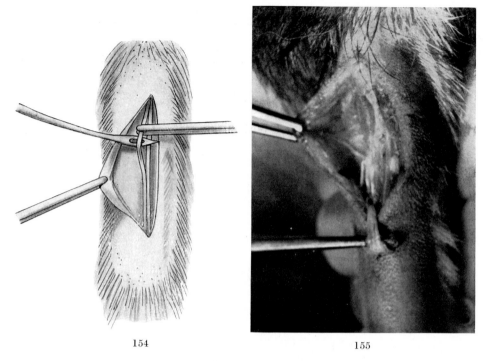

154   155

Fig. 154. Correction of the tail.

Fig. 155. Dissection of the tendon of the lateral erector of the tail (German Shepherd).

only a few days old (4 days), any dew claws present being removed at the same time. If the dog is older than 14 days an anaesthetic must be given. The flap operation is the most useful, the two flaps being brought together by a temporary suture. This technique has the advantage that there is little scarring at the end of the tail and the hair growth is ensured right up to the tip of the tail. In young puppies no bandage or dressing is applied, but in older animals a criss-cross (decussating) bandage is put on. A list of breeds in which the tail is docked is appended, but it is not claimed to be complete. It is always wise to ascertain the owner's wishes as regards length of tail before performing the operation. As a rule bitches are docked with a longer tail than dogs; in any case the docked tail should cover the anus.

A further operation on the tail, correction of the tail carriage, may be combined with docking. The reason for this operation is that the docked or undocked tail is wrongly carried. Among the docked breeds it is usually terriers which carry the tail at too much of a slope format and thus do not comply with the breed standards. In dogs with a sword-shaped trailing tail (German Shepherd, Kuvacz, etc.), it is the so-called curled tail (Fig. 153) which causes the owner to request that

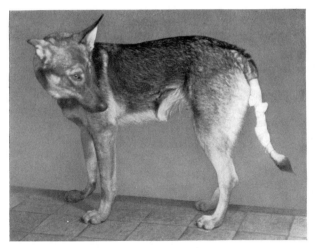

Fig. 156. Condition after correction of the tail. The same dog as that shown in Fig. 153.

ail correction be undertaken. The essence of such an operation is to eliminate ertain groups of muscles which give the tail this faulty position. The lateral rector of the tail, the tendons of which are like a pencil of rays, must be divided, whilst the median erector of the tail must remain untouched, as otherwise the tail would lose its support. The operation is carried out at the point at which the bending of the tail begins. In the curled tail it is sometimes necessary to operate at two or three places.

Technique. Before anaesthesia (lumbosacral epidural anaesthesia) is induced, the site of the operation is determined. Shaving of the site, defatting with ether and painting with iodine is completed. The dog is restrained in the ventral position (Fig. 33). An Esmarch tourniquet is applied to the base of the tail, otherwise bleeding can obscure the field of operation. After making a longitudinal incision for 2–4 cms the outer skin in this area is carefully dissected on both sides from the underlying tissues. This frees the two bundles of tendons in question. As the tendons of the dorsal lateral sacrococcygeal muscle have a great capacity for regeneration, it is not sufficient just to cut them transversely but essential to resect a piece about 1–2 cms long on both sides. All the tendons must be included, so that only the median erector of the tail remains capable of functioning. This is accomplished by pushing a Gerlach needle under the tendon bundle and lifting it from its bed. The Gerlach needle is moved through 90°, so that it lies across under the tendons, which can now be gripped with artery forceps (Fig. 154). Cranial from the artery forceps they are divided and by steady rolling up with the artery forceps are drawn caudally with simultaneous dissection from their non-muscular substratum. About 1–2 cms are resected and then cut off (Fig. 155). The same procedure is repeated on the other side. The Gerlach needle should be inserted from the side towards the middle, because in this way the lateral blood vessels are not in such danger of injury. The wound is closed without making a ridge. It is advisable to instil an antibiotic into the wound cavity in order to protect against secondary infection. As after-treatment the tail is kept in a splint dressing for about 8 days (Fig. 156).

[*Editor's note*. Readers will be aware of the ethical implications in this operation.]

2. Diseases of the ears

When disease is suspected, a careful inspection of both ears must precede treatment. A preliminary assessment is carried out with a sufficiently bright source of light, and in addition an auroscope should be used, with which it is possible to illuminate the deeper parts of the auditory canal. By means of an auroscope fitted with a long speculum, the tympanic membrane can be examined for tension, colour, stratification or perforation. It is necessary to restrain the patient on its side on a firm table and to pull the auditory canal laterally by drawing on the external ear. With the help of the lens in the auroscope, small excoriations in the wall of the auditory canal can be diagnosed.

Diseases of the outer auditory canal (Otitis externa). A predisposition to otitis is said to be dependent on the shape of the ear (pendant, dropped or upstanding ears) but this is not true. The frequency of otitis externa in some breeds has a certain relation to their tendency to eczema and this has been corroborated statistically. There is an increased frequency in breeds having a long and thick hairy covering on the base of the ears, which may also be drawn into the auditory canal by a heavy ear (Spaniel). The production of cerumen in the auditory canal has a certain amount of influence on diseases of the external auditory canal. In normal secretion the canal is protected by an oily film. Chemicals which emulsify fats (soaps) dissolve this film. After bathing, therefore, droplets of water may remain in the auditory canal and initiate inflammatory changes. Overproduction of cerumen (and its retention in the canal) may also be the cause of otitis externa.

Two types of otitis externa must be distinguished. Nonparasitic and Parasitic. **Nonparasitic otitis externa,** which is caused by a wild variety of factors and also occasionally by foreign bodies (husks, grains, splinters), is classified according to the type of inflammation.

In **squamous otitis** there is very marked itching. The dog frequently shakes its head and scratches in the region of the ear. The inner surface of the ear seems to be abnormally warm, and is thickened and reddened. When it is cleaned' fine greyish-black scales are removed.

In **ceruminous otitis** there is a marked accumulation of paste-like, brownish-black cerumen. There is marked itching and shaking of the head, causing an inflammation characterised by thickening, reddening and secretion. If the ear is gently squeezed from the outside, there are squelching noises.

In **squamo-crustaceous otitis** the inner surface of the external ear and the outer auditory canal show clear signs of inflammation. More marked epithelial defects are partly covered by crusts. Itching and head shaking are very marked. The patient scratches the ear and cries in pain.

In **verrucous otitis** there is an enormous thickening of the folds in the external ear and auditory canal. Sometimes this results in the auditory canal being completely occluded (Fig. 157). There is marked itching and head shaking.

Ulcerative otitis is characterised by formation of ulcers in the auditory canal. There is a blood-stained purulent secretion. The intense pruritus causes head shaking, but often this is completely suppressed because of the painfulness of the affection. Palpation of the auditory canal is also painful.

When there is sudden onset of otitis on one side only, one should always consider the possibility of foreign bodies.

Treatment. The auditory canal is cleaned out with a tampon holder, previously moistened with paraffin oil in order to make it as supple as possible. It should not be overcleansed. Vigorous mechanical cleaning may damage the sensitive skin and thus make the otitis worse. After this treatment the auditory canal should be examined with an auroscope, otherwise a foreign body could be driven into the depth of the auditory canal by further probing. During the examination a quiet dog is held by an assistant by the neck and lower jaw grip, the examiner draws the external ear laterally with one hand so that the folds are stretched, and the auroscope is inserted as deeply as possible. Fractious patients must be held in the lateral position, or sedated.

If a foreign body is present the auroscope is inserted and the foreign body removed through the speculum with crocodile ear forceps. If the dog resists strongly, superficial anaesthesia can be produced by instilling a 2 % solution of "lignocaine". In extreme cases general anaesthesia may be necessary: the findings revealed by auroscopy determine the treatment. For conservative treatment a wide variety of drugs has been recommended. In our clinic we use most often cod liver oil and zinc ointment, 10 % sulphathiazole ointment, various antibiotic ointments and occasionally 10 % or 1 % ichthyol ointment. Various powders may be used. If there is marked itching one may instil a few drops of hyoscyamus oil (henbane oil) into the auditory canal and this relieves the irritation by paralysing the nerve endings. Two to 5 % silver nitrate solution may also be used. We obtain good results with 10 % tannin spirit together with Lassar's paste. The following may be recommended:

R.	Boric acid		4 parts
	Glycerine		8 parts
	Distilled water	ad	200 parts

In the acute exudative forms, very good results often follow a single dose of ACTH (50 mg). We also like to give in these cases Prednisone 5 mg tablets, 1–2 tablets a day for 5–10–20 days, but results are variable. For conservative treatment of otitis there is no specific drug, because of the multiplicity of aetiological factors and the variable response of individual patients. In our experience one obtains quicker results if one changes the drug during treatment. If there is chronic otitis externa, which resists conservative treatment, then one must consider whether a better result will be obtained by surgical methods. Surgical intervention is the method of choice for all verrucose and ulcerative otitis. In these cases the auditory canal is partially occluded with ulcers and granulations. This leads to a generalised inflammation further increasing the pressure in the auditory canal, so encouraging formation of granulation tissue. After opening the auditory canal this internal pressure is decreased and so also is the stimulus which led to the inflammation and hyperplastic growth. Foreign bodies are a further indication for surgical measures if they cannot be removed by forceps (see above).

We have obtained satisfactory results by Hinz's method so we prefer this technique to other recommended operative procedures. Zepp's method has several advantages which should not be overlooked, but it requires complete asepsis and also careful after-treatment to ensure healing without too much granulation.

11*

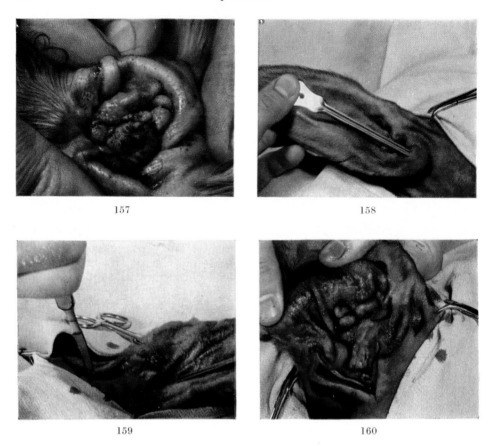

157

158

159

160

Fig. 157. Otitis externa verrucosa (Welsh terrier) (University Dept. of Illustration).

Fig. 158. Hinz's otitis operation. Inserting the director into the auditory canal (University Dept. of Illustration).

Fig. 159. Hinz's otitis operation. Opening the auditory canal with a curved' guarded tenotome (University Dept. of Illustration).

Fig. 160. Hinz's otitis operation. Operation site after opening the auditory canal (University Dept. of Illustration).

Technique of Hinz's operation for otitis. The patient is deeply anaesthetised. This deep anaesthesia weakens the animal's resistance, so the operation should be restricted to essential cases.

The ear to be operated on is cleansed thoroughly with ether. The region between the tragus and the base of the ear is shaved and painted with iodine. The patient is positioned on its side. The ear is held by assistants so as to straighten the auditory canal and allow the surgeon to insert a grooved director (Fig. 158). A curved, blunt-ended tenotome is introduced deep into the auditory canal, guided by the director, and an incision is made through the external wall of the canal (Fig. 159). Blood vessels that bleed copiously are immediately controlled with Pean's forceps. The assistant spreads out the external ear with both hands, so ensuring a good view

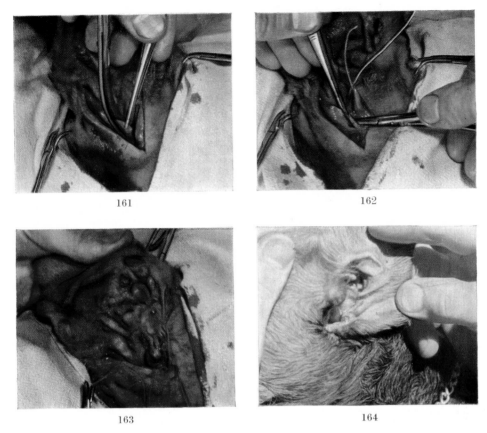

161

162

163

164

Fig. 161. Hinz's otitis operation. Removal of a triangular piece of cartilage on both sides in the lower angle of the wound (University Dept. of Illustration).

Fig. 162. Hinz's otitis operation. Insertion of the suture in the lower angle of the wound with a fully curved needle (University Dept. of Illustration).

Fig. 163. Hinz's otitis operation completed (University Dept. of Illustration).

Fig. 164. Hinz's otitis operation. Condition after healing (Welsh terrier).

of the surgical field by keeping the wound surfaces apart (Fig. 160). Small haemorrhages are controlled with swabs. Careful examination of the auditory canal for a possible foreign body is essential. The operator now seizes with forceps the cartilage on each side in the depths of the wound and with scissors removes a triangular piece (Fig. 161). This brings about a deficiency of substance in the wound so that the tendency to heal over is considerably reduced. Ideally, the sutures should draw together the lining of the auditory canal and the external skin, but in most cases the lining has become too friable from the long-continued inflammation, and it is advisable to pass the suture through the cartilage as well to give it a better hold. The stitches should not be pulled too tight otherwise they will break down in the inflammatory reaction that follows. The suture begins at the wound angle. Two stitches are inserted in the depths with a short, full-curved needle and are drawn together and left untied (Fig. 162). Interrupted sutures are then inserted on each side and finally the two innermost knots are tied (Fig. 163). If there are polypoid growths in the auditory canal, they are removed with scissors, thermo-cautery or electro-cautery (risk of an explosion in ether anaesthesia!), superficial bleeding being controlled with ferric chloride swabs. These swabs should be removed after 24 hours, otherwise the tissues will be cauterised. The wound is covered with antiseptic powder and an ear bandage applied, which should be removed after 24 hours.

After-treatment: From 4–5 days after the operation, the ear is carefully cleansed and then dusted heavily with a wound powder. The area around the wound is covered with cod liver oil and zinc paste to protect against "scalding" by wound discharges. Healing, if it is not by first intention, will take 3–4 weeks.

About 8–10 days after the operation the wound is regularly treated with copper sulphate because, in spite of the excision of the triangular pieces of cartilage, the wound edges still tend to heal together. For this reason one should undertake the after treatment oneself and not leave it to the owner (Fig. 164).

Parasitic otitis is not as common as the non-parasitic type. Ear mites and fungi (otomycosis) are the causal agents.

Ear mange in the dog and also in the cat is caused by the ear mite *Otodectes cynotis*. Cats are frequently affected and in contrast to the dog, there are not always changes in the external ear. Often one can only detect increased formation of cerumen. Despite this lack of visible change in the ear there is always marked itching. Identification of the ear mite is by microscopical examination, and treatment is by a contact insecticide.

Otomycosis is very rare indeed. It is caused by *Mucor, Aspergillus*, and *Verticillium* and the clinical signs consist only of grey or yellowish-grey skin-like deposits on the external ear and auditory canal. Treatment is with salicylate as a 5% spirit or 2% ointment. Nystatin preparations may be especially useful.

In chronic forms of otitis which have been treated by the owner for a long time rupture of the tympanic membrane may occur, with subsequent otitis media. In contrast to Moltzen-Nielsen who considers that about 74% of cases of otitis externa may be preceded by otitis media as the primary lesion (as occurs in man), we were unable to confirm this from the extensive pathological material available to us.

Haematoma of the ear arises in otitis when there is vigorous shaking of the head. By striking the ear against a hard surface a blood vessel is ruptured and a haematoma arises. The breeds chiefly affected are those with pendant or upstanding ears, but quite often haematomata are seen in breeds with cropped ears.

The clinical picture of a recent haematoma is a swelling of the ear flap up to the size of a child's fist. The swelling feels semi-solid and warmer than normal. The affected ear (in breeds with upstanding ears) is bent laterally and held obliquely to the head (Fig. 165). Attempts to shake the head are made very cautiously.

Treatment is initially of an expectant nature and if necessary cold compresses may be applied. The haematoma is left to organise for about 3 weeks, a net (see p. 60) being put round the ear to rest and support it. If after 3 weeks commencing resorption of the haematoma can be detected, further conservative treatment (microwave) should be given. In other cases after an incision into the inner surface of the external ear, the blood clot is cleaned out and the ear is kept bandaged for a prolonged period with a daily change of the bandage. After operative treatment our experience has been that obvious deformation of the affected ear usually resulted, which was not always so with conservative treatment.

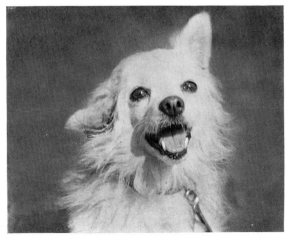

Fig. 165. Haematoma of the right ear of a Pomeranian.

WILLE (Berl. Münch. tierärztl. Wschr. **69**, 456–69, 1956) recommended a modified operation according to Zepp. Under general anaesthesia and with an aseptic field of operation, an S-shaped incision is made through the skin on the inner surface of the ear flap. The blood clot is cleaned out and antibiotics are applied locally. Tension sutures are then inserted transversely to the incision and finally several button sutures are put through the external ear over the whole surface of the haematoma, in order to prevent retention of secretion. A well-padded bandage is applied, first changed after 5 days, and after 9 days the sutures are removed. Any existing thickening of the external ear disappears after some tieme and deformity of the ear should not occur.

GARBUTT (North Amer. Vet. **37**, 1050–59, 1956) recommends the following method: under anaesthesia blood and clot are removed through a tangential incision from the border of the ear to its tip. With a special instrument' small round discs are punched out of the skin and perichondrium, the external ear is padded, laid over the head and bandaged. The dressings should be left on for 3 weeks if possible. Very often, an operation is requested by the owner after a healed haematoma has resulted in a deformed external ear. Surgery in such cases is unsatisfactory and should not be undertaken.

Ulceration of the tip of the ear. In otitis and after dog fights, ulceration of the tip of the ear may occur. The ulcers cause continued shaking of the head so the damaged tissues do not get a chance to rest and heal. A net should be applied to the external ear to immobilise it as much as possible (see p. 60). The ulcerated areas are anointed with ointments that protect and encourage granulation (cod liver oil and zinc ointment).

In some breeds of terriers incorrectly dropped ears occur, the ears remaining upright, giving the dog a bat-like appearance (Fig. 166). By removal of a narrow strip of cartilage from the external ear the upright stance of the ear is lost and correct tilting achieved. The operation can be performed under local anaesthesia, but it is preferable to induce general anaesthesia so that the patient is kept still.

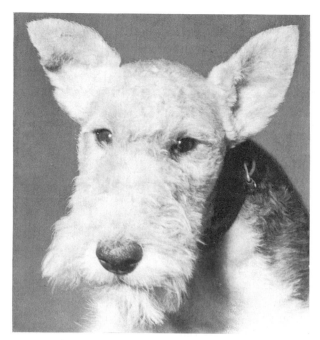

Fig. 166. Fox terrier with upstanding ears.

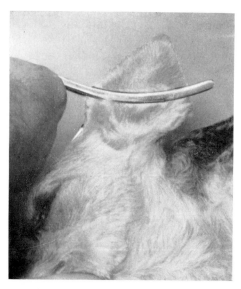

Fig. 167. Applying the Doyen clamp in the ear tilt operation.

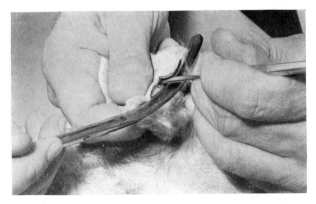

Fig. 168. Undermining the strip of cartilage to be excised.

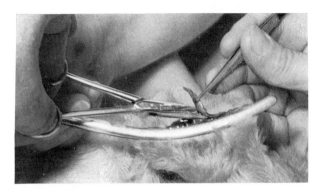

Fig. 169. Excising the dissected out strip of cartilage.

Technique: The dog lies in the lateral position and the operation is done on the inner side of the ear. A Doyen's bowel clamp is placed across the external ear, with the concavity of the clamp turned towards the tip of the ear. At the medial edge of the ear, the clamp is placed about 1 cm from the tip of the external ear and terminates at the lateral edge of the ear at about the upper angle of the Balkon (skin pocket). The portion of ear above the clamp must not form an equilateral triangle but the lateral side must be a little shorter than the medial side (Fig. 167). If this is neglected the ear may show a tendency to be flattened and will not conform to the breed standard. When the operation is successful the tip of the ear should be directed towards the lateral angle of the eye.

After the clamp has been correctly placed, the tip of the ear is stretched over the index finger of the hand holding it. An assistant can adjust the clamp a little more, so that the surface to be incised is stretched as much as possible. The incision is made by drawing a short, pointed scalpel along the concave surface of the clamp beginning about 1 cm from the lateral edge of the ear and ending 1 cm in front of its medial edge. At first only the skin is carefully parted, so that the cartilage underlying it becomes visible (Fig. 168). The first penetration into the cartilage is best done in the middle of the ear flap, because at its edges there is the risk of damaging the blood vessels supplying the ear flap. When the cartilage has been exposed, it is carefully dissected away

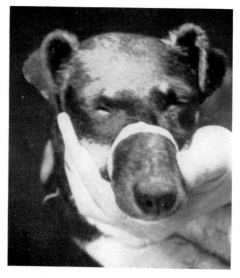

Fig. 170. Condition immediately after the operation (Hunt terrier).

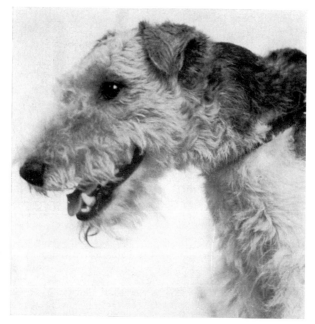

Fig. 171. The same Fox terrier as in Fig. 166 six weeks after the operation to tilt the ears.

from its bed on both sides (on the inner side of the skin covering the external surface of the ear flap). In doing this the greatest care must be taken not to injure the blood vessels already mentioned. If this happens, complete necrosis of the external ear up to the line of the incision may occur. When the cartilage is separated from the outer skin for about 3 mm along the line of the incision, this strip is grasped with eye forceps and removed with scissors (Fig. 169). The head of the patient is now raised in order to check that the ear tilts in the desired manner. If this is not so, a little more must be removed from both edges of the ear. Care must be taken not to remove too much from the medial edge, as otherwise the tilt of the ear is angular.

After doing the same operation on the other ear, both incisions are protected by strips of gauze dusted with powder and bandaged in the desired position. After 24 hours the bandage is removed and the sites are treated as open wounds until final healing occurs (Fig. 171).

In the **German Shepherd dropped ears** are undesirable. An affected dog is usually presented at the age of 5–7 months, with the history that either one or both ears have never stood up, or that they first turned down after teething. Formerly we used various procedures, but none of them brought satisfactory results. The most effective treatment has proved to be regular (daily) massage of the superficial cervico-auricularis and specific accessory scutulo-auricularis muscles. If the ears of a 1-year-old dog are still dropped, it is unlikely that they will ever become erect.

IRWIN (Vet. Med. **52**, 179–184, 1957) corrected badly placed ears as follows: strap-shaped cartilage transplants were aseptically removed from the ears of a sheep dog that had just died. They were sterilised for 24 hours in penicillin solution at 37° and then put in a deep freeze. After localisation of the weakness in the cartilage, these transplants were placed between the perichondrium and the external skin of the faulty ear; several transfixing ligatures secured the transplants. For after-treatment complete immobilisation is recommended.*

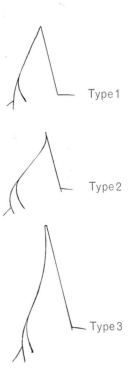

As many veterinarians refuse to crop dogs' ears, it is often undertaken by laymen without anaesthetics. By the Protection of Dogs Law of 29th November, 1933, Section II, paras 2, 7, it is forbidden to shorten the ears or tail of a dog more than 2 weeks old. The shortening is permitted if it is done under anaesthesia. No veterinary surgeon in general practice can be expected to know all the details of the external features of each and every breed. He should, however, know the basic essentials for the carriage of the cropped ear and for the cropping of the ear. By consulting the breeder he should be able to obtain information about any special wishes as regards the ears before embarking on the operation.

Fig. 172. The 3 types of cropped ears.

---

* *Editor's note.* The same ethical considerations apply to these operations as to the operation for correction of a faulty tail carriage.

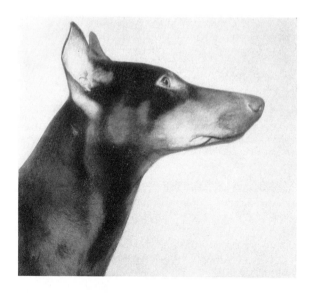

Fig. 173. Well-cropped
Doberman Pinscher.

Accordingly, for general information, we may give some of the rules for cropped ears laid down by the various breed Societies. As a rule, the ears are shortened one-third to two-fifths. Ears of the male should move heavily, those of the female, gracefully. The shape of the ears can be divided also into three types (Fig. 172).

Type 1. The line of the incision is straight with a slightly emphasised end. In general the shape of the cropped ear should be slender. In the Riesenschnauzer and Doberman they are fairly long. In the Mittle-and Zwerg-Schnauzer, the Reh-Zwerg, Affenpinscher and Brabant Griffon they are cropped relatively short (Fig. 173).

Type 2. Line of the incision slightly S-shaped – the tip of the ear runs to a point. This applied to the Boxer (Fig. 174), although recently the ears of the Boxer are given the shape of Type 1.

Type 3. Line of the incision long and S-shaped, especially running to an acute point. The ear should be as long as possible, so that it resembles the shape of a flame. This applies to the Great Dane (Fig. 175).

The ears should be cropped only in healthy dogs, because the stress of the operation is quite severe. Puppies should be starved before operation, otherwise pneumonia due to inhalation of stomach contents may occur and may cause death. Usually the operation is performed when the dog is 8–10 weeks old, but Riesenschnauzers, Dobermans and Boxers should be cropped at 10 weeks, and Great Danes after 12 weeks, because at this age there is a better chance that the ears will be carried correctly after the cropping. Mongrels should not be cropped under 6 months, because usually by then the influence of the father on the external features is evident (Fig. 176).

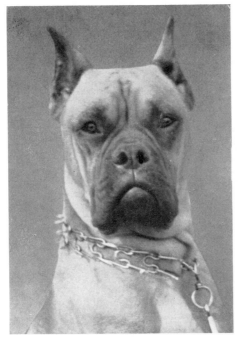

Fig. 174. Well-cropped Boxer.

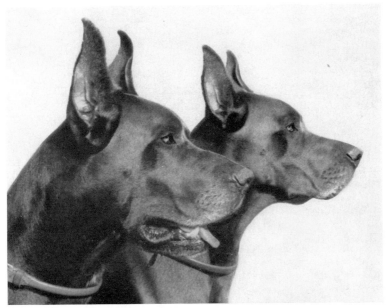

Fig. 175. Two well-cropped Great Danes in which the "flame" shape is well shown.

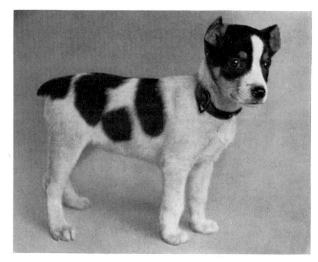

Fig. 176. Badly cropped Fox terrier cross. The tail is too short and the ears should not be cropped.

Technique: Infiltration anaesthesia is sufficient. The ear to be cropped is injected on both sides and a large depot injection is made at the base of the ear to block the auricular nerves. Injection into the line of the incision may cause subcutaneous oedema and lead to difficulty in attaining the correct ear shape.

Different clamps are used for the three types of ear shape described. For Type 1 a straight clamp is suitable. In the second type one uses a clamp bent in an S-shape and for the third type a concave clamp. With practice one can usually attain the desired ear shape with a straight clamp and this is used exclusively in our clinic. In order to be able to tense the ear sufficiently we have provided it with wing-nuts. In this connection Ullrich's ear-clamps may be mentioned. They consist of a straight clamp, which has on one side a hinged joint so that only a screw need be turned to close them. Especially noteworthy is the holder-plate, which precludes injury to the assistant when the overlying external ear is cut off.

The dog is placed in the ventral position. The shape of the ear is carefully studied in order to give the ears a suitable shape (males or females). For this the length of the ears must also be determined. As a rough guide, the tip of the cropped ear, if it is laid over to the other side of the head, should project a little over the middle line. This does not apply to Great Danes, however, because they should be cropped longer. Now both ears are laid together over the head in such a way (Fig. 177) that a notch made with scissors in the anterior edge of the ear flap ensures that both ears are cropped to the same length (Fig. 178). Very occasionally one encounters ears of different lengths and in such cases the notching cut must be corrected. Before the clamp is applied, the animal is placed on its side and a cotton wool plug is inserted into each auditory canal, so that no blood can seep into it during the cropping, as this may be a source of inflammation (otitis externa).

The ear is so placed in the straight half-opened clamp that the notching cut ends directly in the clamp. The lateral edge of the ear should be drawn out of the clamp far enough for the "Balkon" to be cut away as far as possible. If Type 1 ear shape is desired, after screwing up the clamp the part of the ear flap remaining above it is removed. To attain Type 2, before finally releasing the clamp, the ear flap is drawn a little out of the jaws of the clamp in the middle of the line of the incision. If the desired S-shaped variations still appear marked, then the wing-nuts at the notching cut can be repeatedly loosened and the ear flap drawn out to about 2.5–3.0 cm, so that the notching

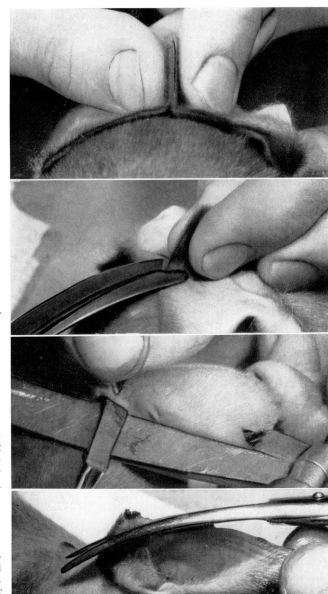

Fig. 177. Cropping the ears. Laying the ears together over the head in order to determine the cropped length (University Dept. of Illustration).

Fig. 178. Cropping the ears. Putting in the notch-cut to mark out the length of the ear (University Dept. of Illustration).

Fig. 179. Cropping the ears. Removing the projecting part of the ear with a scalpel. The notch-cut is readily visible.

Fig. 180. Cropping the ears. Removing the so-called "Balkon" with curved scissors (University Dept. of Illustration).

cut is separated for almost 0.5 cm from the clamp. It will now be very stretched and only the notching cut will be drawn back up to the clamp.

If Type 3 is desired one pulls the ear flap as far as possible out of the clamp in order to achieve the concave variation of the cropped ear.

If by these corrections the desired shapes are attained, the firmly closed clamp is held at both ends by an assistant and the protruding portion of ear flap is cut off with a scalpel (Fig. 179). The direction of this cut is always from the base of the ear to the tip because of the notching cut.

After removing the clamp the still upstanding "Balkon" is removed with curved scissors (Figs. 180, 181). We suture the wounds, with sutures put in at intervals of 1 cm. In doing this it is important that the ear cartilage is not pierced. According to the breed of dog 4–8 stitches are put in. Suturing of the wounds in the ear flap has been retained because it results in minimal scar formation. The other ear is now cropped in the same way. In order to achieve equality in size the excised part of the first ear is used as a guide, when the clamp is applied to the second ear. After removal of the cotton wool from both auditory canals the operation is concluded with a head bandage which is removed after 24 hours (Fig. 182).

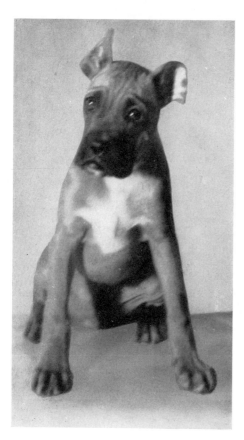

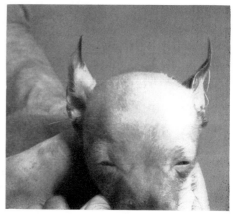

Fig. 181. A badly cropped Boxer. The pinna was not drawn out of the clamp as far the "Balkon" and the "Balkon" was not removed at the end of the operation.

Fig. 182. Cropping the ears. The operation is completed (University Dept. of Illustration).

After-treatment consists of light massage of the edges of the wounds, beginning about 4 days after the operation and continued daily until scar formation is complete. The stitches are removed 4–6 days after the operation. We do not use adhesive dressings or the practice of crossing the ears over one another, as these methods deprive the ears of daily treatment and strictures due to scar tissue contraction may occur.

Strictures due to contraction of scar tissue in the cropped ear may completely disfigure the external appearance of a dog. They arise through neglect of the after treatment of the cropped ear.

Treatment is by the removal of a narrow strip of skin in the region of the stricture with scissors under local anaesthesia.

Sometimes the ears do not stand up after cropping. This occurs in cases in which there is a soft cartilage with a relatively thicker skin (in this regular massage of the erector of the ear may produce good results). It is not seen in dogs which have a strong cartilage and a thick stretched skin. Further cropping of ears that do not stand up (in order to reduce their weight) is not effective.

3. Diseases of the eyes

Examination of the eyes is carried out in accordance with general ophthal-mological principles. The eyes are first inspected from a distance of 1–2 m, in order to detect certain conditions, e. g. strabismus, which may not be apparent at close quarters. Next one examines the eyelids, and the extent and appearance of secretions are noted along with the condition of the conjunctivae. The nictitating membrane may be examined by grasping it with toothed forceps and raising it away from the eyeball (Fig. 183), having first applied a surface anaesthetic and taking care that the cornea is not damaged by the forceps. A careful inspection of the conjunc-tival sac for possible foreign bodies (grass seeds, barley awns, etc.) should be made.

Examination of the eyeball includes an estimation of its position in the orbit, size, shape, mobility and the direction of the axes of vision. In addition the intra-ocular tension can be estimated by light to moderate pressure with the index finger through the eyelid so that the cornea is not damaged. A more accurate estimation may be made by using a Schiotz tonometer, an instrument which records the resistance of the cornea to indentation by movement of a needle on a scale. In co-operative animals instrumental tonometry may be carried out with topical anaesthesia, with the patient in either a sitting position, with the head held so that the eyes are directed upwards, or lying on its back. The eyelids are separated and the tonometer allowed to rest by its own weight upon the centre of the cornea (Fig. 184). The procedure may be rendered difficult, and inaccurate readings ob-tained, if the eyeball is retracted into the orbit, or is rolled, or if the nictitating membrane protrudes. Readings between 15 and 30 mmHg may be considered within the normal range for the dog.

The cornea is examined by artificial light, with focal and lateral lighting which reveal changes in its surface, the radius of its curvature and its transparency. The smallest lesions of the epithelium may be rendered visible by applying fluorescein solution and rinsing with sterile water; defects in the corneal surface will be stained green.

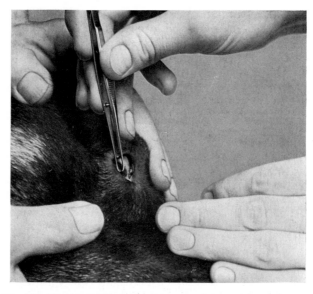

Fig. 183. Picking up the nictitating membrane with eye forceps.

Changes in the radius of curvature are detected by the distortion of the corneal reflection of a small image such as a window or a lamp (Fig. 185). Superficial corneal erosions are detected by the faulty reproduction of an object reflected in it.

The anterior chamber of the eye, the iris and pupil are also examined. The reaction of the pupil to light is of clinical importance, and can be judged by closing and suddenly opening the eyelids, or by illumination with artificial light, with the other eye held closed. The lens is also examined with the naked eye by lateral and focal lighting. The fundus of the eye can be examined with the aid of an ophthalmoscope. To do this efficiently, it may be necessary to dilate the pupil with a mydriatic such as atropine, homatropine or tropicamide.

Homatropine has a much less prolonged mydriatic effect than atropine and is to be preferred for this purpose; tropicamide is probably the most useful agent for preparing the eye for ophthalmoscopy.

In the study of the fundus of the eye the colour of the tapetum, the form, colour, curvature and boundaries of the optic papilla, the number and degree of distension of the blood vessels, any turbidities or other colour changes are all noted. The examination of the fundus should be done in a darkened, or at least, a shaded room (Fig. 186). The visual capacity of the patient is determined by the so-called "stool test", in which the patient is led several times along the same path. A stool is then placed across the path and from the way in which this obstruction is bumped into or avoided, one can make some assessment about the patient's vision. The "stool test" can be varied by placing the stool in front of a clear, dark background and this allows certain nuances in the estimation of visual acuity to be appreciated.

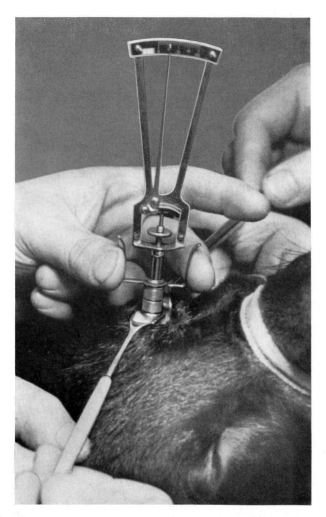

Fig. 184. Tonometry of the eye of a dog with Schiotz's tonometer.

The slit lamp is used for specially detailed investigations. The principle of this method depends on the Tyndall phenomenon. If one illuminates the cornea with a slit-shaped source of light, a light-prism can be seen in which one can examine the different layers microscopically. With the slit lamp it is possible to observe also pathophysiological processes in the interior of the eye (discharge of fluid from the chambers) or in the cornea (flow of red blood cells in pannus). Thus, with the help of this method exact investigations can be made, not only of the transparent parts of the eye (cornea, lens, vitreous humour) but also of other parts (e. g. the iris).

12*

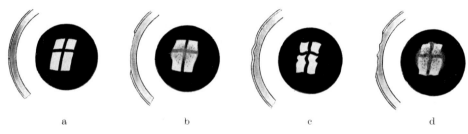

a   b   c   d

Fig. 185. Pictures reflected in the corneal outer layer. (a) Normal outer layer epithelium. The curvature is uniform: the reflected image is sharp, bright and not distorted. (b) Defect in the outer layer of the cornea. Curvature uniform: reflected picture not sharp, dull, but not distorted. (c) Corneal epithelium normal. Curvature not uniform: reflected picture sharp and bright but distorted. (d) Defective corneal epithelium: curvature not uniform: reflected picture dull and distorted.

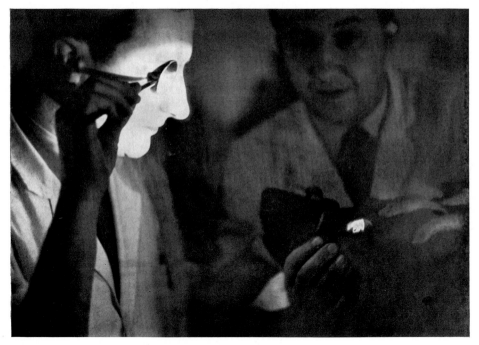

Fig. 186. Examination of the eye with a mirror in a darkened room.

As the focal distance is only 8 cm one must bring the apparatus very close to the patient, and it is therefore necessary to fix the patient with a head-holder (ÜBERREITER model).

Atresia palpebrarum (Coalescence of the eyelids). This condition may also be termed ankyloblepharon. This ankyloblepharon breaks down for the first time approximately 14 days after birth, the eyeball becoming visible.

At birth, both eyelids are firmly joined together. During the first days of life the outer epidermis grows in at the line where the lids will separate and eventually unites with the conjunctiva (Fig. 187). When this union occurs the eyelid opens. As this process takes some time, it is wrong to try to help it by forcibly opening the lids, as scarring and deformity of the lids may result. If after 14 days the lids have still not opened, lukewarm bathing with camomile tea is recommended. The stimulating effect of camomile tea on cells is well known. If satisfactory opening of the lids is not produced in this way, surgical measures are taken.

In **Blepharophimosis** there is a narrowing of the aperture between the eyelids, which can be congenital or acquired (through scar formation), and this also must be surgically treated.

Blepharitis (inflammation of the eyelids) may arise from contact irritants, sarcoptic mange, demodecosis, dermatitis or nutritional deficiencies, or may be associated with conjunctivitis or keratoconjunctivitis, or with tarsal cysts or styes. Treatment consists of thorough cleansing and the application of antibiotic-steroid ointments, together with surgical drainage in those cases where sebaceous or meibomian glands are involved with a purulent infection.

The eyelids are sometimes injured during fights, and it is important to ensure that there are no injuries to other parts of the eye. Small injuries may be treated with antibiotic preparations, but larger wounds may require surgical repair. Injury to the border of the lid may necessitate a blepharoplasty to ensure that accurate closure of the lids is possible. After-treatment consists of the application of antibiotic ointments.

Alterations in the position of the lids appear chiefly as Entropion and Ectropion.

Entropion is the commonest displacement of the eyelids in the dog. In this condition the eyelids turn inwards against the eyeball (Fig. 188). The eyelashes and the hairs of the outer skin cause irritation of the conjunctiva and cornea which ultimately leads to purulent conjunctivitis, keratitis and corneal ulceration. Most cases are congenital in origin, but some may follow cicatricial contraction

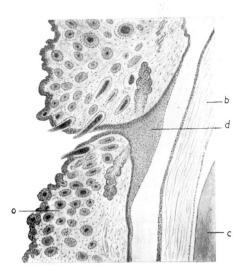

Fig. 187. Transverse section of the eyelids of a dog a few days old. (a) Eyelids. (b) Horny layer of the cornea. (c) Lens. (d) Subsequent split between the lids.

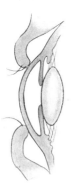

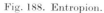

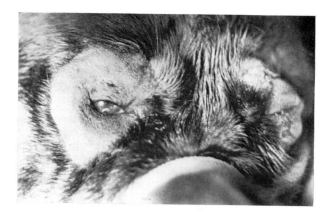

Fig. 188. Entropion.   Fig. 189. Entropion in a Rottweiler.

resulting from lid injuries or may be spastic in origin following chronic conjunctivitis or blepharospasm.

Clinical picture. In most cases only the lower lid is involved, most often in
the lateral segment. The tarsal border rolls inwards and, on occasion, the whole
length of the lid may ultimately become involved (Fig. 189).

Treatment, in cases of spastic entropion, is first directed towards removing
the exciting cause. This may produce resolution in early cases.

If the entropion is not corrected in spite of removal of the exciting cause, or
if the entropion is congenital in origin, surgical measures must be undertaken.

Conservative treatment of entropion by the injection of various drugs (Paraffin,
"Dondren") has been tried, as has the electrocoagulation technique used in human
medicine (SCHULZE, M.hefte Vet. Med. **6**, 57, 1951). Good results were not obtained
by any of these methods, because of the anatomical differences between the eyelids
of the dog and those of man. In the dog there are no tarsal plates, which in man
serve to give the eyelids special support and stiffness, as they form a coherent
connective tissue plate. In the dog these tarsal plates are formed chiefly from
glands and tissues which do not adhere together. The dog also has an incomplete
orbital ring, which in man is closed by the zygomatic process of the frontal bone.
For these reasons the fibrous tissue formation which occurs in the eyelid of the
dog (after a "Dondren" injection, for example) offers no resistance to the bulb
of the eye and does not counteract the pull from the inner skin on the tarsal
border of the turned-in part of the lid.

Technique of the Entropion operation. The hair is shaved off in the region of the lids, the skin
is defatted with ether and iodine applied. Before applying infiltration anaesthesia to the field
of operation, one makes a detailed assessment of the extent of the entropion and the amount
of skin to be removed, because after the infiltration, oedema appears which masks the entropion.

Anaesthesia is performed by inserting the needle about 5 mm from the edge of the lid in the
lateral angle of the eye and pushing it medially from this point into the upper or lower lid as far
as there is any inturning of the lid. As the needle is withdrawn the anaesthetic is injected.

In most cases, it may be found preferable to use general anaesthesia. In such cases, assessment
of the extent of the operation should be made before anaesthesia is induced, and due allowance

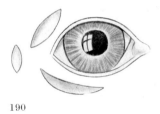

190

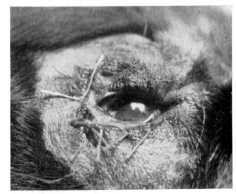

191

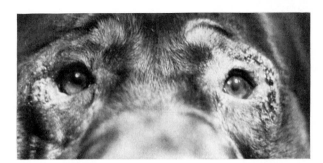

192

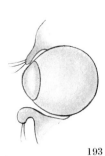

193

194

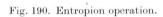

Fig. 190. Entropion operation.

Fig. 191. Condition of the eyelids at the end of the operation.

Fig. 192. Ten days after the operation (the Rottweiler shown in Fig. 189).

Fig. 193. Ectropion.

Fig. 194. Ectropion in a St. Bernard.

must be made for the accentuation of the inturning that may follow retraction of the eyeball under anaesthesia.

The basic idea of the operation is that a larger or smaller elliptical piece of skin is removed from the lid in the inturned region, and the subsequent suturing so shortens the outer skin that eversion of the lid occurs. The skin of the upper or lower lid in the affected parts is pinched up with hooked forceps and a correspondingly elliptical piece of skin is removed with curved scissors (Fig. 190). There is little bleeding and this can be controlled by pressure with a tampon. The distance between the tarsal border and the wound border should be about 3 mm. The edges of the wound are brought together with sutures (Fig. 191). In order to equalise the lateral angles of the eye an elliptical piece of skin lying at right angles to the aperture between the lids and lateral to the angle of the eye is removed. The suture should subsequently be covered with "Noviform" ointment, repeated after 4–5 days. At this time one can now decide whether enough or even too much skin has been removed and whether in extreme cases an ectropion has been made out of an entropion. If this should occur the stitches at specially marked places are removed and the wound is opened until the ectropion has been corrected. Finally, daily massage is applied so that the defect is covered by a broad scar. In such cases subsequent healing must be supervised daily as far as possible. Intractable patients which tend to scratch, are given a neck collar. After 8 days the skin stitches are removed (Fig. 192).

Rottweilers and Chow-chows are especially liable to entropion. In Chow-chows "small eyes" are bred for as a show point and for this reason, and also because of their very loose subcutaneous connective tissue, entropion is often met with in this breed. The operation in these breeds is not always satisfactory.

Ectropion is a turning of the lower lid outwards (Fig. 193). It occurs chiefly in St. Bernards and sometimes also in Newfoundlands (Fig. 194). If it is congenital, continued treatment of the conjunctivitis resulting from it gives more satisfactory results than does an operation. The condition also occurs in dogs which have an undesirably open eye (for example, Setters).

Treatment can only be surgical.

Technique of the Ectropion operation. After shaving and anaesthetising the field of operation (see Entropion) a canthotomy incision is made on the lateral angle of the eye (see p. 202). A triangular piece is removed midway from the margin of the lid and the canthotomy incision (Fig. 195a). The edges of the wound are brought together by sutures in such a way that the tarsal border in the lateral angle of the eye is apposed to the tarsal border of the upper lid (Fig. 195b). This kind of plastic operation is used in order to ensure a constant pull of the lower lid laterally. After-treatment is given with suitable ointments. The skin sutures are removed after 8 days.

Ptosis, i. e. a drooping of the upper lid, has been observed in the dog in space-occupying lesions of the brain. It may also occur in the course of rabies.

Tumours of the Eyelids (Tumori palpebrarum) occur in older dogs and arise from the border of the lid (Fig. 196). They may cause inflammation of the cornea mechanically, so that it is advisable to remove them.

Treatment must be restricted solely to ligating or cauterising them, because these tumours are not only on the margin of the lid but extend deeply into the lid. Radical removal can only be achieved by a wedge-shaped excision (Fig. 197). In after-treatment the greatest pains should be taken to see that the tarsal border assumes its former shape.

Diseases of the Conjunctiva. The main condition is so-called conjunctivitis. In its simplest form it occurs as **catarrhal conjunctivitis (Conjunctivitis simplex),** consisting of a superficial inflammation of the conjunctiva. The causes are multifarious, mechanical causes playing a large part in the aetiology. Dust and dirt

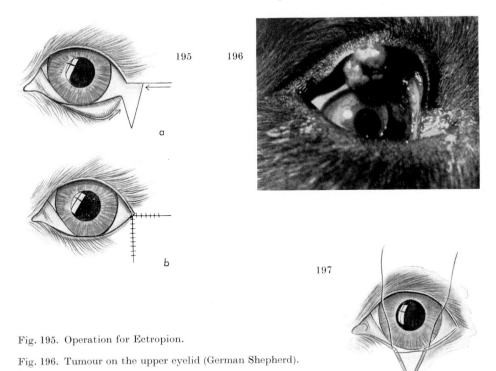

Fig. 195. Operation for Ectropion.

Fig. 196. Tumour on the upper eyelid (German Shepherd).

Fig. 197. Wedge-shaped excision in tumour of lower eyelid.

may irritate the conjunctiva of the lids in the large breeds either when they are at work or romping about. In the smaller breeds this also occurs by way of dust stirred up by the owner as he walks along. Other causes of conjunctivitis are chemical (ammoniacal kennel air, SO_2, gases, smoke, chalky dust, etc.). The use of old decomposing eye drops (for example, of atropine) may also cause conjunctivitis. Infectious diseases (distemper) and a deficiency of vitamin A (degeneration and loss of epithelium) are also frequently involved in the aetiology.

The *clinical picture* of catarrhal conjunctivitis shows at first a serous and later a more mucoid discharge from the eyes. The conjunctiva may be reddened and slightly oedematous. Slight tenderness and photophobia are usually elicited during the history of the case.

Treatment. Slightly astringent drugs, such as 0.25% solution of zinc sulphate, may be used. Silver solutions should not be used over long periods, however, for this might lead to argyrosis of the conjunctiva or cornea. Various antibiotic preparations are recommended. One should always remember that foreign bodies, such as grass seeds or barley awns, may be embedded in the conjunctival sac and may cause conjunctivitis at any rate in the early stages. If the foreign body is discovered, superficial anaesthesia is given and the foreign body is carefully removed with a swab soaked in physiological saline. Sometimes forceps may have to be used to remove the foreign body.

If the cause of the conjunctivitis is a deficiency of vitamin A, which is quite rare, the vitamin must be applied directly to the conjunctiva in the form of drops, with additional internal administration of vitamin A or of the provitamin in the form of raw carrots.

Catarrhal conjunctivitis may develop into **purulent conjunctivitis (conjunctivitis purulenta).** It is caused either by the entry of pyogenic bacteria into a serous conjunctivitis or by general diseases (distemper).

The *clinical signs* comprise a purulent discharge, sticking together of the eyelids in the morning, and accumulation of a purulent exudate in the conjunctival sac. The mucous membrane at first usually looks quite pale but later becomes markedly injected.

Treatment of purulent conjunctivitis is by frequent irrigation of the conjunctival sac with suitable cleansing lotions, followed by instillation of astringent and antibiotic drops or ointments.

Good resolution may sometimes be obtained if the conjunctival sac is superficially cauterised with a 1 % silver nitrate solution. After it has acted for about 1 minute, the excess of silver nitrate is neutralised with physiological saline.

Follicular conjunctivitis is very often seen. In our experience it occurs in many breeds in up to 30 % of dogs examined for eye disease. It is chiefly a disease of the lymphatic tissue on the bulbar surface of the nictitating membrane (Fig. 198). This tissue consists of about 50 individual lymph follicles, which protrude as a result of inflammation and rub on and abrade the cornea, due to continual movement of the nictitating membrane (Fig. 199). Probably, during the cleaning action of the nictitating membrane on the cornea, very small particles of dirt get under the nictitating membrane and then cause the inflammation described. From this combined irritation a chronic conjunctivitis develops, which may result in a spastic entropion and finally lead to keratitis and corneal ulceration.

The *clinical signs* are similar to those seen in the various kinds of conjunctivitis.

Treatment in the milder cases (in which no follicles are formed) is as described for purulent conjunctivitis. If there are large follicles, these are surgically removed. Indications for the extirpation of the nictitating membrane sometimes described are very restricted and should not be used in any of these cases. Extirpation of the nictitating membrane robs the eye of a very important organ. From the anatomical point of view, it also results in a space between the conjunctiva and the cornea, in which particles of dirt may accumulate which are not removed by marked flow of tears and may lead to development of a chronic purulent conjunctivitis. In addition, absence of the nictitating membrane and especially of its pigmented border gives the dog a "dead-eye" appearance. Extirpation of the nictitating membrane is therefore indicated only when tumours develop with a broad base in the nictitating membrane.

Technique of Removal of Follicular Conjunctivitis. Under general anaesthesia the nictitating membrane is grasped with eye forceps (with broadened tops) and everted. The follicles are then scraped off with a sharp spoon, drawing the spoon away from the eye (Fig. 200). Using it in a reverse direction will not remove all the follicles quickly, because of the elastic suspension of the nictitating membrane. Blood clots must be washed out with boric acid solution. Before the operation 2–3 drops of 1/1000 adrenalin are dropped into the conjunctival sac so that the subsequent bleeding is very slight.

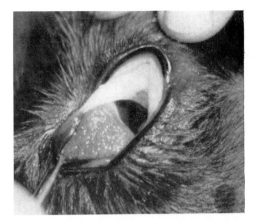

Fig. 198. Conjunctivitis follicularis (German Shepherd).

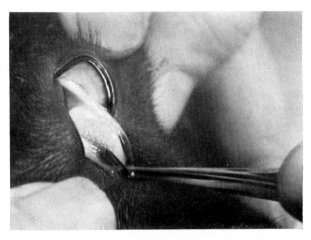

Fig. 199. Conjunctivitis follicularis. The nictitating membrane is drawn forwards with forceps.

Later, antibiotic ointment is put into the conjunctival sac. After-treatment is given by the owner by instilling such ointment 2–3 times daily for 8 days. After 8 days a repeat examination is made and, if there are no complications, astringent zinc sulphate drops are instilled to the conjunctival sac for a week.

Disease of the naso-lacrimal duct is revealed by a continual flow of tears and possibly the formation of a secretory tract. In every case of chronic conjunctivitis one should make sure that the naso-lacrimal duct is patent. The simplest way of doing this is to drop a coloured solution, such as fluorescein, into the conjunctival sac and after a while to swab out the corresponding nostril. If the nasal secretion is coloured, the patency of the duct is demonstrated. Inflammatory

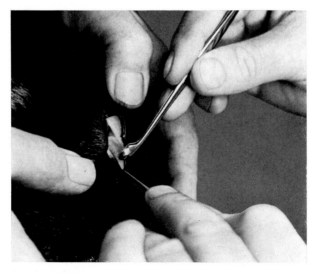

Fig. 200. Starting position for removal of the follicles.

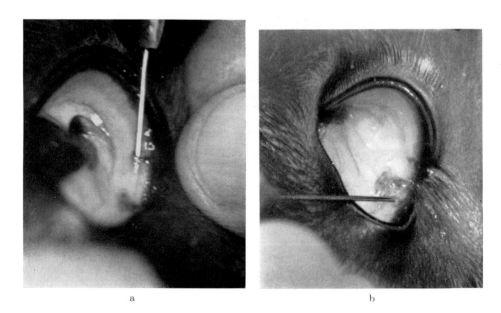

a   b

Fig. 201a. Division and irrigation of the naso-lacrimal duct. Position of the cannula in the upper
punctum lacrimale.

Fig. 201b. Division and irrigation of the naso-lacrimal duct. Position of the cannula in the lower
punctum lacrimale.

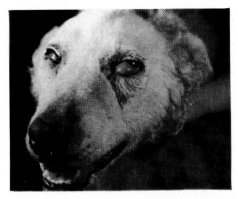

Fig. 202. Hyperplastic Harderian gland which is covered by the nictitating membrane (Kuvacz).

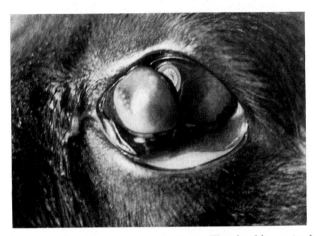

Fig. 203. Hyperplasia of the Harderian in a young Boxer. The gland has extruded itself between the eyeball and the nictitating membrane.

processes may cause closure of the naso-lacrimal duct. Both lacrimal punctae lie on the tarsal border and are found at about 2–4 mm from the medial angle of the eye. The naso-lacrimal duct is explored with a fine blunt-ended cannula and it is thoroughly irrigated (Figs. 201a and 201b). For this irrigation one uses diluted solution of adrenaline, saline, acridine dyes, boric acid solution, sulphonamides, zinc sulphate or antibiotic solutions. The irrigation is repeated as many times as necessary.

Malformations of the naso-lacrimal duct (atresia, partial or total) are occasionally observed.

Prolapse of the nictitating membrane (Protrusio membrana nictitantis) is sometimes seen in cachectic patients with severe diseases. Shrinkage of the orbital pad of fat allows the eyeball to fall back into the orbit (Enophthalmus cachecticus)

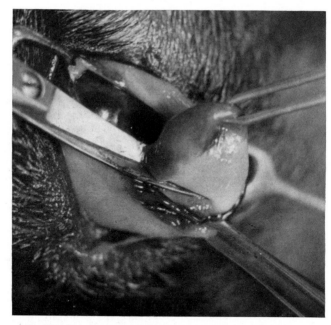

Fig. 204. Removal of hyperplastic Harderian gland.

thus exerting pressure on the anchor-shaped process of the nictitating membrane and forcing the membrane out forwards. Prolapses of this kind can only be corrected by improvement of the general condition.

Hyperplasia of the Harderian gland (Fig. 202). In this condition the nictitating membrane is displaced away from the eyeball by a white spherical structure protruding between the membrane and the eyeball (Fig. 203). *Treatment* is by removal of the hyperplastic glands.

Technique. Under general anaesthesia the membrane is pulled out with eye forceps and fixed with two mosquito forceps. The hyperplastic gland is seized with forceps and dissected out with finely pointed scissors (Fig. 204). The slight resultant haemorrhage can be controlled with a swab soaked in adrenalin. Suture of the defect in the mucous membrane is not necessary.

Extroversion of the cartilage of the nictitating membrane is sometimes seen from the outside (Fig. 205). The cartilage is everted at about a distance of 2–3 mm from its outer border. As this prevents the nictitating membrane from fully discharging its function, a conjunctivitis occurs which disappears only with the removal of the extroversion. Surgical treatment is given preserving the border of the nictitating membrane intact, so that it can again discharge its functions of clearing away particles of dirt from the cornea.

Technique. Under general anaesthesia of the nictitating membrane in addition to superficial anaesthesia. The nictitating membrane is drawn out and fixed with two mosquito forceps. With a small pointed scalpel a cut is made into and through the crown of the curvature in the cartilage The curved part is dissected away on both sides and excised. The nictitating membrane is sutured.

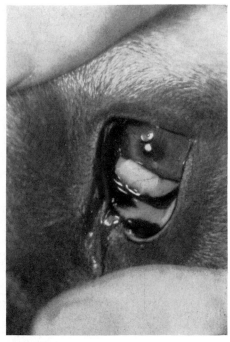

Fig. 205. Extroversion of the cartilage
of the nictitating membrane.

with 2 catgut sutures to the conjunctival sclera of the upper half of the eye. Catgut is used which will be absorbed after 5–6 days. During this time the area of the wound has begun to heal, so that the nictitating membrane remains in the desired position. To prevent secondary infection during the first few days after the operation, penicillin drops are instilled into the eye several times a day.

Dermoid cysts are often seen on the bulbar conjunctiva. They arise from foetal ectodermal transplants. Usually they are in the temporal canthus where they obstruct complete closure of the eyelids. They extend over the conjunctiva of the eyeball to the cornea and being part of the outer skin are usually markedly hairy (Fig. 206). This causes permanent irritation of the conjunctivae and also of the cornea, from which conjunctivitis and keratitis may result.

Treatment is by surgical removal of the dermoids. Under general anaesthesia the dermoid is carefully removed with scissors.

If it extends to the cornea, it is carefully removed from this using a Graefe's cataract knife. One must be especially careful not to perforate the cornea, and for this reason the incision is made tangentially to the eyeball. The eyeball may be fixed with a stay suture. Suture of the mucous membrane is not necessary, although a plastic operation may be needed to close the lateral angle of the lids.

Prolapse of the eyeball may occur after dog fights and accidents. Usually in these the eye muscles are so damaged that the eyeball can no longer be held in the orbit and there is a tendency for it to prolapse (Fig. 207). Nevertheless, one should try to replace the eyeball in the orbit in every case of prolapse of the eyeball diagnosed immediately after its occurrence. This should only be done if no extensive damage to the eyeball itself can be detected.

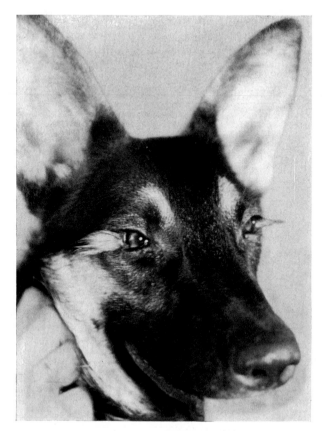

Fig. 206. Bilateral dermoid cysts in a German Shepherd.

Technique. It is necessary first of all to cool the prolapsed eyeball with ice-cold boric acid compresses, in order to reduce any inflammatory swelling that has occurred. With a moist swab, pressure is exerted to try to replace the eyeball in the orbit. It may be necessary to widen the eyelid opening by a temporal canthotomy to allow the swollen eyeball to pass through. Finally, the canthotomy incision is sutured and the eyelids are brought together with catgut stitches in order to prevent repetition of the prolapse. For 4–5 days wet dressings are applied and the patient is protected by an antibiotic cover. During this time the patient is given only soft food because during active chewing the temporo-maxillary joint acts directly on the orbital cavity thus disturbing this area and delaying healing.

If the eyeball has not recovered its original form on the 5th day after the operation, or if purulent processes (Panophthalmia) have occurred, one should not hesitate to remove it.

If the prolapse persists for a longer time, so that the cornea dries up and fissures, or even ulceration occurs, extirpation of the eyeball is indicated. Experience has shown that the dog cannot endure a prosthesis, because the dog feels it as a foreign body and always tries to remove it. For this reason, in the dog it is only a question of evisceration of the orbit with an artificial ankyloblepharon. The marked develop-

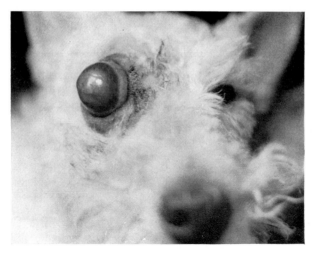

Fig. 207. Prolapse of the eyeball.

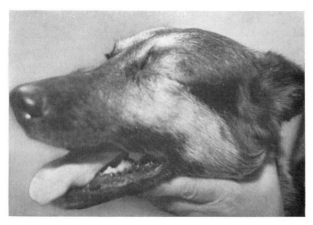

Fig. 208. Condition after evisceration of the orbit (artificial ankyloblepharon). The withdrawal of the eyelids into the orbit can be adjusted after injection of "Dondren" (German Shepherd).

ment of hair on the dog's eyelids gives quite a good cosmetic effect. If the retraction of the closed eyelids into the empty orbital cavity is considered unpleasant, sub-cutaneous injection of "Dondren" into the upper and lower lids can compensate for this to some extent (Fig. 208).

Technique of evisceration of the orbit. The patient is fixed on its side under general anaesthesia, the eyelids are shaved, defatted with ether and iodised. An incision is made 2 mm from the margin of the lid through the skin as far as the submucosa. The conjunctiva is carefully separated from the skin. The conjunctiva, the tarsal border, the eyeball and the lacrimal glands constitute a whole and must not be separated from one another during the evisceration. The eye muscles are severed with scissors. It is recommended that the eyeball enclosed in the conjunctival sac should be grasped with hooked forceps and traction applied during the dissection of the orbital cavity. Finally, the retractor bulbi muscle and the optic nerve are severed. Only in a few cases can one succeed in ligaturing the optic nerve before severing it, so there is a moderate amount of haemorrhage (Art. ophthalmica ext.) which can be controlled by pressure with a tampon. Before the edges of the wound are sutured together, one should make sure that the lacrimal gland, which lies in the region of the temporal canthus, has been removed. If this has not been done it must be dissected out from the orbital area with scissors. The edges of the wound are united so that a narrow slit is left in the nasal canthus through which is inserted a tamponade soaked in penicillin. Alternatively, iodoform gauze can be used. Recently "Vasenol" tampon strips have been found to be very useful. These have been treated with "Vasenol" base as a paste, with the advantage that it does not adhere to the depths of the wound, as may occur when iodoform gauze is used. The tampon is removed after 24 hours; because of its pliability the "Vasenol" strip does not cause any delayed haemorrhage. If this should occur, another tampon must be put in for another 24 hours and this often causes marked pain to the patient. The operation is completed by putting on a monocular bandage. Subsequently, the bandage and tampon are removed. If there is marked secretion, the surrounding skin is anointed with protective cream and the wound cavity is treated with iodoform ether. In 2–3 weeks the wound has healed sufficiently for the patient to be discharged. The eyelids are markedly drawn into the orbital cavity and this is especially disfiguring in short-haired dogs. The use of the sclero-therapeutic substance "Dondren" can compensate for this by stimulating new formation of connective tissue. It is injected into the upper and lower eyelids, the dose being assessed according to the degree of the defect (0.5–1 ml). This treatment should only be given when all reactions in the wound area have subsided (about 6 weeks after the operation). Formation of connective tissue commences after 2–3 weeks and is completed after about 8 weeks (Fig. 208).

Retrobulbar Tumours can also produce the clinical picture of exophthalmus. In these cases the eyeball can be replaced only with difficulty because of the presence of the tumour (Fig. 209). *Treatment* is also by evisceration of the orbit.

Enlargement of the Eyeball (Megalophthalmus) is in most cases related to an increase in the aqueous humor and subsequent increase of internal pressure (Fig. 222). In contrast to megalophthalmus is **congenital microphthalmus** where the eyeball is too small. This condition cannot be treated therapeutically.

Enophthalmus appears in the form of a Phthisis bulbi. As the result of protracted panophthalmia, softening processes occur in the eyeball which lead to

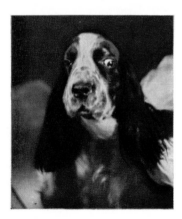

Fig. 209. Exophthalmus in a Spaniel caused by a retrobulbar tumour.

degeneration. In addition, the retrobulbar fat is broken down, so that the enophthalmus sinks back into the orbit. Purulent conjunctivitis and entropion are
always seen in this condition.

Treatment is by evisceration of the orbit.

Squint (Strabismus) appears when the antagonistic action of the eye muscles is
deranged. *Treatment* is by strabotomy of the muscles of the opposite side. Some
cases are so slight that surgical intervention is not required.

Nystagmus often occurs, especially in the form **"Nystagmus oscillatorius"** as in
nervous distemper and after accidents. In the latter it gives us indications of the
possible existence of brain damage. In general anaesthesia, nystagmus is seen
mainly when the depth of anaesthesia is reduced. There is no known treatment of
nystagmus.

Panophthalmitis may occur following penetrating wounds of the eyeball caused
by dog fights, road accidents or after perforation of a corneal ulcer. Conservative
methods of treatment always result in a phthisis bulbi, so evisceration of the orbit
is indicated. This should be done as early as possible otherwise septicaemia may
occur.

Among **diseases of the cornea** those caused **by injuries** will be considered first.
Such injuries occur during play with other dogs and cats, or by blows from twigs
and branches springing back into the eye when the dog pushes its way through
low bushes. The history reveals that the dog has suddenly closed one eye, later
rubbing it with a paw.

It is investigated by the method described above (p. 177).

Treatment is governed by the degree of the injury. As a basic principle patients
should be kept in a darkened room. With slight superficial injuries, the conjunctival
sac is irrigated daily with boric acid solution and then penicillin oil is introduced.

Keratitis (inflammation of the cornea) may be caused by external (trauma) and
internal agencies (disturbance of metabolism, distemper).

In **superficial keratitis (Keratitis superficialis)** there is degeneration of the corneal
parenchyma due to purulent inflammation of its superficial layers. The cornea
becomes opaque and steel-grey in colour in places. The surface appears dull and
grey (Fig. 210). A **corneal ulcer (Ulcus corneae)** may then develop, by break-down
of the tissue and formation of a crater-like depression, the bottom of the ulcer
being covered with yellow pus (Fig. 211). Subsequently, the epithelial defect is
filled in and cicatrised. The scar tissue causes transient or more often permanent
opacity. The patient avoids light and there is irritation. The eyes are kept closed
and are carefully rubbed with the paws because of the marked pain.

Keratitis parenchymatosa affects the deeper layers of the cornea. There is an
accumulation of fixed corneal cells between the lamellae and also infiltration of
leucocytes. This causes a diffuse steel-grey colour which may appear overnight.
In contrast to superficial keratitis, the corneal surface is smooth. Irritation and
photophobia are present, but the pain does not seem to be so marked. If there is
no degeneration of tissue in parenchymatous keratitis, months later it may sometimes completely clear up without scar formation.

Treatment is directed towards removal of the cause (foreign bodies, conjunctivitis,
entropion). The patient is nursed in a darkened room, the diet being mostly semi-
fluid. Antibiotic or sulphonamide eye drops are used locally.

13*

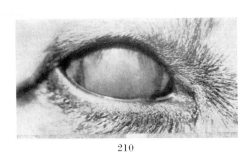 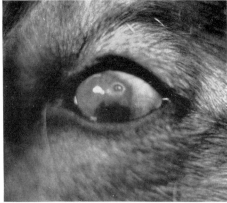

210   211

Fig. 210. Superficial keratitis (German Shepherd).

Fig. 211. Corneal ulcer and keratitis pigmentosa (Dachshund).

If there is a corneal ulcer with a risk of a perforation, the intraocular pressure can be reduced by prescribing eserine eye drops.

If there is not a favourable response, corticosteroids may be given as eye drops or possibly by subconjunctival injection, provided there is no corneal ulceration.

In addition to these drugs, hot, moist fomentations should be used in keratitis, given several times a day. Good results may be obtained by subconjunctival injection of 2 % saline solution (0.5–1 ml) in conjunction with the other drugs. Nonspecific protein therapy is a useful adjunct to treatment (see p. 138). For this purpose the intramuscular injection of milk (1–4 ml) has proved satisfactory.

Chronic superficial conjunctivo-keratitis (Conjunctivo-keratitis, superficialis chronica) was described by ÜBERREITER (10th International Veterinary Congress at Madrid **2**, 307–309, 1959). He observed this disease especially in Alsatians, but also in dogs of other breeds. The disease begins with a reddish spot on the cornea, usually temporal in position, near the limbus. As the disease progresses, thick, well-vascularised and obvious granulation tissue spreads towards the middle of the cornea. This tissue becomes pigmented in the later stages. The surface of the cornea is uneven, but its epithelium is intact. If the condition is not treated, blindness results.

Treatment consists of removal of the affected part of the cornea with a cataract knife, after which the area is carefully and precisely cauterised. After-treatment is carried out with 2 % silver nitrate solution, 4 % "Collargol" ointment and adrenalin/boric acid solution. In addition, antibiotics and cortisone preparations can be given periodically, and finally nonspecific stimulant treatment should also be given. The condition clears after about 6 weeks.

Pigmentation of the cornea (Keratitis pigmentosa) cannot be influenced therapeutically.

If there is a corneal ulcer and this deepens, perforation may occur. The aqueous humor escapes and the iris prolapses, so that **prolapse of the iris** occurs. On the other hand, Descemet's membrane may withstand the internal pressure of the eye and a **Keratocoele** is formed.

Treatment consists of the replacement, as far as is possible, of the iris within the eyeball. On occasion, it may be necessary to excise part of the prolapse, but this is likely to result in excessive haemorrhage. The defect in the cornea may sometimes be sutured, and, in any case, should be covered with conjunctival membrane. Anterior synechiae are likely to form, and may sometimes be avoided by regular instillations of atropine.

Before treatment of prolapse of the iris, the conjunctival flap is prepared sufficiently to enable it to be applied immediately after excision of the iris.

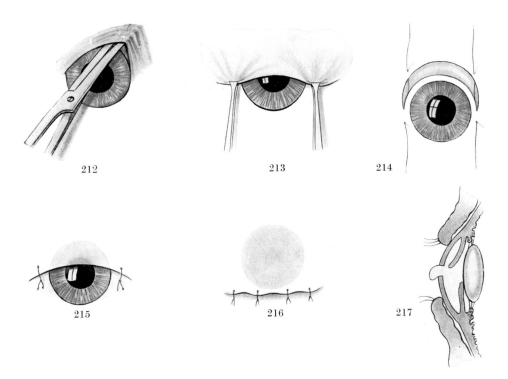

212

213

214

215

216

217

Fig. 212. Separation of the conjunctiva from the sclera to make a conjunctival flap.

Fig. 213. Drawing the conjunctival flap over the eyeball and estimation of the correct sites for the insertion of stay sutures.

Fig. 214. Position of the sutures for the conjunctival flap.

Fig. 215. The sutures for a partial conjunctival flap are tied off.

Fig. 216. Complete conjunctival flap.

Fig. 217. Staphyloma of the cornea.

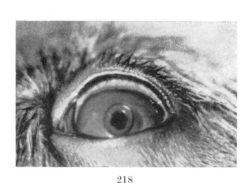 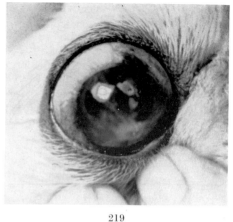

218   219

Fig. 218. Acute staphyloma (Dachshund).

Fig. 219. Corneal staphyloma with lower right quadrant. Reflected images of the cornea clear but distorted (Pekingese).

Technique of application of a conjunctival flap. Under general anaesthesia the scleral conjunctiva should be carefully separated to about one-third in the immediate neighbourhood of the edge of the limbus (Fig. 212), then the conjunctiva is bluntly undermined and drawn over the cornea (Fig. 213). Two catgut stitches are put in lateral to the keratoplast (Figs. 214, 215, 216). After 4–5 days these fixation stitches give way and the conjunctival flap retracts, but in the meantime the corneal defect has healed. After the operation a monocular bandage is applied.

Staphyloma of the cornea develops after a prolapse of the iris and forms a bulging scar on the cornea (Fig. 217). Owing to faulty closure of the eyelids a conjunctivitis develops. Sometimes the tip of the staphyloma is broken down by sepsis (Figs. 218, 219).

Treatment is by ablation of the staphyloma. In contrast to recent prolapse of the iris, the ablation leads inevitably to anterior synechia. By anterior synechia we understand adhesion of the iris to the cornea.

Treatment is conservative with mydriatic drugs in order to dilate the pupil and break down the iris adhesions. For this, atropine, scopolamine and "Eumydrin" are used.

When the synechia is accompanied by increase of intra-ocular tension (glaucoma), then treatment with atropine is contraindicated.

Glaucoma occurs through increase of the pressure in the eyeball. For primary cases it is not always possible to determine the cause, but hereditary factors are responsible in some breeds. Secondary glaucoma arises in association with synechiae, dislocations of the lens (Terriers), etc. Unfortunately, glaucoma is first detected when the owner notices marked changes in the eyeball or disturbances of vision (Fig. 220). The changes in the eyeball are such that, because of its greater elasticity as compared with that of the sclera, the cornea takes on a shorter curvature radius. The scleral blood vessels are markedly injected and the pupil is usually

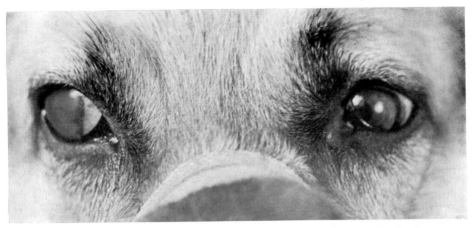

Fig. 220. Right glaucoma with parenchymatous keratitis (German Shepherd).

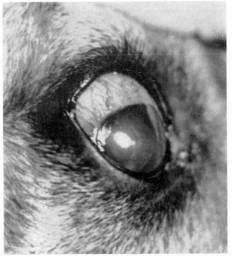

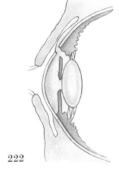

221   222

Fig. 221. Injection of the episcleral vessels in glaucoma (German Shepherd).

Fig. 222. Mode of action of the formation of a fistula in glaucoma. The aqueous humor runs
through the fistula under the conjunctiva and forms there the so-called "trickle-pads".

widely dilated (Fig. 221). Sometimes diffuse turbidities are apparent in the cornea.
The interior of the eye must be examined for changes with mirrors. Dislocation
of the lens into the anterior chamber of the eye can be diagnosed best by lateral
illumination. With some experience one can estimate the increase of pressure in
the eyeball by palpation of the lower eyelid with the fingertips. Tonometry (see
p. 177) is more accurate. An internal pressure of over 30 mm of mercury is regarded
as pathological. The sight is tested by the "stool test".

Treatment of acute cases is directed towards decrease of pressure or the return to normal of the factors governing the intra-ocular tension. The pupil is contracted with miotics to increase filtration in the region of the canal of Schlemm. Suitable miotics are Eserine, Pilocarpine, Arecoline and Muscarine.

Once the acute stage has subsided the so-called fistulaforming operations are undertaken. These act on the principle of a wick allowing excessive aqueous humor to drain away (Fig. 222). Trephining of the globe is carried out according to Elliot, while others (Prof. ÜBERREITER, of Vienna) prefer cyclodialysis.

Technique of Elliot's operation. The patient is securely tied in lateral recumbency under general anaesthesia. At 10 mm from the upper margin of the limbus an incision 1.5 cm long is made with scissors in the conjunctiva and the latter is then separated from the sclera up to the limbus (Fig. 223). The flap of conjunctiva thus freed is drawn over the cornea with a small hook. Elliot's trephine (1.5 mm in diameter) is applied so that part of the cornea and sclera is punched out (Fig. 224). The trephine is placed at right angles to the eyeball and introduced into the tissues by rotatory movements. Pressure on the trephine should be lessened as the operation proceeds to prevent the instrument suddenly bursting through into the eyeball. When it has been opened up, the aqueous humor escapes and the iris is flushed out with it. A piece of the iris is removed from the base and the rest is replaced with a spatula (Fig. 225). The flaps of conjunctiva are drawn back over the trephine opening and fixed to the conjunctiva with sutures (Fig. 226). No bandage is needed. The excess of aqueous humor is now discharged under the conjunctiva producing a swelling, the so-called drainage pad (trickle-pad).

Disease of the iris (iritis) is rarely seen alone. Usually, it is associated with cyclitis (iridocyclitis) and can be recognised by careful examination of the eye with mirrors. The pupil is contracted and the iris seems to be covered with mucoid deposits. There is photophobia and injection of the ciliary blood vessels. Conjunctivitis and injection of the sclera vessels occurs and the aqueous humor may be cloudy **(fibrinous iritis)** or may even contain blood **(haemorrhagic iritis)**. There is a possibility of absorption of the exudate but a panophthalmia may develop or at least a synechia.

Treatment. Atropine, "Eumydrin" and scopolamine are recommended. As iritis often follows various diseases (distemper, tuberculosis, etc.), the basic diseases must be treated. In addition, wet, hot compresses and injections of milk are used.

If the choroid is inflamed, the condition is called **choroiditis.** The history reveals that the owner has noticed that the dog can no longer see as well as formerly. Ophthalmoscopic examination shows that the fundus cannot be seen as distinctly as normal. *Treatment* is similar to that described for iritis.

Persistently adherent pupillary membrane of the cornea is a deformity of the eye which was fully described by ÜBERREITER (Dtsch. tierärztl. Wschr. **64**, 507–509, 1957). The membrane is attached to the anterior surface of the iris. This inherited anomaly may appear in conjunction with a congenital cataract.

Among **diseases of the lens,** alterations of its position must be distinguished from changes in the lens itself.

Changes of the position of the lens appear as dislocations of the lens from its suspensory apparatus, in which the lens falls either into the anterior chamber of the eye **(anterior dislocation of the lens),** or into the vitreous chamber **(posterior dislocation of the lens)** (Figs. 227, 228).

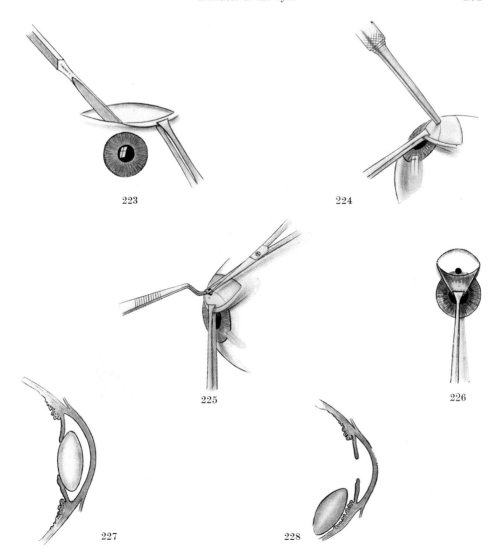

Fig. 223. Trephining according to Elliot. Incision into the conjunctiva and its separation up to the margin of the limbus.

Fig. 224. Trephining according to Elliot. Erection of the trephine at the transition from the cornea to the sclera.

Fig. 225. Trephining according to Elliot. Basal excision of the iris.

Fig. 226. Trephining according to Elliot. Situation before closure of the conjunctival flaps.

Fig. 227. Anterior dislocation of the lens.

Fig. 228. Posterior dislocation of the lens.

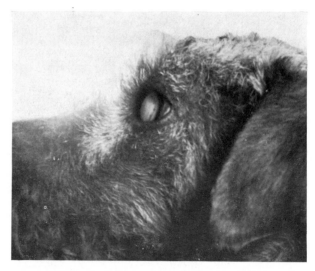

Fig. 229. Glaucoma and anterior dislocation of the lens in a Welsh Terrier. The lens is completely turbid.

The causes of a dislocation are not always apparent from the history. Rarely injuries are the cause. Dislocations of the lens are frequent in rough-haired terriers (especially the Fox terrier) and are almost always due to inherited weakness of the suspensory apparatus. In these dogs dislocation of the lens of the other eye usually occurs immediately after the detection of the first dislocation. Very often with a unilateral dislocation, loosening of the lens of the other eye is seen, so that an early second dislocation can be predicted. In glaucoma dislocation of the lens may occur as a result of the altered pressure conditions; enlargement of the eyeball resulting in increased stress on the zonal fibres resulting in their separation from the lens.

The *clinical picture* in a recent dislocation is shown by serous conjunctivitis combined with marked injection of the scleral blood vessels and photophobia.

Fig. 230. Posterior dislocation of the lens. The lens is turbid (Spaniel) (photograph by the University Department of Illustration).

Fig. 231. Anterior dislocation of the lens as a primary disease with secondary parenchymatous keratitis (Spaniel) (photograph by the University Department of Illustration).

Fig. 232. Canthotomy. Insertion of the scissors into the lateral angle of the eyelids (photograph by the University Dept. of Illustration).

Fig. 233. Condition after canthotomy (photograph by the University Dept. of Illustration).

Fig. 234. Putting in the stay suture under the tendon of insertion of the superior rectus muscle (photograph by the University Dept. of Illustration).

Fig. 235. The upper and lower stay sutures (photograph by the University Dept. of Illustration).

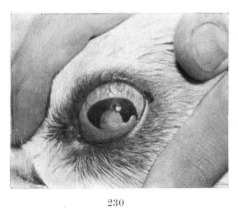

230

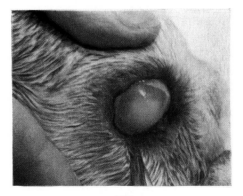

231

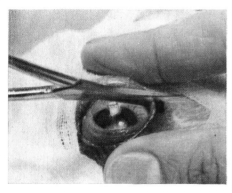

232

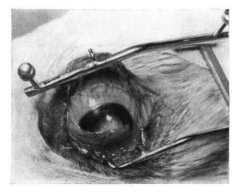

233

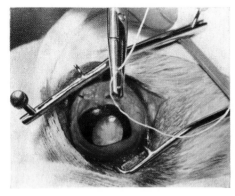

234

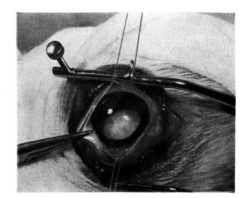

235

Usually the dogs are presented when these symptoms have subsided and signs of loss of sight are evident.

If the edge of the lens is damaged it soon becomes opaque. The lens is then visible as a greyish-white disc in the anterior chamber of the eye (Fig. 229). If there are no injuries to its capsule, the lens may remain clear for a long time. In these cases, the edge of the lens in the anterior chamber can be detected by its different refractive index when viewed by oblique light. Dislocations into the vitreous chamber are less often seen.

Treatment of anterior dislocation of the lens is essential as it appreciably reduces the dog's vision, and will lead to glaucoma and hydrophthalmos. With a posterior dislocation, where the lens is wholly within the vitreous, complications are less likely to arise, provided the lens does not subsequently move into the anterior chamber. This may sometimes be avoided by maintaining the pupil in a contracted state with the use of eserine.

Technique of extraction of the lens. The patient should be well secured in deep general anaesthesia. The surgeon should ensure that he has a good support for his arms during the operation (this applies to all operations on the eyeball). In this connection the operating table recommended by ÜBERREITER (Arch. wiss. Prakt. Tierhk. **72**, 239, 1938) is the best. The eyes must be prepared by rendering the conjunctival sac as free as possible from bacteria by instillation of penicillin eye oil for several days before the operation. The hairs are shaved from the eyelids and the surrounding area. The pupil is contracted with eserine because the vitreous humor may protrude when the incisions are made. Dogs (especially the terrier breeds) often have a narrow eye opening and in these cases a canthotomy must be done with scissors to widen the angle of the lids (Figs. 232 and 233). In order to be able to control the eyeball so that it is clearly visible, two stay sutures are inserted. These have the advantage over fixation with forceps in that they stay firm, so that during the operation continual adjustments do not have to be made. In order to insert the upper stay suture, the tendon of the superior rectus muscle is grasped with surgical forceps through the conjunctiva in the 12.0 o'clock position (Fig. 234). The suture to be inserted is drawn through under the tendon. If one has not taken in the tendon and the suture lies only in the conjunctiva the ball of the eye cannot be directed by it. The lower stay suture is inserted in the 6 o'clock position into the conjunctiva in the immediate vicinity of the margin of the limbus (Fig. 235).

The nictitating membrane may protrude and obscure the field of operation, so it should be grasped with mosquito forceps and drawn forwards and downwards. This causes a fold in the conjunctiva in the median angle of the eye and often in its lateral angle. This fold is notched with fine scissors so that the cornea and the limbus are free.

The next stage in the operation is to pierce the prolapsed lens with a fine, straight needle (Fig. 236). The puncture is made through the sclera in a medio-lateral direction near to the margin of the limbus. Fixation of the lens before the eyeball is opened is advisable, as a mobile lens may

---

Fig. 236. The scleral flap incision. The point of the knife is directed to a point on the inner half of the cornea near to the limbus, in order to begin a puncture (photograph by the University Dept. of Illustration).

Fig. 237. Scleral flap incision. The point of the knife penetrates immediately behind the margin of the limbus and is pushed forward in the same direction and is simultaneously drawn upwards, so that the incision can be made with little traction (photograph by the University Dept. of Illustration).

Fig. 238. Scleral flap incision. After cutting through the sclera the knife is turned in order to separate off the conjunctival flaps (photograph by the University Dept. of Illustration).

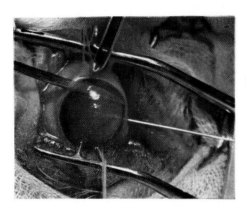

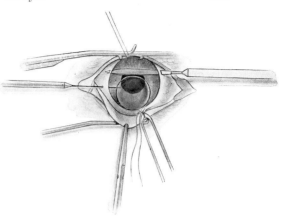

236

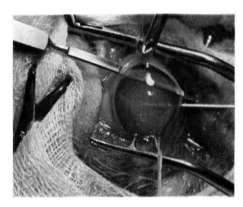

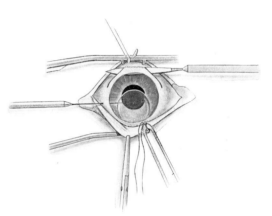

237

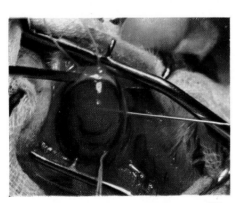

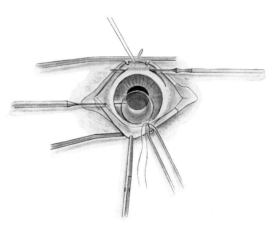

238

slip back into the posterior chamber once the eye is opened. When the lens has been transfixed, the flap incisions to open the eyeball can be made. A Graefe's cataract knife is inserted from the side at the lateral margin of the limbus with its edge directed upwards. The cut is made in the sclera close to and along the cornea, the eyeball being fixed by the surgeon with forceps in the region of the lower stay suture and slightly drawn forward. Assistants should exert a slight pull on the upper stay suture from above forwards. The upper eyelid is drawn upwards with a Desmarres eye hook or with an eyelid separator (Arruga). The incision should be big enough to enable the lens to be released without difficulty (Fig. 236). Very often one tends to make the incision too small because the anterior chamber of the eye is greatly reduced by the prolapsed lens and it must then be carefully enlarged with iris scissors. The cataract knife is now inserted into the sclera, its point is carried rapidly parallel to the iris through the anterior chamber and pushed through medially on the corresponding side close behind the limbus (Fig. 237). Whilst it is pushed through, the cataract knife is also pulled up, so that with a few pulls the sclera is pierced behind the limbus (Fig. 238). After the sclera has been cut through, the knife is directed under the conjunctiva towards the body and a flap of conjunctiva is detached. If this flap seems big enough, the knife can again be advanced and the conjunctiva severed (Fig. 238). The conjunctival flaps are useful in the closure of the flap wounds.

In making the flap incisions, certain errors can arise which may lead to difficulties. The incision should describe a half-arc which penetrates the sclera exactly along the margin of the limbus. The commonest fault is that the cataract knife is wrongly directed in the anterior chamber of the eye. Refraction causes the point of the knife to appear closer to the cornea than it actually is, with the result that one directs it deeper so that it is now too near the ciliary body. The result is an incision which is not shaped like the arc of a circle. The incision is medially too deep into the sclera and comes to lie above in the cornea (Fig. 247). A further disadvantage is that in this way ciliary blood vessels are damaged, which causes undesirable haemorrhage into the anterior chamber, thus obscuring the field of operation.

If one pays attention to the other refraction conditions in the anterior chamber, the point of the knife should lie in such a position as if one wished to thrust it through the cornea. The knife is thus nearer to the cornea. One should also take care that the iris is not injured. This readily occurs if the anterior chamber becomes too flat after the puncture, the resultant escape of aqueous humor pressing the iris forwards. If the flap incision is quickly and efficiently made, this accident can be avoided. Incision into the cornea (corneal flap incision) has certain advantages, but also disadvantages. Certainly, this method does not cause any haemorrhage during the operation and this is always welcomed by surgeons unaccustomed to the operation (Figs. 239–242). The main disadvantage is the post-operative partial corneal opacity around the incision which needs intensive after-treatment. If the flap incision is made as described above, the eye forceps are removed and the tension on the upper stay suture is relaxed a little. The operator now puts the Weber's loop into the anterior chamber so that it lies behind the lens and presses it gently against the cornea. The needle transfixing the lens can now be carefully removed (Fig. 243). In extracting the lens the action of the Weber loop is supported from the outside by light pressure with a strabismus hook (Fig. 244). If the lens has become adherent to the cornea or the iris, it must be carefully separated before the extraction. Forcible extraction may lead to undesirable sequelae.

Prolapse of the vitreous humor is not important, but before closing the flap wounds any prolapsed vitreous humor must be removed. In order that the iris does not prolapse into the wound and disturb the healing, and to avoid synechia (risk of glaucoma), an iridectomy must be done before the wound is closed. Basal excision has proved to be the most beneficial, as the screening action of the iris remains intact. The iris is grasped at its periphery with Arlt's iris forceps and slowly and carefully drawn out of the flap wound (Fig. 248). With iris scissors the tip of the iris immediately on the forceps is removed (Fig. 249). Total iridectomy is performed by grasping the iris with iris forceps at the margin of the pupil and carefully drawing it out of the wound (Fig. 250). Excision goes quite deep so that a broad coloboma is formed which involves the whole of the iris (Fig. 251). By this disruption of the iris screen the dog's ability to see may be restricted. When iridectomy has been done the flap wounds can be closed by smoothing down the portion of cornea hanging on the flaps and attaching them to the conjunctiva by two stay (temporary) sutures (Fig. 245).

Finally the stay stitches are removed and the canthotomy is closed. By this time the anterior chamber has usually resumed its normal shape (Fig. 246). The conjunctival sac is cleaned and treated with penicillin eye oil. Bandaging of the eye is not absolutely essential, but our post-operative patients are kept in total darkness during their stay in the clinic.

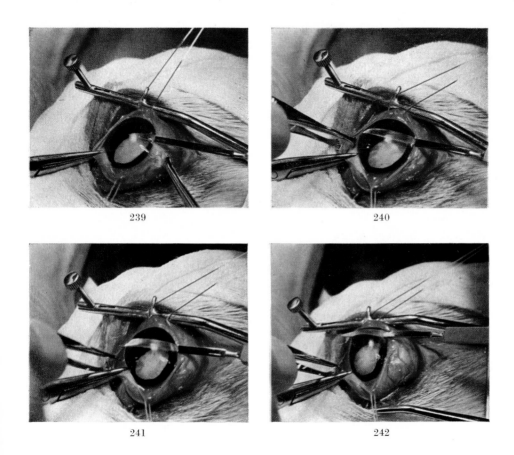

Fig. 239. Corneal flap incision. Insertion of the cataract knife. The fixation of the globe is supported from the right by eye forceps (photograph by the University Dept. of Illustration).

Fig. 240. Corneal flap incision. Commencing withdrawal of the cataract knife (photograph by the University Dept. of Illustration).

Fig. 241. Corneal flap incision. The cataract knife has been withdrawn on the corresponding side and is now pulled up by simultaneous to and fro movements (photograph by the University Dept. of Illustration).

Fig. 242. Corneal flap incision. The incision is completed (photograph by the University Dept. of Illustration).

For *after-treatment* antibiotic eye ointment is used. If the pupil is very constricted, atropine is given. Sometimes corneal opacities may appear which remain for weeks and are treated with the recognised drugs (at first intramuscular injection of milk combined with moist, warm compresses and later iodoform or "Dionin").

Opacity of the lens is called **Cataract.** The opacity may be accompanied by sclerosis, disintegration, shrinkage or separation of the lens fibres, the formation of

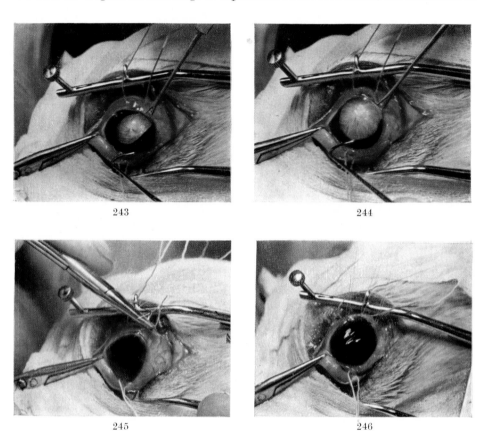

243

244

245

246

Fig. 243. Removal of the lens. As this was a case of posterior dislocation Weber's loop had to be inserted carefully into the posterior chamber of the eye (photograph by the University Dept. of Illustration).

Fig. 244. Removal of the lens. The lens is brought forward out of the posterior chamber of the eye with the Weber's loop. To prevent it slipping back a strabismus hook is held lightly against it from beneath (photograph by the University Dept. of Illustration).

Fig. 245. Corneal flap incision. Insertion of the closure sutures (photograph by the University Dept. of Illustration).

Fig. 246. Corneal flap incision. The operation completed. The eyeball already begins to assume its former shape (photograph by the University Dept. of Illustration).

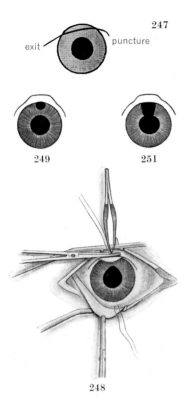

247

exit — puncture

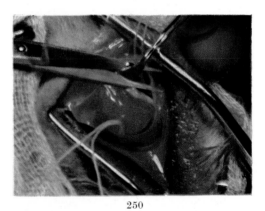

Fig. 247. Faulty exit of the suture from the sclera.

Fig. 248. Basal excision of the iris.

Fig. 249. Result of basal excision.

Fig. 250. Total iridectomy. The extruded portion of iris is excised with scissors (photograph by the University Dept. of Illustration).

Fig. 251. Result of total iridectomy.

249   251

248   250

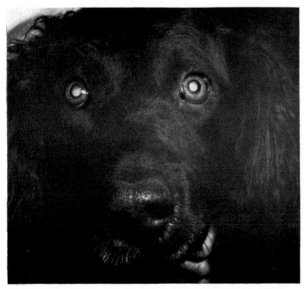

Fig. 252. Bilateral cataract in a 4-year-old Spaniel.

areas of cleavage or collections of fluid. The disintegration brings with it degeneration of connective tissue and deposits of opaque substances. In the dog the main types are **cataract of old age (senile cataract), juvenile cataract** and **congenital cataract. Traumatic** and **diabetic cataract,** which are symptomatic, are rare. In the clinical picture discoloration of the pupil is striking, and this, plus the restriction of vision, causes the owner to seek veterinary advice. Total cataract is thus the type usually recognised. **Cataracta partialis** and **Cataracta punctata** are often accidentally diagnosed during a basic general examination. In **total cataract** the lens is usually like frosted glass (Fig. 252). The pupil is widely dilated and does not react to light. In **senile cataract** vision may remain for a long time in spite of obvious changes in the lens. The "stool test" (see p. 178) gives good results in testing the ability to see. *Treatment* must be surgical because conservative methods to clear a lens are not yet available. IVY, PARK and DOLOWY (Vet. Med. **54**, 205–213, 1959) have sought a conservative treatment of cataract. They repeatedly injected a preparation made from horse serum, after the donor of this had previously been injected with a culture of *Actinomyces bovis* previously cytolysed. This preparation contains a polysaccharide and a carbohydrate or fatty acid. It is not toxic. These workers hoped to influence the permeability of the cells with this extract and to be able to intervene in the growth of the cells and the regeneration of the normal structure. In animals in which the cataract was of recent standing, the opacity of the lens was improved in 26 out of 27 eyes after an average of 2.4 (1–6) months and in cataracts of longer duration in 19 out of 21 eyes after 3.3 (1–7) months. The blood vessels of the retina were visible after seven (2–17) months in 21 out of 48 eyes (45 %). It was possible to increase this percentage to about 75 % by continued treatment. In most cases the owner reported a return of visual capacity or improvement of it. On average there was 43 % clearing of the lens and in 12 % of the dogs there was 90 % or more. The lens cleared either from its periphery or diffusely.

If the lens is still soft, which is in general to be expected in cataracts up to the age of 6–8 months, discission of the capsule of the lens can be done in order to bring about absorption of the lens. When the lens is hard, extraction of the lens must be attempted.

Technique of discission (needling) of the lens. Mydriasis of the pupil is effected with atropine (commencing the day before operation). The eyelids must be maximally separated with an Arruga lid-spreader and the eyeball fixed by assistants with forceps in the region of the origin of the tendon of the superior rectus muscle. The surgeon does the same to the lower limbus border. Now with the discission knife a posteriorly directed incision is made from the side, at the level of the eyelid opening, through the sclera into the anterior chamber of the eye and parallel to the anterior surface of the iris (Fig. 253). One passes the little knife upwards and back to the upper border of the widely dilated pupil, directs the edge of the knife somewhat towards the lens, and with a lever movement opens the lens capsule with a vertical incision. Finally, incisions as small as one chooses can be made in order to destroy the capsule over as large an area as possible. In doing this care should be taken not to damage the posterior wall of the capsule or the vitreous humor. The operation is ended by turning the knife parallel to the iris and finally withdrawing it. Penicillin eye oil is instilled into the conjunctival sac; a bandage is not necessary, the patient is kept in a dark kennel for a few days.

After-treatment consists of maintaining dilation of the pupil with atropine. The anterior chamber is almost filled with the cloudy mass of the lens. Its absorption

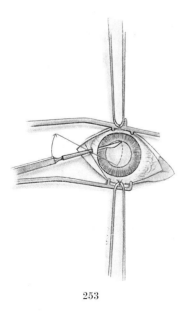

253

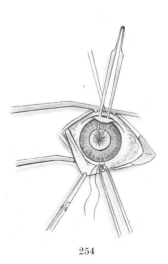

254

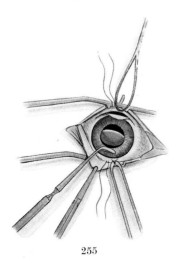

255

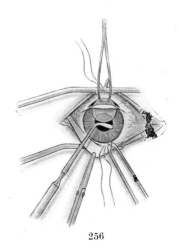

256

Fig. 253. Discission of the lens.

Fig. 254. Tearing the lens capsule with capsule forceps.

Fig. 255. Dislocation of the lens forwards.

Fig. 256. Removal of the lens can be helped by Weber's loop.

14*

can be hastened by non-specific protein therapy, but it requires about 7–8 weeks until it is completely clear again and the ability to see begins to be restored. If the capsule wound has closed prematurely the remains of the lens may remain in it and a secondary cataract occurs. For this another discission has to be done.

Technique of extraction of the lens. The patient is securely fixed under deep surgical anaesthesia. The preparation of the patient (canthotomy, insertion of the upper and lower stay sutures and the flap incision) proceeds as described on p. 204. It is necessary to dilate the iris with atropine. In our experience extra-capsular extraction of the lens is the method of choice. If the capsule is especially tough, however, one must attempt intra-capsular extraction. In extracapsular extraction the closed capsule forceps (Hess) are introduced through the flap wounds as far as the middle of the lens. The forceps are then opened and the lens capsule is grasped (Fig. 254). By light rotatory movements the capsule is rent and a large piece of its anterior border can be removed. Dislocation of the lens occurs at the same time. By light pressure with a strabismus hook the lens is brought edgewise to the lower part of the cornea (Fig. 255). In this way the lens can be more easily guided through the flap wounds, the edges of the scleral wound being depressed with the Weber's loops. Often one can also extract the lens with the Weber's loops after it has been brought edgewise and has already been displaced upwards (Fig. 256). Finally, a basal excision of the iris is done (see p. 206). The iris is smoothed down with a spatula and the flap-wounds are closed (see p. 206). If the extracapsular extraction of the lens does not succeed, it is advisable to do a total iridectomy beforehand and to divide the zonule fibres carefully with a spatula. Then the lens is brought into the edgewise position and is released. The operation is concluded with the instillation of atropine and penicillin eye oil.

After-treatment is as described (p. 207) for extraction of the dislocated lens.

The eye operations described are by no means simple and the necessary technical skill should be acquired by practice on a dead animal.

4. Diseases of the respiratory system

Clinical investigation of the respiratory tract covers the nose, larynx, trachea, lungs and the thorax. Observation of the type and frequency of the respiratory movements will often provide useful information in certain conditions. We differentiate three different types of respiratory movements. The usual type is costo-abdominal breathing, in which at inspiration the ribs are first moved outwards, expanding the thorax followed by enlargement of the abdomen. The latter is due to the contraction of the diaphragm pushing the abdominal viscera caudally and thus expanding the transverse section of the abdomen. Costal or pectoral type of respiration occurs when the diaphragm plays no part in the respiratory process. This is seen when there are painful or inflammatory disease conditions of the diaphragm, e. g. acute diaphragmatic pleurisy, hepatitis, etc. Mechanical factors may also be involved in the production of this type of respiration. Increased abdominal pressure due to ascites, gastric torsion and tympany, pyometra, neoplasia, final stages of pregnancy, etc. may counteract the contraction of the diaphragm. Abdominal type breathing is shown by excessive respiratory movements of the abdominal wall, due to a reduction in the activity of the intercostal muscles of the thorax This may be due to any painful or inflammatory condition affecting the chest wall such as pleurisy, intercostal myositis, fracture of ribs, etc. or to partial transverse section of the spinal cord in the region of the first intercostal nerve, etc. Respiration is then dependent on the movements of the diaphragm, with consequent displacement of the abdominal wall and marked depression of the intercostal areas during inspiration.

In the normal dog the respiratory rate is fairly regular at about 10–30 inspirations per minute. Inspiration is always shorter than expiration. Disturbances of respiratory rate and rhythm occur in all disease conditions of the respiratory passages, although these may be smoothed out intermittently by inhalation or exhalation. In cases of neurogenic shock after accidents and also in uraemic coma, "Cheyne–Stokes breathing" may occur. Here there is a period of apnoea followed by shallow respiration, which becomes progressively deeper until it is almost dyspnoeic in character. This is followed by another period of shallow breathing and then an apnoeic period of 15–30 seconds. "Kussmaul's respiration" (Bradypnoea, "heavy respiration") may occur in conditions of acidosis and is manifested by deep inspirations at fairly long intervals usually accompanied by loss of consciousness. Tachypnoea ("shortness of breath") occurs in parturient eclampsia, pyrexias, sepsis, respiratory disease, etc.

If the frequency of respiration cannot be ascertained by visual inspection, a whisp of cotton wool or a feather is held in front of the dog and its movements during inspiration and expiration noted. The fact that respiration is still occurring can be detected by holding a mirror close to the nose where it will be clouded with moisture at expiration.

Palpation of the thorax. In the dog this is performed by placing the two hands flat one on each side of the chest. The elasticity of the thorax is estimated by compression between the two hands. In the young animal the elasticity is much greater than in the old dog. After accidents or dog fights, compression of the thorax may reveal whether it is still intact. Where there is suspicion that there may be fracture of ribs, the individual ribs are palpated with the finger laid flat on them, and similarly painful conditions of the intercostal muscles can be determined.

Percussion of the lungs. The middle or index finger of one hand is placed firmly against the chest at the site under investigation and is then struck between the nail and the phalangeal joint with the middle finger of the other hand bent like a hook. The blows should be brief, springy and light and made from the wrist, so that the percussing finger can be quickly withdrawn to avoid obstructing the induced vibrations. This finger to finger technique has the advantages that it can be performed without any other aids, that it is possible to distinguish quite

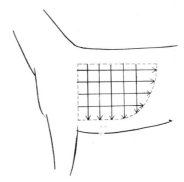

Fig. 257. Percussion field of the lungs. The arrows show the direction in which percussion is done in order to determine the extent of the percussion area.

sharply between tissues containing air from dense ones, and that it provides the best conditions for evoking the resonance of air-containing organs. The field of effective lung percussion is demarcated caudally by the 11th intercostal space on the level of the iliac tuberosity, by the 9th intercostal space in the middle of the thorax and by the 6th intercostal space at the lowest level. Above it is limited by the musculature of the back and in front by the shoulder. By drawing forward the forelimb one can increase the area available for percussion on that side. For exact determination of the percussion field it is always percussed from within outwards (Fig. 257). In the normal animal a good resonant note is elicited by percussion over the lung especially in lean dogs.

Auscultation of the lungs. Auscultation may be performed by placing the ear directly against the thoracic wall, but preferably with the aid of a stethoscope or phonendoscope. It is essential that the examination should be carried out in a quiet room. The contact between the instrument and the skin of the patient gives rise to crackling noises, and it is important that these should be recognised. These noises can be minimised by parting or moistening the hair. During respiration the entry of air into the lungs and the movement of the latter within the chest produces sounds. Alteration in the character or sites of these sounds allows conclusions to be drawn about the condition of the air passages, the lung tissues and the pleural membranes. The stronger the respiratory movements, the louder the respiratory

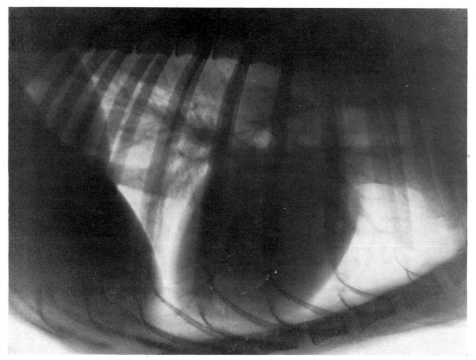

Fig. 258. Normal picture of the lung with latero-lateral irradiation.

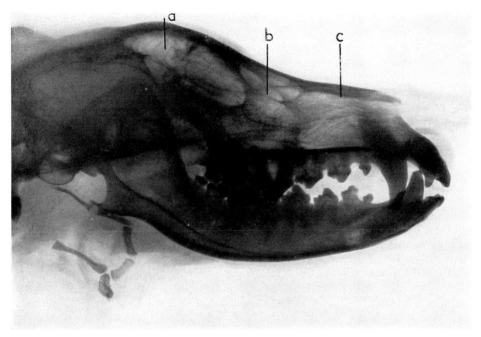

Fig. 260. Radiograph of the skull. (a) frontal sinus; (b) maxillary sinus; (c) nasal cavity.

lent unilateral rhinitis the possibility of a foreign body must always be borne in mind. Additional symptoms are rubbing the affected side of the nose with the paws, or against objects in order to get rid of the irritation or pain. Rhinitis produced by infection or other causes is almost always bi-lateral. Clinically, initially there is sneezing, snorting and rubbing of the nose with the paws. There may be sufficient swelling of the nasal mucosa that the passages are occluded, and the patient must breathe through the mouth, the cheeks being blown out during expiration. There is seldom any pyrexia in the simple catarrhal rhinitis. The discharge which is at first serous becomes more profuse and more viscous, later becoming purulent. There is a crusty deposit in the nasal cavities which may completely occlude the nostrils, resulting in mouth breathing.

Treatment. In rhinitis the underlying disease should be treated specifically where possible. The inflamed nasal mucosa may be treated by inhalations, suitable prescriptions being as follows:

R.	Turpentine oil	} āā	5 parts
	Pumilio pine oil		
	Eucalyptus oil		3 parts
	Olive oil	ad	100 parts
R.	Iodine		0.5 part
	Potassium iodide		2.5 parts
	Glycerine	} āā	100 parts
	Distilled water		

The inhalation fluid can be either atomised in an electrically heated inhaler (it is essential to cover the patient's eyes) or a simpler method may be used at home, in which the patient is put on a chair, the seat of which is made of tubular mesh. Under the chair there is an electrically heated vessel containing saline to which the inhalation fluid is added. A covering is put over the patient and the chair so that the vapour rising through the seat must be inhaled by the patient.

Aerosol treatment has been used with very good results. By aerosols we mean atomised fluids which have a particle size of 0.5 to 5 μ. Particles bigger than 5 μ will not reach the alveoli and the smallest bronchioles, and particles smaller than 0.5 μ are expelled with the expired air without settling and thus are valueless. In contrast to human medicine, where the patient inhales the aerosol, in dogs a respirator must be used. There is considerable risk of cross infection where only one inhaler is available. Bartels solved this problem by using cardboard or plastic disposable drinking cups which can be destroyed after use. To the nozzle of the atomiser a short piece of rubber tubing is attached and this is pushed through a hole in the bottom of the cup. Treatment should be given daily, at least once a day, over a period of five to ten minutes. If there is no response after fourteen days the aerosol treatment should be discontinued. Bartels administered agents which had a spasmolytic, mucolytic or secretolytic effect, and to each aerosol were added 200,000 units of an aqueous mixture of penicillin and streptomycin. In milder types of rhinitis the dog's nose may be sprayed with chlorine powder, so that it is forced to breathe in the chlorine particles. This irritates the mucosa, increasing the secretion and producing a flushing out of the irritant agent, the disinfectant action of the chlorine being also valuable. A brisk reaction may be produced by instilling a few drops of eucalyptus oil into the nasal cavity, the resultant marked irritation causing continual sneezing by the patient. This may be of special value in the purulent forms of rhinitis, as it produces a clearing out of the nasal passages. The inflamed nostrils may be anointed with a bland ointment to obviate cracking.

Linguatula serrata. The nasal worm (*Linguatula serrata*) occurs chiefly in the dog. We have only seen the parasite in one case. The worm, which is actually an arthropod, is 2–12 cm long and from 3–10 mm broad. It is tongue-shaped and its surface is ringed transversely. Clinical signs of infection are chronic nasal catarrh, lasting for up to one year, with an abundant nasal discharge of a variable kind. There may be epistaxis, frequent sneezing and rubbing of the head, obstruction of breathing and swelling of the submaxillary lymphatic glands. Diagnosis can only be made either by finding the worm itself or its eggs in the nasal discharge. Quite often also the eggs are swallowed and then it may be possible to find them in the faeces.

Treatment. The only treatment is the removal of the parasite from the nasal passages. According to ENIGK and DUWEL (Dtsch. tierärztl. Wschr. **64**, 401–403, 1957) contact insecticides in an aerosol form are the most effective treatment.

Laryngitis (Laryngeal catarrh). The causes of laryngitis are similar to those of rhinitis, viz. infection (chiefly distemper) and mechanical factors. Often continuous barking or, in excitable dogs, continued pressure of the collar or chain round the neck due to pulling, are found to be precipitating factors. The clinical picture is one of frequent spontaneous attacks of coughing which appear to be painful. The larynx is extremely sensitive to pressure and this causes a coughing spasm, which may also be produced by eating. The cough is at first dry, later becoming moist in character. Sometimes râles develop in the larynx but auscultation of the lungs reveals no clinical signs of disease. Inspection of the throat will show diffuse reddening (laryngo-pharyngitis).

Treatment. The patient should be rested as much as possible and any causal factors should be removed, e. g. the collar being replaced by harness, and the patient should be allowed as much fresh air as possible. To alleviate the cough. the following prescriptions are recommended:

R.	Codeine phosphate	0.3 part
	Althaea syrup	10.0 parts
	Distilled water	ad 100.0 parts

Dose. One teaspoonful several times daily

or

| R. | Ethylmorphine hydrochloride | 0.5 part |
| | Distilled water | 20.0 parts |

Dose. 10–20 drops 2–3 times daily

It is also possible to suppress a marked irritative cough by the injection of oxy-codone hydrochloride. The dose is 2–20 mg, the injection being repeated after two hours if necessary. Oxycodone should be used only if codeine or dionin (ethyl-morphine hydrochloride) have proved ineffective. Inhalation treatment may be given several times a day, or aerosol treatment.

Tracheitis. Inflammation of the trachea usually arises as an extension from laryngitis so that the causes and the treatment of the condition are as given for laryngitis.

Foreign bodies in the trachea. These are rare but they do occur occasionally. A correct diagnosis is probably possible only by radiography. GEHRING (Kleintier-praxis 3, 92–93, 1958) described a case of a German shepherd dog which had irregular respiration accompanied at each inspiration and expiration by a snapping sound, which was readily heard without a stethoscope. Radiography revealed a stone, the size of a walnut, in the trachea which was tossed up to the bifurcation of the trachea and during expiration to the larynx. The stone was successfully removed with elongated bullet forceps under general anaesthesia. SAVAGE and ISA (Cornell Vet. 46, 216–218, 1956) describe an actinomycotic granuloma in the trachea of a hound which died of asphyxiation.

Bronchitis. The aetiology of this condition is similar to that of laryngitis and it is seen chiefly in distemper. Almost all cases of pneumonia in the dog are accom-panied by bronchitis. The inflammation of the mucosa acts as an irritant and pro-duces frequent coughing attacks which may be productive. Swelling and exudation of the mucosa of the smaller bronchioles may produce obstruction to the passage of air.

Clinically the condition may be recognised by râles on auscultation, a loud percussion note and cough. Dullness and bronchial respiration are not symptoms of bronchitis. There is a scanty nasal discharge and the cough may be either marked and moist in character, or weak and dry (bronchiolitis).

Pneumonia. Pneumonia may occur as a complication of bronchitis when it is termed bronchopneumonia. In the dog, pneumonia usually occurs during the course of distemper and is rarely found as a primary condition.

Clinically there is at first a high temperature which later drops to around 39.3 °C where it remains fairly constant during the course of the disease. There is general malaise with loss of appetite. If the degree of lung consolidation is slight, then dullness on percussion and bronchial breathing are usually absent, but may appear later. Invariably there is an increase in the respiratory rate with râles on auscultation. Nasal discharge is either catarrhal or purulent, and the cough is moist in character and occurs in spasms. Radiography will reveal the consolidated areas of lung by obliteration of the blood vessels, which are now of the same radiodensity as the affected lung tissue. On the other hand, the bronchi being full of air appear as branched lighter areas against the darker background of the lungs. Sometimes the interlobular divisions are also visible. The localisation of the consolidated areas may be so marked as to make it possible to differentiate the affected areas from the neighbouring normal tissue.

Bronchopneumonia may have a long drawn out course, sometimes persisting for 2–3 weeks.

Treatment. The treatment of bronchitis, bronchopneumonia and pneumonia is the same, so they can be described together. Initially antibiotic therapy should be prescribed for several days and the sulphonamides are also useful. Priessnitz compresses should be applied to the thorax once or twice daily and left on for 1–1½ hours at a time. To loosen the cough expectorant mixtures may be prescribed, e. g.

R.	Apomorphine hydrochloride	0.015	part
	Dilute hydrochloric acid	2.0	parts
	Glycerine	10.0	parts
	Distilled water	ad 150.0	parts

Dose. One teaspoonful every 3–4 hours

or

R.	Potassium iodide	3.0	parts
	Sodium bicarbonate	6.0	parts
	Distilled water	150.0	parts

Dose. One teaspoonful 3 times daily

Inhalations may also be recommended. A formulation of quinine 3%, camphor 2.5%, eucalyptus oil 18% and peppermint oil 8% in olive oil may be used successfully in cases of inflammatory or catarrhal conditions of the respiratory tract. The quinine is retained in the diseased areas of the lung tissue and therefore exerts a local action, the concentration of the drug being 8 times greater in the lungs than in the liver. The greater part of the essential oils are inhaled into the lungs, where they act by inhibiting inflammatory change and by way of their secretolytic and secretomotor effects. The camphor increases the pulmonary circulation, thus improving the transport of the other two agents to the diseased tissues. The usual dose is 1–5 ml injected intramuscularly.

Massaging mustard oil into the chest wall then covering it with woollen bandages is often beneficial, and leukocytosis may be improved by the injection of turpentine oil to form a sterile abscess. Non-specific therapy as outlined on p. 138 should also be used. The dog should be kept at rest as much as possible in a well-ventilated, draught-free room.

Ascaris pneumonia. This condition is mainly seen in puppies. It is essential to treat the underlying helminth infestation in addition to the pneumonia.

Bronchial asthma. A condition resembling bronchial asthma in man may be seen in the dog, especially in the toy breeds in their later years. In man there is an allergic hypersensitivity affecting the respiratory tract. This engenders a severe, chiefly expiratory dyspnoea, due to constriction of the small bronchi.

Clinical signs. The dog is agitated and there is a severe dyspnoea, interspersed with attacks of moist coughing. The cough may be very distressing and may persist for months or even years, often being more marked at night, or in wet periods of the year.

Treatment. The most effective treatment is by the use of antispasmodic drugs, e. g. ephedrine, which relax the constricted bronchi.

Good results have been obtained with aerosol treatment (see p. 218). Often a change of climate, e. g. mountain air, will produce a remission of the attacks, but relapse occurs when the dog returns to its former environment.

Haemorrhage. Pulmonary haemorrhage is usually seen after road accidents. Bright red frothy blood escapes from the nose and mouth of the victim, and there is frequent coughing to clear the trachea of blood. Auscultation of the chest will reveal râles. The only possible treatment is rest.

Pulmonary oedema. This occurs only shortly before death in the dog.

Pulmonary emphysema. Emphysema is a condition in which the alveoli of the lungs are overdistended due to obstruction to the passage of inspired or expired air. This may occur in the brachycephalic breeds when a tape muzzle is applied for purposes of restraint.

Tumours of the lungs. Neoplasia of the lungs occurs mainly in older dogs. Usually the tumours are metastases, primary lung tumours being rare in the dog (Fig. 261). In some cases acropachia (Marie's disease) may be found on radiographic examination of the skeleton.

Clinical signs. Usually there is little or no pyrexia, the main symptoms being listlessness and dyspnoea of varying degree. Percussion of the chest may reveal dullness, but this is dependent upon the number and size of the growths. Variation in the respiratory sounds may be detected by auscultation. These commence with weakened vesicular sounds and terminate with complete disappearance of the sounds. On occasions there may be mixed bronchial and vesicular sounds present. Diagnosis can be confirmed by radiography combined with the clinical signs (Fig. 262). Prognosis is unfavourable in view of the fact that most tumours are secondary.

Treatment. Where the tumours are confined to one lung or lobe, then surgical removal of the affected part should prove successful where the tumour is primary, or where the primary tumour is accessible to surgery.

Tuberculosis and streptotrichosis. These conditions affecting the lung are considered under the section dealing with "Infectious Diseases".

Pleurisy. Inflammation of the pleural membranes is almost exclusively due to infection of the pleural cavity by bacterial agents. Usually infection occurs by direct spread of a pneumonic process, or by rupture of an inflammatory focus into

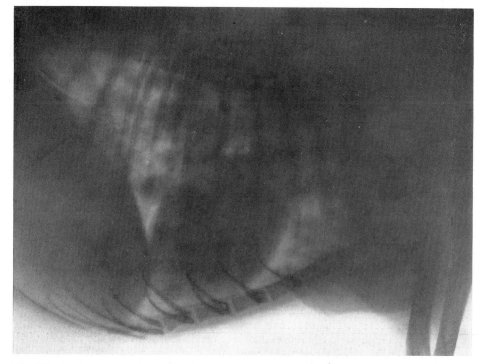

Fig. 261. Carcinomatosis of the lung arising from the thyroid gland with metastases in the lungs, spleen and kidneys.

the thoracic cavity. Most of the latter are due to impaction of foreign bodies in the thoracic oesophagus. These are usually pointed bones which perforate the wall of the oesophagus by pressure necrosis.

Clinical signs. Initially the dog is listless and there is fever. The inflammation of the pleural surfaces produces pain, so any pressure on the chest wall is resented. The respirations are shallow and mainly abdominal in character and sometimes there is guarded coughing. Auscultation of the thorax in the early stages may reveal friction sounds, but these usually disappear when effusion occurs. Exudation into the pleural cavity causes dullness to percussion and a muffling of the respiratory sounds on auscultation, and the apex beat of the heart is weakened or completely absent. Respiratory movements become superficial, strained and abdominal and the dog attempts to increase the vital capacity by expanding the ribs outwards, so that the chest becomes barrel-shaped (Fig. 263). The level of fluid in the chest can be determined by radiography and the presence and nature of the fluid confirmed by thoracocentesis.

Treatment. In the early stages cold compresses are useful, but in the later stages, warm, wet wraps are to be preferred. Massage of the chest wall with spirits of mustard, then covering the thorax with woollen cloths may be beneficial. Most important is systemic treatment with sulphonamides and broad spectrum anti-

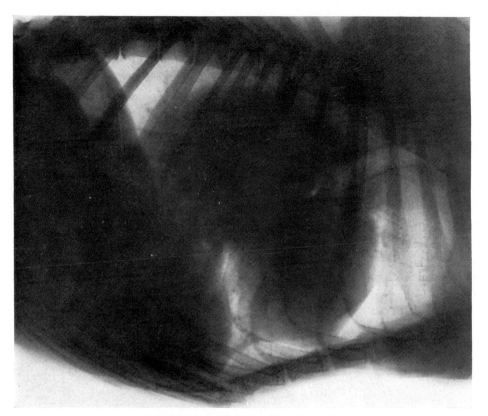

Fig. 262. Tumour in the lungs of a Setter.

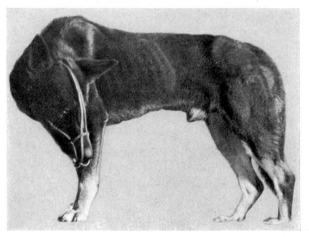

Fig. 263. Exudative pleurisy (German Shepherd).

biotics. The local instillation of antibiotics into the thoracic cavity by thoracocentesis also gives good results.

Pneumothorax. Atmospheric air enters the thoracic cavity as a result of penetrating injuries of the thoracic wall or tearing of the lung tissues. The pressure of the
air causes collapse of the lung and severe embarrassment of the respiration and
circulation. Where the pneumothorax is open, the air still gains access to the
thoracic cavity so the pressure remains constant or increases. In a closed pneumothorax, the imprisoned air is gradually absorbed over a period of about four
weeks. A valvular pneumothorax may occur in which the air is sucked in during
inspiration and on expiration the opening closes, so that there is an increasing
pneumothorax.

With regard to the possible use of a therapeutic pneumothorax in canine medicine, it must be remembered that it is difficult to localise pulmonary conditions
to one side of the chest or the other. Added to this is the fact that the mediastinum
of the dog is usually patent, so that it is not possible to establish a unilateral
pneumothorax in most cases.

Clinical picture. An extensive pneumothorax always induces respiratory difficulties. The thorax is widened by the raising of the ribs and the respirations are
abdominal in character. Percussion gives an overloud or hyper-resonant note and
no respiratory sounds can be detected on auscultation. Lateral radiography will

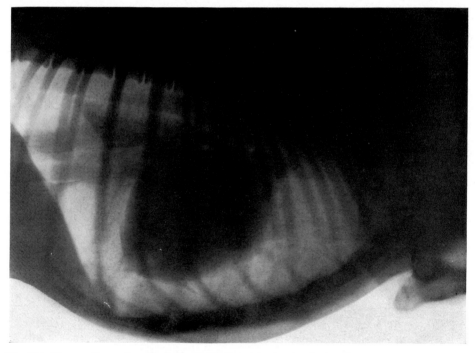

Fig. 264. Pneumothorax in a Dachshund. The heart is clearly displaced away from the sternum.

reveal that the heart is separated from the sternum (Fig. 264) and that radio-
lucent air has gathered in the upper portion of the thorax. A dorso-ventral radiograph shows the atelectic nature of the lungs and the lobar demarcations of the
lungs are very clearly defined.

Treatment. In closed pneumothorax, treatment consists of ensuring absolute
rest for the patient in an oxygen-rich atmosphere. Anoxia may be countered by
the subcutaneous injection of oxygen. The imprisoned air may be removed by
suction applied through a water drain. In an open pneumothorax, the penetrating
wound of the thorax must be closed as soon as possible. Anaesthesia should be via
an endotracheal tube, so that the lungs can be fully inflated before the chest wound
is closed.

Hydrothorax. In this condition fluid collects in the pleural cavity due to various
causes. Neoplasms in the mediastinum may exert pressure on the great vessels
and cause transudation of fluid. Congestive heart failure and certain diseases,
such as tuberculosis and streptotrichosis, may also lead to accumulation of fluid
in the chest.

Clinical picture. It must always be remembered that hydrothorax is invariably
a secondary condition; it develops slowly and has an afebrile course. Percussion
of the chest shows increased dullness with a horizontally delineated upper border

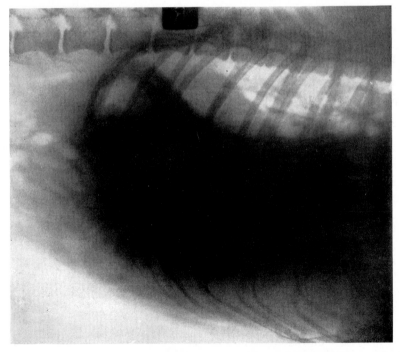

Fig. 265. Hydrothorax. With the patient standing up, the upper horizontal level of the fluid is
parallel to the vertebral column.

with the dog in the normal standing position. Auscultation reveals muffling of the heart and lung sounds, and the apex beat of the heart may be undetectable. Respiration is difficult and abdominal in character and the thorax becomes barrel-shaped due to expansion of the ribs. Radiography is of great value in arriving at a diagnosis in these cases. The dog is first radiographed laterally in the standing position (Fig. 265) and then sitting down (Fig. 266). In both positions the fluid level remains horizontal. The nature of the fluid can be determined by thoraco-centesis and may be of a serous, haemorrhagic, or chylous (milky) character. A chylous transudate indicates a high fat content and may be due to rupture of the thoracic duct. A similar appearance is seen where the transudate contains a high albumin or globulin content. The two types can be differentiated by shaking up the fluid with a little ether. The latter dissolves the fat so that a chylous transudate becomes clear, whilst the albuminous one remains milky.

Treatment. The underlying cause of the transudation should be treated where possible. Removal of as much fluid as possible can be achieved by thoracocentesis and the application of suction through a hypodermic syringe fitted with a two-way

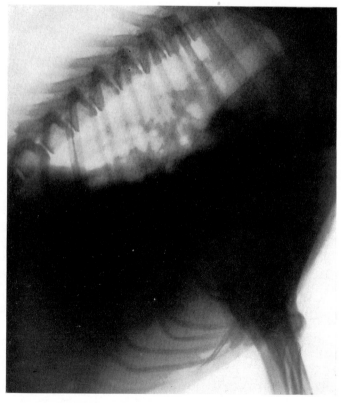

Fig. 266. Hydrothorax. When the patient sits down the upper border of the fluid remains horizontal.

valve. The closed cannula is carefully inserted into the pleural cavity in the 5th or 6th intercostal space at the level of the elbow, the operation site having been prepared in the usual manner. It is advisable to mark the depth to which the needle is to be inserted so as to avoid damage to the lungs or heart. After removal of as much fluid as possible, the needle is withdrawn whilst negative pressure is applied by withdrawing the plunger of the syringe. A considerable quantity of protein is removed with the transudate and emaciation of the patient may occur with repeated tapping of the fluid. To counter this, amino acids must be given for a long period, e. g. methionine (0.5–1 g 3 times daily). On completion of aspiration, the respirations and the cardiac action immediately improve in the majority of cases.

Haemothorax. Bleeding into the thoracic cavity usually occurs after a road accident and presents a nice problem in therapeutics, as thoracocentesis to remove the blood may stimulate further bleeding. If haemorrhage is obviously severe it is probably best to perform thoracotomy, identify the torn vessels and arrest the haemorrhage if possible.

Removal of the vocal cords (Devocalising, Debarking). This procedure is some-times necessary where large numbers of dogs are kept or where dogs disturb neighbours in high density population areas. It may also be indicated where there are neoplasms of the vocal cords.

Technique for excision of the vocal cords. The patient is restrained on its back with the thorax raised above the level of the larynx to minimise the risk of aspiration of blood or mucus during the operation. The operation site is prepared in the usual way and the field anaesthetised with local anaesthetic. The head is then extended to stretch the throat area as much as possible, a 5 cm incision is made over the larynx and the subcutaneous fascia separated. The omo-hyoid and sterno-hyoid muscles are divided at their raphe to minimise haemorrhage, thus exposing the larynx. Haemostasis must be effected before the larynx is opened. Capillary oozing is checked by the application of adrenaline-soaked swabs. The crico-thyroid ligament is nicked with the point of the scalpel blade and a probe-pointed tenotome is introduced and moved caudally, dividing the cricoid cartilage and the crico-tracheal ligament up to the first tracheal ring. Cranially the crico-thyroid ligament and the thyroid cartilage are divided, leaving only a narrow bridge of cartilage remaining. The opened larynx is then sprayed or painted with 2 % lignocaine solution, spread with wound retractors and the mucosa then anaesthetised in the same way. After waiting for 2–3 minutes for the anaesthetic to take effect, one of the vocal cords is grasped with forceps and is completely removed using fine curved scissors. The resultant haemorrhage is controlled by the application of adrenaline-soaked swabs. The other cord is dealt with in the same way. Finally the larynx is closed with catgut sutures through the muscles and silk button sutures through the skin incision. The wound is bandaged for some days and given the usual post-operative care.

5. Diseases of the circulatory system

Inspection of the cardiac region is performed with the dog in the standing position and with the left leg drawn forwards. In young and lean dogs, the apex beat of the heart can now be clearly seen in the 5th–6th intercostal space just above the sternum. In older dogs the apex beat only becomes visible after exercise or excitement. Examination of the visible mucosae may provide valuable evidence about the condition of the circulation, e. g. cyanosis, capillary filling, etc.

Palpation of the thorax provides information concerning the position of the heart (from the apex beat), its rhythm and possibly changes in its action, e. g.

15*

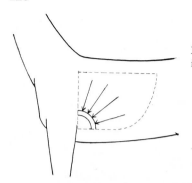

Fig. 267. Direction of percussion
in investigation of the heart.

fremitus. The clinician stands behind the dog with his hands on both sides of the
chest in the cardiac region compressing the chest slightly. Normally the heart
beat occurs more strongly on the left side, but in conditions in which the heart
is enlarged, the beat may be equally discernible on both sides, or even more strongly
on the right. Fremitus is due to turbulences in the blood flow caused by defective
heart valves. The pulse can be palpated at the femoral artery in the mid third
of the inner aspect of the thigh. Normal pulse frequency in large and adult dogs
varies between 70–100 beats per minute, and in small or young dogs between
90–120 beats per minute. Male animals tend to have a slower beat than bitches
and pregnant bitches a more rapid rate than non-gravid females. The pulse rate
accelerates in conditions of excitement and after exercise. Simultaneous auscultation of the heart and palpation of the pulse will provide valuable information.
The aorta can also be palpated in lean or slender dogs by placing the animal on
its back, with the hindlimbs fully flexed to relax the abdominal muscles; the
fingertips are then pressed in towards the midline just under the lumbar muscles.

It is very difficult to map out the outlines of the heart by percussion due to the
variations in the shape of the thorax in individuals and in breeds, but it may be
possible in the larger dog. The technique is performed by finger to finger percussion
as described earlier and should be done towards the elbow joint (Fig. 267). Radiographs give a more accurate assessment of the size and shape of the heart.

Auscultation of the heart sounds is an important part of the clinical examination.
Two types of heart sounds must be differentiated; the systolic sound – dull, deep,
more prolonged and usually louder, probably arising from the closure of the atrio-
ventricular valves and the contraction of the cardiac muscle; the diastolic sound is
brief, more high pitched and sharply delineated, quieter and sometimes of a
clicking or ringing character; it is produced by the stretching and closure of the
aortic and pulmonary semilunar valves. The optimum sites for cardiac auscultation
are as follows:

Left side. 1. The apex of the heart (mitral valve area). 2. In the 4th intercostal
space (below the flexure line – the aortic valve area). 3. In the 3rd or 4th intercostal space (between the flexure line and the margin of the sternum – the pulmonary valve area).

Right side. The tricuspid valve area is to be found in the 4th intercostal space at
the level of the costo-chondral junction. A pulmonary valve sound may often be
detected in the 3rd intercostal space immediately over the sternum.

If the sounds are very loud, a fremitus (thrill) may be felt at the *punctum maximum*, but accurate determination of this point is very difficult in small dogs. Sometimes it is only possible to say whether the sound is audible only on the left or the right side, or is in the region of the base or the apex of the heart.

The foregoing clinical examination can be supported by instrumentation, chiefly in the field of radiography. The shape of the heart can be determined by plain lateral and dorso-ventral radiography. Assessment of the heart action can be performed by fluoroscopy, preferably by way of an image-intensifier. Electrocardiography can be used to diagnose such diseases as myocarditis, myocardial infarction, arrhythmias, etc. There is a good deal of variation in the ECG of normal dogs of different breeds.

Measurement of blood pressure in dogs is very difficult due to the conical shape of the thigh. A certain degree of accuracy in estimating the pressure from the feel of the pulse can be achieved with practice. The systolic pressure should be between 120–160 mm of mercury.

In all cases of disease of the circulatory system a complete haematological examination should be performed.

The causes of cardiac disease may lie in mechanical defects of the valves, or functional or organic conditions of the myocardium. Occasionally the nervous control is disturbed and there are arrhythmias. In diseases of the circulatory system, the cause may be defective cardiac action, or disease or dysfunction in the blood vessels. Some cardiac diseases may be described as an insufficiency in that the cardiac output cannot meet the requirements of the body. Such insufficiency may be acute or may slowly develop as a chronic condition.

Acute insufficiency. This may be caused by sudden, excessive physical exertion, e. g. hunting, severe training schedules, etc., but it may arise during the course of severe pyrexial diseases. In the latter case, a chronic insufficiency may occur especially where large parenchymatous organs, such as the liver or kidneys, have been damaged.

The insufficiency of the myocardium results in a diminished cardiac output so that the uniform exchange processes (body-blood-body) become upset. A resultant acidosis may lead to dysfunction of the water balance of the body with the transudation of fluid into the body cavities and subcutaneous tissues – cardiac ascites.

Clinical picture. The dog shows a palpitating heart beat with a weak, rapid pulse, the artery not being completely filled and the pulse waves almost indistinguishable one from another. This may give rise to insufficient oxygenation and lead to cyanosis of the visible mucosae. Dyspnoea may be a sign of a defective pulmonary circulation. A sudden, severe insufficiency may lead to immediate collapse of the animal followed by death within a few minutes.

Chronic insufficiency. This is first revealed by a discrepancy between the heart beat and the pulse, viz. a palpitating heart beat with a weak pulse. These signs appear after exertion and may be accompanied by dyspnoea, so patients should be examined both at rest and after exercise. Chronic insufficiency causes defective circulation and this is especially important with regard to effective oxygenation of the central nervous system. The affected animal may suffer from slight fainting fits, ataxia, and staggering. If the insufficiency is associated with disease of the liver or kidneys, ascites may occur, making differential diagnosis difficult.

Treatment. The first essential measure is to ensure immediate rest. Working animals must be kept off work for at least six months. The diet should be highly nutritious but of low bulk, and the dog should be given several small meals daily to avoid congestion of the abdominal organs. The tone of the myocardium may be improved by the administration of digitalis or strophanthus. The latter is given as a weekly dose of $1/4$–$1/16$th mg of strophanthin made up to 5–10 ml with 10 % dextrose and injected intravenously. The dose of strophanthin should be assessed with moderation, but there is no cumulative effect and, if necessary, the drug may be given daily. Usually about 6–10 injections are necessary before any improvement is noted. Digitalis may be given orally in the form of digitalis tincture (5–15 drops once or twice daily over a period of 4–6 weeks). Because of the cumulative effect of this drug we dose the dog from Monday to Thursday only, allowing Friday to Sunday free of medication. If signs of gastric irritation occur, the oral form is discontinued and digitalis suppositories are substituted.

Where the cardiac insufficiency is a secondary condition, the primary underlying disease must be treated at the same time. If ascites is present then paracentesis must be performed (see p. 299) and methods of producing diuresis instituted (see p. 330). It is also advisable to counter the loss of albumin by the administration of amino acid mixtures (see p. 227).

A condition of insufficiency of the vascular system is said to occur when the blood flow to the heart is so small that the circulation rate (minute volume) is decreased and the arterial pressure falls. Vascular insufficiency can be divided into neurogenous and peripherally-caused types.

Neurogenous. The most harmless form of insufficiency in this group is syncope, a form of circulatory shock in which the oxygen requirements are drastically reduced by loss of consciousness and muscle tone. The arterial pressure in these cases is almost normal but the minute volume is extremely low. The condition is also termed stress collapse. Treatment is by application of peripheral stimuli, e. g. cold compresses and the administration of centrally-acting analeptics such as caffeine, leptazol, etc. The circulation should be controlled for a few days by the oral administration of 5–15 drops of liquid leptazol 2–3 times daily.

Another type of vascular insufficiency of neurogenous origin is the paralysis of the vasomotor centres produced by certain narcotics and poisons. As there is a general loss of vascular tone in this condition, so that the blood tends to stagnate in the circulation, this type is known as relaxation collapse. In this condition there is a palpitating heart beat with a scarcely discernible pulse. The venous return to the heart may be so small that the heart chambers are almost empty. Treatment is aimed at restoring the tone of the vessels especially in the blood storage organs. As the cause of the condition is central one must try to re-establish central control by centrally-acting analeptics. It may be necessary to use peripherally-acting vasopressors (sympathomimetics) such as Pholedrine sulphate, etc.

Vascular insufficiency due to interference with the regulating stimuli in vasomotor nerves as occurs in epidural anaesthesia, ganglion blockade, etc., is of little significance in the dog. In these cases restoration of the vessel tone should be effected by the peripherally acting vasopressors.

Reflex vascular insufficiency may occur where there is stimulation of the vasodilator nerves, or where they are hypersensitive. Barbiturate anaesthesia is probably the most common cause in the dog, but the condition may also occur where operations are performed in the region of the carotid sinus, e. g. neck, ear, etc. A typical clinical feature of the condition is slowing of the heart rate due to vagal stimulation. Small doses (5–10 mg) of atropine are the most useful treatment. Where the insufficiency is severe, the centrally acting analeptics or the peripherally acting vasoconstrictors should be employed.

Collapse due to insufficient blood volume is an important feature of vascular insufficiency due to peripheral causes. It arises through injury to the vascular area, particularly of the capillary bed, breaching of large vessels, or an increase in capillary permeability. Collapse due to haemorrhage is indicated by considerable loss of blood and pallor of the mucous membranes, a fall in blood pressure with a thready pulse but a distinct heart beat. The blood in these cases is watery or hydraemic. Another form of collapse is due to capillary atony and increased permeability. Here there may be escape of plasma into the tissues (oedema) or into the intestine, where it gives rise to a bloody diarrhoea. In this form the blood is thickened due to loss of plasma (hypervolaemia). Treatment consists of replacing the loss in blood volume. With haemorrhage, transfusion of whole blood is indicated, and with loss of plasma this should be replaced by serum or plasma. Transfusion is not always practicable in canine medicine so substitute fluids have to be used. Ordinary saline solutions are of no use for this purpose as they are of small molecular size and soon leave the vascular system, so blood volume expanders, such as "Macrodex" or "Dextran", should be used.

Acute peripherally induced vascular insufficiency is not of great importance in the dog, in contrast to collapse due to blood volume deficiency.

Hypertrophy and Dilatation of the Heart. These two conditions must be considered together as the one usually merges into the other and they are not easily distinguishable clinically. Hypertrophy or increase in the cardiac muscle, develops when a dog with a normal heart is subjected to continual heavy work, e. g. racing greyhounds. Dilatation, or increase in the lumen of the heart, develops from fatigue of the heart muscle, where the work exceeds the organ's functional capacity. This often occurs in diseases which damage the myocardium. The dilated heart is unable to meet the demands of the body, the output is decreased, and passive congestion results. An hypertrophied heart can become dilated if the work load proves too much for the increased musculature of the organ.

Clinical picture. There are no clear-cut clinical signs in cardiac hypertrophy. The apex beat may be displaced and visible in lean dogs, and the heart sounds are changed in that the first sound is louder than the weakened second sound. If dilatation supervenes, then the clinical signs of cardiac insufficiency appear. The dilatation may be severe enough to cause incompetence of the heart valves, with the production of turbulence in the bloodflow which can be detected on auscultation as vibrations or murmurs.

Diagnosis of hypertrophy or dilatation of the heart can be confirmed by radiography but the differential diagnosis of the two conditions can only be made after due consideration of the clinical findings. For radiography we position the patient on the left side, otherwise distortion of the cardiac outline may occur. In a lateral radiograph, the right ventricle lies cranially and the left ventricle caudally between the 3rd and 7th ribs. In many cases of dilatation of the right ventricle the cranial limit is extended into the 2nd intercostal space up to the 2nd rib. In left ventricle dilatation the heart outline may extend beyond the 7th rib.

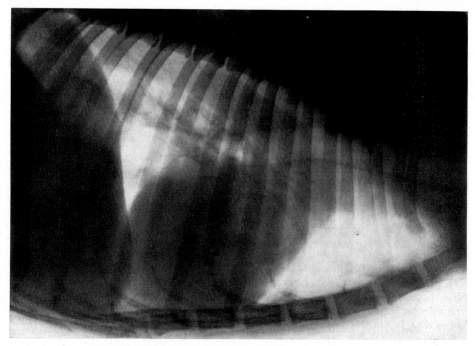

Fig. 268. Dilatation of the heart, especially in the right side.

The actual size of the heart is closely related to its function, so that, for instance, the heart of a racing greyhound is larger in relation to the body size than that of a lap dog. It is very difficult to distinguish certain forms of dilatation or hypertrophy by radiography as they may represent physiological rather than pathological variations. If, however, one or more of the heart cavities enlarge beyond the average diastolic volume, then the shape of the heart becomes more globular, the apex more rounded and the right heart becomes greatly increased ventrally (Fig. 269).

Dilatation can be divided into the so-called Tonogenic and Myogenic dilatation. In tonogenic dilatation, the increased volume may be regarded as a physiological adjustment of a healthy heart to increased demands, or as an active or compensatory dilatation, and is reversible. Only when the increased demand is prolonged is there any growth of the cardiac muscle and the condition should thus be regarded as a precursor to hypertrophy. Myogenic dilatation, on the other hand, is due to disease or weakness of the heart muscle fibres. The weak contractions lead to a passive over-dilatation of the heart in diastole. Myogenic dilatation is usually not reversible. The heart chambers in this case are enlarged on all sides, especially in a transverse direction, whilst in tonogenic dilatation there is more of an elongation of the ventricle, particularly in the apical region.

A systematic study of the radiography of the canine heart showed that the majority of the dogs investigated showed a variable degree of dilatation of the right

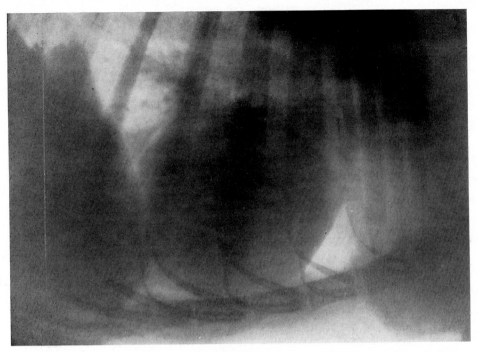

Fig. 269. Globular heart.

heart. This was detectable by a moderate cranio-ventral pouching of the contour of the heart extending back to the apex, the ventricle lying more anteriorly. The condition was therefore, in most cases, one of tonogenic dilatation. Clinical examination of such patients reveals no signs of cardiac insufficiency as the condition is basically physiological in character. The hypertrophy can also be recognised radiographically in the considerably enlarged and dense shadows of the left side of the heart. The cardiac output is strong and regular. Such a heart often shows an eccentric hypertrophy in which the shadow is not so distinct as it is in simple hypertrophy. In the latter the contractions are rapid and productive and the heart seems more tense than usual. This type of condition is found especially in the racing greyhound in training, the condition being comparable with the so-called "athlete's heart" in man. As noted earlier, when estimating the relationship between the load on the body and the damage to the heart, the constitutional type of the dog should be borne in mind. The heavy breeds of working dog (Rottweiler, Boxer, German Shepherd, Airedale, etc.) suffer much more frequently from cardiac insufficiency than the racing breeds. This is due to the facts that regular training leads to hypertrophy of the right heart in the racing dog and also the bodily conformation is such that the extra effort does not cause overstrain. The large body build of the Rottweilers or Boxers is a disadvantage when the dog is subjected to strenuous effort in short bursts, such as may occur during training. In these cases hypertrophy may pass rapidly into dilatation with consequent cardiac insufficiency.

Treatment. Treatment of cardiac dilatation is essentially the same as that for insufficiency. Hypertrophy being a physiological response requires no treatment.

Valvular Disease of the Heart. The majority of valvular defects of the heart of the dog consist of incompetence of the valves due to dilatation of the ostia. Whilst the valvular defect is compensated, the activity of the heart is not impaired and the dog is clinically normal, but eventually the compensation breaks down and insufficiency results.

Clinical signs. It is important to determine which set of valves is affected but this can be very difficult. In the compensated defect the clinical picture is expressed entirely in the heart sounds, which are either altered or additional murmurs occur. In the normal course of events, a compensated heart defect is only found accidentally, as there are no general clinical signs and the dog appears quite healthy. Only when the compensation breaks down do clinical signs of insufficiency occur.

Treatment. Treatment of compensation consists essentially of rest. Where decompensation has occurred, treatment is as for insufficiency.

Disturbances of Frequency and Arrhythmias. These are not of great importance in canine medicine and treatment is as for insufficiency.

Tumours of the Heart and Pericardium. Neoplasia of the heart and pericardium is rare and is usually only diagnosed at postmortem examination. If diagnosed during life, treatment will be symptomatic.

Malformations of the Heart and Great Vessels. Again these are rare in the dog. Probably the most common defect is persistent ductus arteriosus and this gives rise to characteristic clinical signs. PALLASKE (Dtsch. tierärztl. Wschr. **66**, 203–207, 1959) describes a case in a 1½-year-old German Shepherd dog which had been ill for 8 weeks before death with signs of pulmonary disease. In the latter stages of the illness, abdominal distention occurred and ascites and cardiac insufficiency were diagnosed. As a result of the increased pressure in the pulmonary circulation there was severe congestion leading to a marked degree of hydrothorax, hydropericardium and ascites. According to LINTON (J. Amer. vet. med. Ass. **129**, 1–5, 1956), persistence of the right aortic arch combined with persistent ductus arteriosus leads to strangulation of the oesophagus. Clinically there is oesophageal stenosis with dilatation extending forwards from the level of the base of the heart (Figs. 295 and 296). LINTON was able to treat one case surgically with success, the persistent ductus being divided.

Endocarditis. Inflammation of the lining membrane of the heart may appear during the course of infectious diseases, e. g. distemper, but usually passes undetected.

Treatment. Treatment consists of complete rest and the administration of drugs as indicated for cardiac insufficiency. Full therapeutic doses of broad-spectrum antibiotics should be given.

Cardiac Necrosis (Infarction). TEUSCHER (Dtsch. tierärztl. Wschr. **65**, 409–410, 1958) described a case of this condition in a 5-year-old Collie. The dog was quite normal in the morning but dyspnoea developed during the early part of the evening. Clinically there was evidence of severe pain in the thoracic region, the abdomen was soft, and the heart sounds were markedly altered in that they seemed to have somersaulted. Body temperature was 38.5 °C. Symptomatic treatment consisting of penicillin and cardiac stimulants was administered but the dog died the following morning. Postmortem examination revealed that there was a tear about 7 cm long in the pericardium through which part of the heart protruded. The extruded portion of the myocardium was necrotic.

Pericarditis. Inflammation of the pericardium is usually bacterial in origin. We have seen it in a chronic exudative form in a dog with tuberculosis.

Clinical signs. In exudative pericarditis there is an extension of the area of cardiac dullness on percussion of the thorax and the heart beat is weak and barely palpable. Radiography will reveal enlargement of the heart shadow with a general blurring of the outline. Fluoroscopy shows that the heart contractions are obscured but they produce undulatory movements in the surrounding fluid which cause flickering movements of the edges of the outline.

Treatment. Where possible treatment should be specific for the underlying disease condition. If there is marked effusion, pericardial puncture should be attempted.

Technique of Pericardial Puncture. The instruments for this operation have already been described on p. 226. The hair is clipped or shaved from the 3rd to 6th intercostal space and disinfected in the usual way. A needle attached via a two-way valve to a syringe is inserted in the lower portion of the site with the dog in the standing position. After traversing the thoracic wall one can detect friction sounds on the point of the needle. These arise from the pericardium and are not pathological but occur in every puncture of the thorax as soon as the needle touches the pericardium or heart muscle. At this first contact with the pericardium the piston of the syringe must be withdrawn to suck in fluid as closer contact may cause perforation of the heart. If no fluid appears in the syringe the needle is deflected so that it lies close to the pericardium at its apex in order that it may then be pushed in with a brief sharp push. If the puncture is not successful the attempt should not be repeated.

Filariasis of the Heart (Dirofilaria immitis). This condition occurs mainly in tropical and sub-tropical regions and is seen only in isolated cases in Europe in dogs imported from such areas. This is due to the fact that *Dirofilaria immitis* can only be transmitted by certain mosquitoes (*Culex, Aedes* and *Anopheles* spp.) and not by flies.

Clinical signs. The clinical picture in this condition is sometimes rather vague. There may be endocardial sounds, reduplicated heart murmurs, irregular pulse, an increase in the areas of dullness of the heart and the liver, anaemic mucous membranes, ascites, weakness and diminished functional capacity.

Diagnosis. Angiocardiography will show that there is a diminished blood supply to the pulmonary arteries. In heavy infections the microfilariae may be demonstrated in fresh smears of the peripheral blood, but in light infections, concentration and special staining methods are necessary. Other microfilariae of the dog occur in the blood and these must be differentiated before a positive diagnosis can be made.

Treatment. The use of substituted piperazines and organic antimonial compounds is effective. The organic arsenical compounds are active against the sexually mature worms as is "Filarsen" (Dichlorophenarsine hydrochloride). This drug is well tolerated by the dog and 2–3 daily doses will kill the adult worms. One mgm of arsenic per kg bodyweight given 3 times daily removes adult worms within 10 days. Where the infection is heavy it is unlikely that medical treatment will be successful, in which case surgical removal of the worms will be necessary.

6. Diseases of the digestive system

Description of diseases in this section can be divided into oral cavity, oesophagus, and stomach and intestine.

Oral cavity. Investigation of the oral cavity is done chiefly by inspection and palpation. X-rays are useful only when there are diseases of the teeth. A preliminary inspection is made with the mouth closed in order to detect possible swellings (dental fistula). These will be excluded by careful palpation of the closed jaws and the regional lymph glands. By lifting up the lips the gums and the mucosae of the cheeks are investigated and also the state of the teeth (for wear and tear and the presence of tartar, etc.). The jaws are now opened in the manner described (p. 30) and the tonsils and pharynx are inspected (Fig. 270) by pressing down the tongue with a spatula.

Diseases of the teeth are most commonly the reason why the mouth cavity must be investigated. Very often extraction of persistent milk teeth is required. The milk teeth are clearly differentiated from the permanent teeth (see p. 17). In the upper jaw they are always behind the permanent teeth and in the lower jaw lateral to them – the owner often thinks that the persistent milk tooth could affect the position of the permanent tooth, but in our experience this does not happen (Fig. 271). However, frequently it does lead to the trapping of food particles with the risk of initiating a circumscribed gingivitis.

The extraction of milk canines is carried out with incisor extraction forceps. The gum is first carefully pushed back with a Bein's elevator so that as much as possible of the neck of the tooth can be grasped with the forceps. The tooth to be extracted is grasped and is carefully moved in the alveolus by rotatory movements

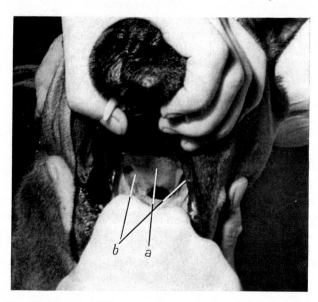

Fig. 270. View into the open mouth. (a) soft palate; (b) tonsils.

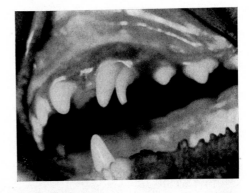

Fig. 271. Persistent milk canine in the upper jaw.

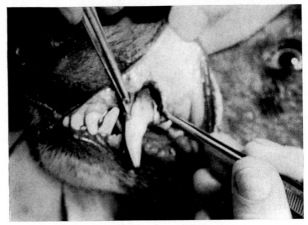

Fig. 272. Extraction of the canine tooth. The gum is dissected away on both sides and the alveolar wall is opened up with a chisel.

in order to loosen its hold in the socket. Then extraction follows. Very often the tooth is broken off at the level of the gum, because absorption of the root has already occurred. Splinters of the root remaining in the alveolus are removed with root forceps or a Bein's elevator. The possibility of infection after extraction of a tooth is slight because the saliva is bacteriostatic in action.

Extraction of permanent teeth rarely presents any difficulty because these teeth are usually extracted because they are loose.

Extraction of the canines and carnassial teeth requires a special technique. As the roots of the canines do not lie vertically in the upper or lower jaw and because they are distinctly curved, they cannot be removed by the usual method (Fig. 260). Extraction is done under general anaesthesia. A curved incision is made with a scalpel into the gum lateral to the canine (corresponding to the curve of the root). The gum is carefully dissected away on both sides so that the wall of the alveolus is exposed (Fig. 272). Then a section of the bony wall is removed with a slender curette so that the tooth can be lifted out laterally. The wound is considerable and is closed by suture of the flaps of gum.

Before extraction of the carnassial (because of its 3 roots) the tooth must be split across with a bone chisel. For this it is necessary to use a plastic or wooden hammer,

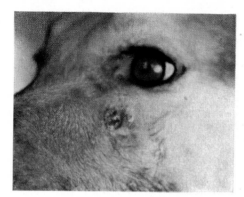

Fig. 273. Dental fistula.

otherwise the alveolus may be fractured. The force of the blows should also be checked by a hand placed on the jaw. Roots that break off are loosened with a Bein's elevator and removed with root forceps.

Dental Fistula is another condition which may be overcome by tooth extraction. Clinically this is seen as a fistula opening which always appears on one side of the head below the eyes (Fig. 273). In spite of thorough treatment, healing cannot be obtained. The secretions from the fistula opening go chiefly downwards and pain can rarely be produced by pressure. The fistula is caused by disease of the root tips. By careful introduction of a sound it is possible to make out the direction of the fistula canal and also identify the affected tooth. The carnassial and first molar are chiefly affected. Light blows with a metal spatula on the affected tooth cause pain which is shown by the patient flinching.

Extraction of the affected tooth presents few difficulties. To complete the operation a strip of gauze is drawn through the fistula canal and tied off outside. This is removed after 24 hours and the fistula will heal up within a very short time without further treatment.

Parodontal disease (inflammation of the alveoli) begins with gingivitis, as a result of which small pockets are formed in the gums which increase in size. The introduction of pathogenic organisms is favoured by foreign bodies which get into these pockets (e. g. grains, hairs, etc.) and readily cause haemorrhages; tartar and food remains are also involved. With the increasing depth of the pockets and retraction of the gums, inflammatory disintegration of the alveolar bone occurs. This results in a loosening of the affected teeth due to a loss of their bony support.

Clinically there is marked salivation, fetor from the mouth and a disturbed intake of food (aversion to cold drinks). The gums are reddened and retracted. Pus may frequently be pressed out of the pockets in the gums.

Treatment consists of removal of the exciting causes. Very often there are foreign bodies causing a circumscribed parodontitis. In addition, the owner should be instructed to wash out the mouth cavity with dilute solution of potassium permanganate. This washing out can be carried out with an enema bulb. The therapeutic effect is better if a wooden rod, wrapped with a cloth soaked in the fluid used for the wash out, is pushed transversely across the mouth of the patient, compelling it to bite round the cloth, and so there is a uniform and intensive

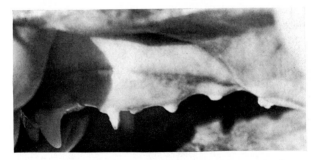

Fig. 274. Half retention of the premolars and molars of the upper jaw.

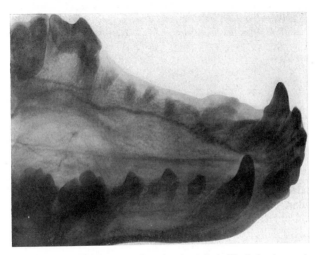

Fig. 275. Faulty development of the premolars in the left half of the lower jaw, apparent half
retention.

distribution of the cleansing fluid in the mouth. In addition, vitamin C should be
administered.

Caries of the Teeth is a process which destroys the hard substance of the teeth
(enamel, dentine and cement) in a chemicoparasitic way mostly from without
inwards. The dog shows the highest incidence of dental caries of all the domesticated
animals. It always appears as moist caries and as occlusion caries involving the
masticatory surfaces in about 5% of cases. Brachycephalic breeds are only rarely
affected because of the incorrect relationship of their teeth, whilst the dolicho-
cephalic breeds suffer more frequently. The Fox terrier is the most frequently
affected breed (14%). The teeth of the upper jaw are usually affected, the disease
being confined to the molars. Caries occurs much less often in the lower jaw
(chiefly in the carnassials).

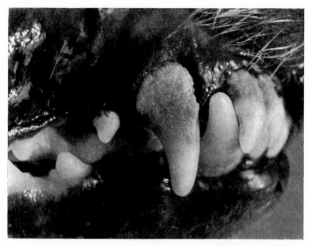

Fig. 276. Tartar formation. The gum is retracted especially in the region of the canine.

Treatment is by excavation of the carious hard substance of the tooth with a drill and possibly filling with an artificial substitute (inlay). Severely affected teeth are extracted.

Tooth retention and half-retention are also seen in the dog. These terms refer to an anomaly in which the tooth does not erupt although it is present, or only half of it erupts (Fig. 274). Retention can only be shown by the veterinary surgeon if the presence of the tooth can be determined by X-rays. Loss of the premolars occurs very often and the owner maintains that the dog has itself bitten out a premolar. This can only be shown if the premolar bitten out is present but not erupted, or if at least there is in its place an injury to the gum and an alveolus is visible in the X-ray. The so-called half-retention is usually only apparent because there is a faulty development of the half-retained tooth. X-rays will show that the crown, neck and root are malformed (Fig. 275). The owner's request that the gum should be incised in order that in this way the tooth may erupt more easily should only be granted if it has been possible to determine the half-retention by X-rays. If there is such an anomaly, then removal of the obstruction to eruption by such an incision is usually effective.

Tartar plays an important part in dental pathology. One must distinguish between hard and soft deposits on the teeth. Soft deposits can be regarded as a precursor of tartar. It consists of deposits of fibrin, bacteria, desquamated epithelial cells, saliva and the smallest particles of food.

Clinically tartar lies directly on the tooth and exhibits different degrees of hardness. Its colour may be yellowish-grey or brown or black. It is found near the outlets of the salivary glands (buccal surface of the carnassials and molars of the upper jaw, on the canine and lingual surface of the carnassial of the lower jaw) (Fig. 277). Sometimes the deposits are so heavy that they form a bridge between several often very loose teeth, thus giving them a better hold. At first there is only a hyperaemia or slight inflammation of the gum (Gingivitis). As the condition

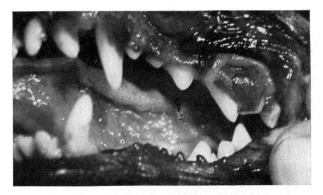

Fig. 277. Tartar in a Dachshund.

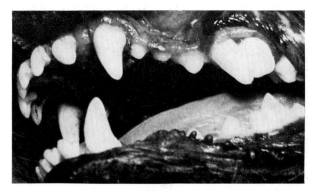

Fig. 278. Teeth of Fig. 277 after treatment.

progresses extensive exposure of the neck of the tooth occurs and with this is associated a break-down of the alveolar ridge. The surface of the tartar deposits may be very rough and may cause inflammatory patches on the mucosa of the cheek, which can be very easily confused with the erosion found in uraemia.

Treatment consists of mechanical removal. For this, hooked, curved, sharp instruments are used. If there are loose teeth which require extraction, this should only be done when the tartar is removed from the other teeth, because haemorrhage obscures the view, the patient is upset, and complete removal of the tartar can no longer be ensured. The more thoroughly the tartar is removed, the longer new formations can be delayed (Fig. 278). The owner should rub the teeth with prepared chalk or cigar ash once a week.

Conservative treatment may be used in the dog, but only to a limited extent. The crowning of fractured teeth (canines) and insertion of inlays are left to the dental surgeon (Fig. 279). The veterinarian will only administer and supervise anaesthesia. Crowning the canine is serviceable only if the crown is considerably smaller than the original tooth and is firmly anchored in the tooth tissue by a

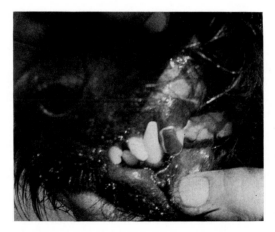

Fig. 279. Gold inlay in the canine of a Schnauzer.

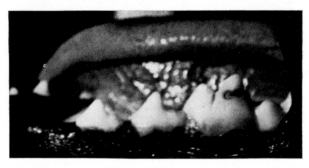

Fig. 280. Hypoplasia of the enamel of the lower left carnassial tooth after recovery from distemper.

transverse peg. Inlays which must be inset in the tooth to a slight degree are more successful. Treatment of the root tip has in our experience given doubtful results.

Hypoplasias of the Enamel appear in the course of distemper if the patient is infected during dentition. They consist of symmetrical quantitative and qualitative changes in the structure of the enamel. It is accepted that the virus of distemper acts on the parathyroid glands (which control the mineralisation of the hard tissues of the teeth) and injury occurs to the components of the enamel, thus causing this condition.

Clinically the teeth show a dull, chalky or a coloured (dark brown) surface. Sometimes there are excavations due to loss of enamel. Hypoplasia of the enamel must not be confused with tartar (Fig. 280).

Treatment. The uneven areas may be ground down with a carborundum stone (drill) and then polished. The coloured parts of the enamel are best rubbed with an oil free from acid.

Gingivitis (Inflammation of the Gums) may arise alone or as part of a general stomatitis.

Clinically it is shown either by simple reddening, swelling, ulceration or gangrenous disintegration of the gum (see stomatitis).

Treatment consists of removing or combating the known causes. If there is only a simple catarrhal inflammation, a cure may often be rapidly achieved by frequent painting with Lugol's iodine. In addition, 2 % Tannin solution or washing with sage tea is useful.

Stomatitis is inflammation of the mucosa of the mouth. It is caused by unsuitable preparation of the food, foreign bodies, vitamin deficiency or infections and is associated with certain disease complexes (uraemia).

The condition commences with a simple reddening and swelling, followed in more severe cases by the formation of vesicles, nodules or ulcers. Prominent features are marked salivation, fetor from the mouth and a greyish-white, dull deposit on the tongue. There may be inflammation of the angles of the lips or the outer skin in certain cases.

Treatment. The causes must be removed as quickly as possible. Tartar is removed and loose teeth are extracted. The mouth is examined for foreign bodies. Strong ointments used externally may cause stomatitis if they are licked. The mouth should be washed out after each feed with fluids named on p. 238 or oak bark tea. One % hydrogen peroxide or 2 % alum solution are also recommended. For painting the affected area of the mucosa, in addition to Lugol's iodine, tincture of myrrh or tincture of krameria may be used. Administration of vitamin C (intravenous or per os) and nicotinamides is advisable.

Noma is a virulent, deeply-penetrating, inflammation resembling moist gangrene affecting the mucosa of the mouth. It is caused chiefly by spirochaetes and fusiform bacteria. Clinically there is a gangrenous breakdown of the mucosa and the tongue. Sharply circumscribed, ulcerated surfaces appear on which there is a greyish-green, soft deposit (Fig. 281). The mouth gives off a putrid odour. There is diminished desire for food, so that the patient becomes emaciated. Noma is usually associated with a severe generalised infection. Palpation reveals enlargement of the submaxillary lymph glands.

Treatment is local painting with a 1 % alcoholic solution of trypaflavin, or 10 % copper sulphate, but systemic treatment must also be given with high doses of vitamin C neoarsphenamine and broad spectrum antibiotics. Very often spontaneous cure follows the extraction of all the teeth.

Glossitis (Inflammation of the tongue) may be caused similarly to stomatitis and is treated in the same way. Ulcers and necrosis of the margin of the tongue appear in various diseases (uraemia, "thrush", etc.). Necrosis of the tongue requires no special treatment as sloughing occurs spontaneously.

Macroglossia (Enlargement of the tongue) may suddenly appear if a ring-shaped foreign body should get wrapped round the tongue during eating. This causes rapid, gross swelling, so that the tongue becomes so enlarged that it no longer has room in the mouth. In such cases one should immediately consider likely ring-shaped foreign bodies given with the food, such as tracheal rings or cross sections of large blood vessels.

Clinically the tongue is dark bluish-red and so much enlarged that it hangs out of the mouth. There are often on its surface bleeding areas where it has been

16*

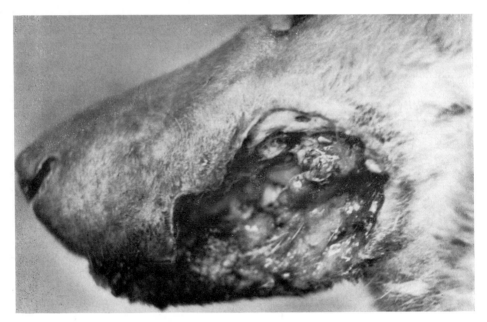

Fig. 281. Noma. The process has caused very extensive destruction of the tissues of the upper
and lower lips. With such extensive tissue destruction treatment is hopeless.

damaged by the teeth. The patient paws at the mouth and there is marked salivation. By palpation a ring-shaped constriction can be made out in the depth of the
mouth cavity.

Treatment consists of immediate removal of the foreign body. If necrosis has
occurred, then there is demarcation between healthy and diseased tissue at the
site of the foreign body. Loss of part of the tongue is justified so long as the prominence (base) of the tongue remains. The patients quickly adapt themselves to
altered conditions in the mouth. If the tongue prominence is absent, however,
the patient can no longer swallow normally and sooner or later aspiration pneumonia
occurs and the animal dies.

Injuries of the tongue after dog fights may be treated surgically if they are
cases of longitudinal injuries. In transverse injuries, on the other hand, there is
always demarcation with loss of the distal portion.

New growths (tumours) of the tongue are rare. Provided that the new growth is
distal to the base of the tongue it can be removed by a wedge-shaped excision.
The edges of the wound are then brought together with deep, closely placed
stitches.

New growth of the Gum (Epulis) may arise either from the mucosa, the periosteal
alveolar process or from the bones. Boxers and terriers are the breeds chiefly
affected.

Clinically there are different forms of epulis; they may be stalked or sessile,
and sometimes displace the teeth. Often multiple fibromas appear which wall in

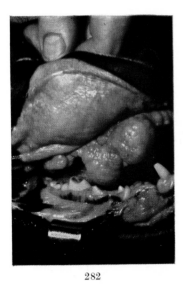

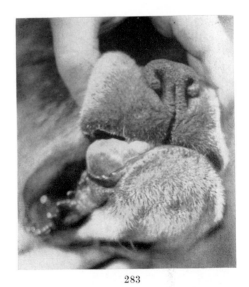

282   283

Fig. 282. Epulids in a Boxer (photograph by the University Dept. of Illustration).

Fig. 283. Epulis in a Boxer.

displace or loosen the teeth (Fig. 282). Desire for food is frequently diminished. Epulids may sometimes reach such a size that they appear between the lips when the mouth is closed (Fig. 283).

Treatment is by complete removal of the new growths. As this operation is very painful we recommend general anaesthesia of the patient. If the broadly sessile epulids affect only the gum there is no difficulty in removal. Occasionally, some teeth must first be extracted. If the new growth reaches the bone or arises from it, then a corresponding lamella of bone must be chiselled out. The wound surfaces caused by the extirpation have a marked tendency to bleed and this can be controlled by the usual surgical methods. Surgical diathermy has proved the method of choice, but if this cannot be used, excision may be done with a knife and the haemorrhage controlled with iron perchloride solution.

New growths of the soft palate are rare.

Clinically the patient can no longer swallow normal food but can take only fluids. The animal is emaciated and has an exhausted appearance. Marked saliva- tion and continued swallowing and gulping indicate a disease of the mouth cavity. The new growth can be seen on the soft palate by inspection of the opened mouth, and depression of the tongue. Sometimes part of the hard palate is involved (Fig. 284).

Treatment consists of radical excision of the new growth. This may involve loss of much of the soft palate and this in turn leads to difficulties in swallowing, because the food particles tend to be drawn into the nasal passages by the base of the tongue. For this reason one should do this operation only at the express wish

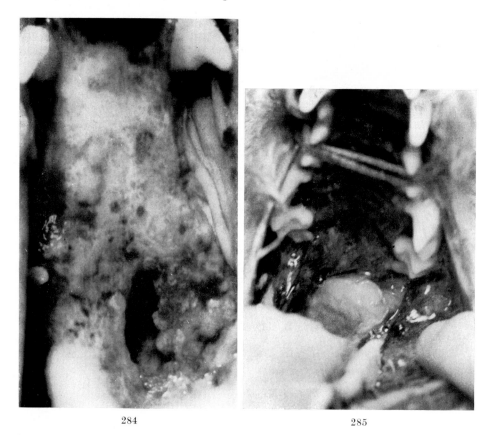

284   285

Fig. 284. Inoperable carcinoma of the upper jaw. Most of the soft palate is already destroyed.

Fig. 285. New growth in the pharynx of a German Shepherd (Alsatian).

of the owner, stressing the possibility of such complications, otherwise euthanasia should be advised (Fig. 285).

Tonsillitis is an inflammation of the palate – less often of the tongue and pharyngeal tonsil. It may be acute or chronic. It has been said that it could be caused by chills (eating snow, drinking cold water, open air bathing, sudden changes of climate, etc.) and bacterial infection. Streptococci, staphylococci, coliform organisms, *Pasteurella multiscida* and *Clostridium welchii* A have been isolated from the tonsils of dogs affected by tonsillitis. Some workers are of the opinion that there is a relationship between a septic focus in the tonsils and other lesions in the body, e. g. nephritis, arthritis, etc. Therefore one should pay special attention to the examination of the tonsils in other diseases, especially those of a chronic recurrent nature.

Clinically the acute form occurs especially in dogs aged 1–3 years. As a result of the sudden onset of pyrexia (up to 41 °C) the patient is prostrated and looks dull. There is no desire for food. Swelling of the tonsils narrows the tonsillar ring and this causes choking and attacks of coughing. Yawning is another common sign. Light pressure on the larynx causes coughing. Inspection shows that both tonsils are greatly enlarged and reddened and protrude from their crypts. In distemper the peri-tonsillar tissues are definitely reddened. Frequently, a viscous white mucus surrounds the tonsils.

In the chronic form there are recurrent attacks of fever, the tonsils are prolapsed and reddened and often dotted over with small, purulent specks. In the afebrile stage the hypertrophic tonsils look rather paler. Loss of appetite, prostration, cough and salivation of a viscous mucus may also be seen.

The treatment of acute tonsillitis consists of the administration of appropriate sulphonamides or antibiotics. In addition, the tonsils are painted with sulphon-amides or iodised glycerine.

R.	Iodine	1 part
	Potassium iodide	3 parts
	Glycerine	ad 30 parts

All factors that might irritate the tonsils (drinking cold water, eating snow, feeding with bones or hard bread) are withheld from the patient. A harness is put on in place of a collar. Priessnitz compresses round the neck are helpful. Affected animals should be nursed in a well-warmed room and allowed out only to relieve themselves. Clinically acute tonsillitis in its early stages closely resembles the early stage of distemper, so we give a suitable amount (10–20 ml) of distemper hyper-immune serum in the first day of the disease. This has often protected us from unwelcome surprises. The serum is also beneficial by virtue of its albumin content as a non-specific stimulant in cases of tonsillitis.

The treatment of chronic tonsillitis, which is characterised by its relapsing course, consists of tonsillectomy.

Technique of Tonsillectomy. The patient lies on its back under general anaesthesia and is tied down diagonally in such a way to obviate aspiration of blood from possible haemorrhage. One in 1,000 adrenalin solution and enough swabs must be at hand. The mouth is opened with tapes and the tongue pulled forwards with forceps. The tonsil is grasped with Pean's forceps carefully (because the glandular tissue is extraordinarily friable) and drawn out of the crypt. A round atraumatic needle (carrying a double catgut suture) is passed between the anterior and posterior strand of tissue. The posterior strand of tissue is ligatured with one suture and the anterior portion with the other. Then the gland can be carefully cut out. If there is secondary haemorrhage (due to slipping of the ligature) it is controlled with swabs soaked in adrenaline. The tonsillotome of BAUER (Hauptner Catalog No. 3350) may also be used and this greatly simplifies and shortens the operation. This tonsillotome combines the haemostatic action of Blunk's forceps with that of the Emasculator. After opening the mouth (see above) the tonsillotome is applied to the tonsil to be removed and closed. The tonsillotome remains in place for 2–3 minutes. The operation is repeated on the other side. Possible haemorrhage is controlled with swabs soaked in adrenaline.

After-treatment consists of restricting the patient to soft food during the succeeding days.

Pharyngitis (Inflammation of the mucosa of the throat) has the same causes as those described for stomatitis and laryngitis. Often a secondary tonsillitis occurs. Treatment is analogous to that of the diseases described.

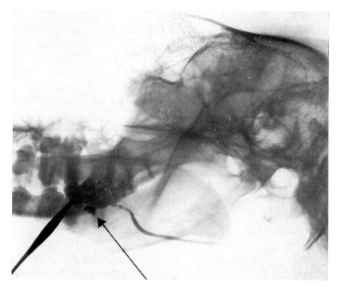

Fig. 286. Radiograph of the parotid duct with a diverticulum at the level of the first premolar
tooth, caused by a splinter of wood.

Diseases of the salivary glands or their ducts are relatively rare in the dog.
Nevertheless, sometimes syndromes occur which cannot be accurately classified
in the differential diagnosis.

Diseases of the Parotid may arise by extension of inflammatory processes which
occur near this gland. Underlying causes are the effects of choke chains such as
those used on guard dogs or on hunting dogs when they are crawling. The inflammation occurs in the subcutaneous tissue and extends to the parotid, so that a secondary parotitis is established. Finally, an abscess is formed and under treatment
this bursts or, when it is sufficiently ripe, can be incised. We have not yet observed
the formation of a fistula as a result of such a process.

Further, secondary parotitis may occur in otitis externa in which flat or circumscribed ulcerations occur down to the deepest layers of the external auditory
canal, the epithelium being macerated and the papillary body exposed. This
form of parotitis subsides with treatment of the basic disease without further
measures. If the primary disease is surgically treated, one must ensure that the
angle of the wound, which is very deep, granulates well, so that a fistula is not
formed extending to the parotid. A fistula of this kind would be revealed by a
relapse of the otitis and the presence of a watery, colourless secretion in the auditory
canal.

Salivary stones (sialoliths) which may be met with as a pathological condition
chiefly in the duct of the parotid gland, are, in contrast to the horse, quite rare in
the dog. KRÄMER (Berlin. Personal communication) encountered a salivary cyst in
the parotid duct of a long-haired Dachshund. After radical extirpation of the cyst
he found a stone about 1 mm in size in the parotid duct. We ourselves removed a

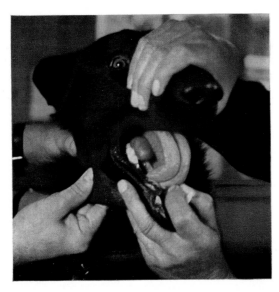

Fig. 287. Ranula.

foreign body from the parotid duct (Fig. 286). The rare occurrence of a stone in the canine parotid duct is probably due to the fact that dogs bolt their food greedily without previously chewing it, whilst the Equidae deliberately grind up their food in the mouth. In the latter there is every possibility that food particles may enter the parotid duct through the salivary papilla and there act as nuclei for the crystallisation of salivary stones of this kind.

Diseases of the Mandibular and Sublingual Salivary Glands. Inflammatory processes in the lumen of BARTHOLIN's duct may cause stenosis, and this results in thickening of the saliva dammed up there so that ultimately the duct may be blocked. Due to the obstruction (salivary stasis), the duct becomes dilated and a salivary cyst is formed. Such a cyst may also be caused by concretions and con- glomerations which block the duct and these are true retention cysts. According to the site of the obstruction, the retention cysts may be in different places in the lower jaw or intermaxillary space. If the obstruction is near the opening of the duct the salivary duct is dilated lateral to the tongue in the mouth. We call this a Ranula (Frog tumour) (Fig. 287). It represents a classical retention cyst also known in man. In the dog, the ranula lies lateral to the frenum of the tongue, and depending upon the degree of dilatation may displace the tongue to the other side (Fig. 288). In our experience the swelling has been invariably unilateral.

If the obstruction of the ducts is nearer to the gland, then the stasis of the saliva shows as a swelling that is fluctuating, or hard as a board, in the region of the submaxillary space or the neck (Fig. 289). Differential diagnosis between a sub- maxillary or neck cyst from other diseases is difficult.

Retention Cysts may develop very slowly. When there is stenosis of the salivary duct they may last for weeks. If the cyst becomes visible in a few days, the duct has suddenly become obstructed. Usually, there is no general disturbance in the animal's condition, but when there is a ranula, feeding may be cautious or delayed.

Treatment. Conservative treatment does not give satisfactory results, only operative treatment being successful. Incision into the cyst can only be done in the case of ranula, because the fistula that results delivers the saliva into the

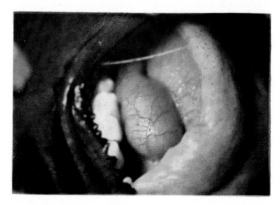

Fig. 288. The ranula pushes the tongue to the opposite side.

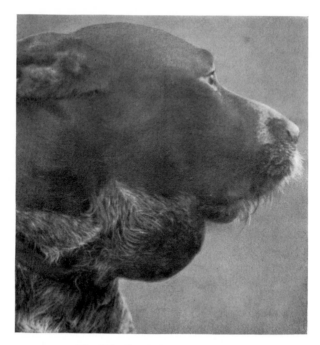

Fig. 289. Cervical cyst in a hound.

mouth, whilst in cases of submaxillary or cervical cysts, incision leads to an undesirable fistula opening to the exterior with unpleasant results. The glands which
may lead to the persistence of a fistula must be extirpated. According to our
experience it is always the Bartholin's duct that is affected, so that the sublingual
gland must be removed. As it is technically impossible to remove this gland alone,
the mandibular and the sublingual glands are removed together.

Technique of the extirpation of the mandibular and sublingual salivary glands. The operation is
performed with the patient under general anaesthesia. After shaving, cleansing and disinfection
of the field of operation, the jugular vein is compressed so that the maxillary veins become
clearly visible. The glands to be removed lie in the fork of these veins. An incision into the skin
about 5–7 cm long is made and the platysma myoides muscle is divided. After dissection of the
connective tissue from the large vessels, the capsule of the mandibular gland lies under the
connective tissue. The capsule is divided and the firm nodules of the gland, which can be recognised
by its lobular structure, are shelled out of its capsule. At its cranial end is attached the sublingual
gland and this is now shelled out of the same capsule (Fig. 290). In these manipulations the vessels
which supply the glands and enter the glands medially must be identified or ligatured to minimise
haemorrhage. When the glands have been removed from the capsule far enough, the sublingual
gland is tied off with a deep catgut ligature and cut away. The tampon is removed after 24 hours.
Only at the end of this operation is the cervical cyst opened (Fig. 291). Bandage for 24 hours.

A ranula and a cervical cyst may also occur together. In such cases a connective
tissue strand formed by the affected duct leads from the ranula to the cervical
cyst. The contents of the cyst consist of mucous, thickened saliva which has a
colour resembling that of albumin, or it is brownish-yellow and this gave rise to
the name Meliceris (honey tumour) formerly used.

Foreign Bodies are found **in the mouth** or pharynx in the form of bone, or wood
splinters stuck between the teeth, or the teeth of the upper jaw, in the hard palate,
or between the teeth and the cheeks. The animals avoid their food, show marked

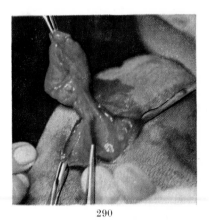

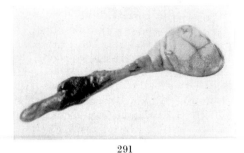

290   291

Fig. 290. The mandibular gland and sublingual gland have been completely dissected out of
their capsules and can be tied off.

Fig. 291. Operation specimen of the extirpated salivary glands. The dark coloration of part
of the sublingual gland shows the starting point of the cervical cyst, because the cyst contents
have been coloured with methylene blue.

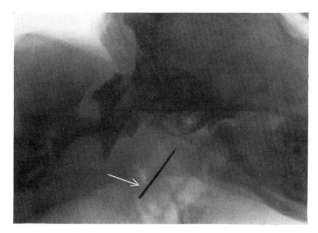

Fig. 292. A needle in the neck muscles in a Fox terrier puppy 6 weeks old.

salivation and sometimes the jaws cannot be closed. The patient tries to get rid of the foreign body by wiping the mouth with its paws, or rubbing its head on the floor. Inspection of the mouth readily reveals the foreign body and it is removed with dressing forceps or dental forceps.

Other foreign bodies often found in the mouth, pharynx or beginning of the oesophagus are impacted needles. Such needles are ingested when the dogs, mostly young ones, play with a thread on to which the needle is hanging. The thread is swallowed and when the needle has passed the base of the tongue the dog reacts against it by retching or gulping, the result of which is that the needle is pressed in in an oral direction usually at the base of the tongue. The animals show salivation, retching, avoidance of food and are very sensitive to palpation in the pharyngeal region. It is possible to palpate an impacted needle by careful digital exploration of the pharynx if it is not completely embedded, or at least make out the thread attached to it. A certain diagnosis is made by X-rays. As the needle does not always penetrate parallel to the direction of the food canal, radiographs must be made in two planes in order to ensure accurate removal of the foreign body (Fig. 292). The removal is done with the patient anaesthetised, the eye of the needle being fixed with a finger nail, and a slightly curved dressing forceps introduced and closed on it. The needle is removed in the direction opposite to that in which it entered. If necessary, this operation is done with a (X-ray) screen control.

If needles without any threads are ingested (pins and sewing needles), they usually cause little or no trouble and pass through the food canal without penetrating the mucosa. In the gut, pins are drawn along with the heads, and sewing needles with the blunt ends, directed towards the anus, their long axis is directed parallel to the gut and thus they pass through a coil of the gut. This phenomenon can be explained by the fact that, when the gut mucosa makes contact with a pointed object, the part of the muscularis mucosae under the point of contact relaxes, the part touched falls back and the adjacent parts are drawn together to a corresponding degree like walls round the point of the needle. The object is thus

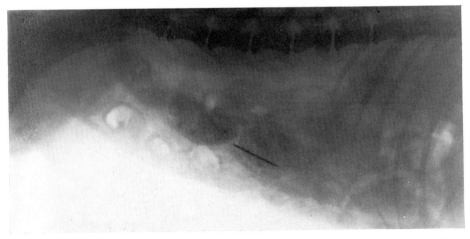

Fig. 293. A needle in the rectum. The blunt end of the needle has become directed towards the anus, so that most of it has wandered through the intestine.

held firmly at its pointed end and the blunt end is moved by peristalsis, so that it goes first in the progress down the food canal (Fig. 293).

Rarely, young dogs during their play swallow a thread in such a way that the free end lies in the oesophagus and the loop is under the tongue. These patients are presented with the complaint that they cry out when they swallow solid food. When solid food is swallowed the free end in the oesophagus exerts a pull on the loop round the base of the tongue and this slowly cuts into the base of the tongue. On inspection of the mouth a transverse, linear reddening can be seen under the tongue. Palpation of the sides of the root of the tongue reveals the thread which is deeply embedded in the tissue anteriorly. On removal of the thread the clinical symptoms disappear immediately.

Examination of the oesophagus by palpation is restricted to the neck region. Radiologically of interest are foreign bodies in the oesophagus. Contrast demonstrations of them succeed only when there is occlusion. Patency of the oesophagus (when a foreign body is suspected) can be demonstrated by the passage of a stomach sound.

Various sized capsules of barium sulphate may be used for the diagnosis of occlusions of the oesophagus. These are given during screening and are very useful in the elucidation of doubtful cases.

Stenosis of the oesophagus is encountered as a congenital condition. It occurs chiefly in the cardiac region (idiopathic dilatation of the oesophagus) (Fig. 294).

Clinically the history is that the puppy, after changing to artificial feeding, would vomit part of the solid food immediately after taking it. X-ray examination shows that on ingestion of the contrast medium, only a small part of it goes into the cardiac part of the stomach, most of it remains in the oesophagus, which is greatly dilated (Fig. 294). In many cases it is impossible to pass a stomach sound through the stenosis.

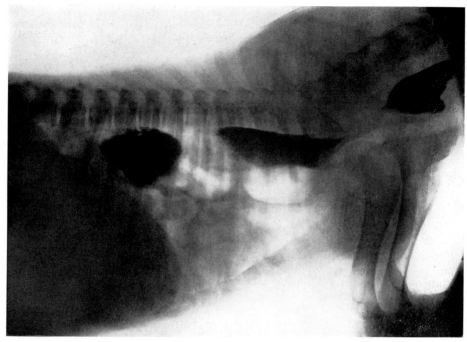

Fig. 294. Dilatation of the oesophagus in cardiospasm. The contrast medium has remained in the
oesophagus.

Treatment is prolonged and should be given only to cases in which the stenosis
is not too pronounced. First the diet is rigorously controlled (small amounts of
fluids given frequently throughout the day). We have obtained encouraging
results with tetraethylammonium bromide (TEAB – a ganglion blocking agent)
administered over a period of several weeks. The drug is given in a dose of 7 mg
per kg bodyweight mixed with dextrose and administered by slow intravenous
injection. Caution is necessary as overdosage may cause collapse.

Forced dilatation of the cardia with increasing sizes of bougies has been recommended by some workers, as has crushing of the left phrenic nerve.

Stenosis of the oesophagus and trachea. This condition may occur if the aorta
develops abnormally (Fig. 264). Being a congenital disease it is only seen in young
dogs. The puppies often vomit immediately after taking food. In suckling puppies
milk may appear at the nostrils as the supply of milk may be too rapid to percolate
past the stenosis. Dilatation of the oesophagus gradually occurs anterior to the
obstruction so that the ingested food is regurgitated after a varying period of
time. This is usually noted at the time of weaning, a characteristic feature of the
condition being the ravenous appetite combined with loss of condition without
malaise. The stenosis may also lead to strangulation of the trachea, resulting in
respiratory difficulties. The cause of the condition is persistence of the right
aortic arch combined with persistent ductus arteriosus.

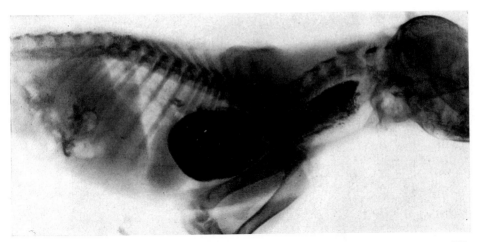

295b   295a

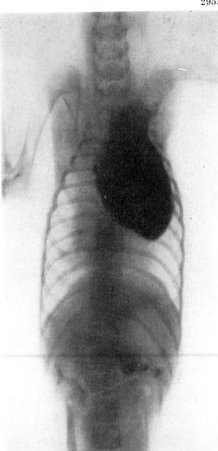

Fig. 295a. Diverticulum of the oesophagus due to persistence of the ductus arteriosus. The contrast medium has accu-
mulated in the oesophagus and only a little
of it has flowed into the stomach. Latero-
lateral radiograph.

Fig. 295b. Oesophageal diverticulum. Dorso-ventral radiograph.

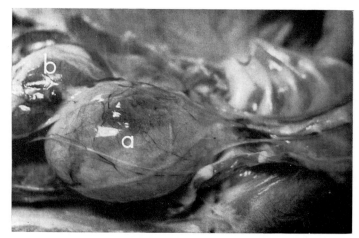

Fig. 296. Persistence of the ductus arteriosus and resultant diverticulum of the oesophagus.
(a) the oesophageal diverticulum; (b) the heart. (Postmortem preparation.)

Radiographic diagnosis depends upon the demonstration of oesophageal stenosis at the base of the heart with oesophageal dilatation anterior to it (Figs. 295 and 296).

Treatment is entirely surgical and consists of division of the persistent ductus arteriosus via a thoracotomy incision.

Foreign bodies in the oesophagus occur mainly in the shape of large pieces of meat or bones. These usually result from the dog jealously gulping down food in large lumps without breaking it up in the mouth. In the oesophagus of the dog there are predilection sites at which foreign bodies are especially likely to stick. They stick firmly at the entrance to the chest because here the oesophagus makes a slight bend and its elasticity is compressed by the bony ring formed by the first pair of ribs, the sternum and the cervical vertebrae (Fig. 297). The second predilection site is in the anterior part of the thorax, a little above the heart, and the third site is before the oesophagus passes through the diaphragm (Fig. 298). At these two latter points there is a natural narrowing of the oesophagus.

Clinically if there is obstruction of the oesophagus there is fairly immediate vomiting of swallowed food and fluids are returned with choking and retching of nothing more than a glassy, colourless mucus. If an obstructive foreign body (vertebral bones of a rabbit) has stuck fast in the oesophagus, the same symptoms are seen, but in this case sometimes small quantities of fluids can be retained.

Diagnosis is supported by the history that the symptoms appeared suddenly after eating a bone or pieces of meat and the characteristic symptoms just described. Passing a stomach sound will usually confirm the diagnosis, but errors may occur in that sometimes the foreign body presents no distinct resistance to the sound which may by-pass it. In such cases the most certain method is X-ray examination. A non-radio-opaque foreign body above the heart may be misinterpreted as the large vessels leaving the heart. Where radiography is indefinite a stomach sound is introduced under fluoroscopic control. A foreign body will be seen to move in concert with the sound due to the elasticity of the oesophagus.

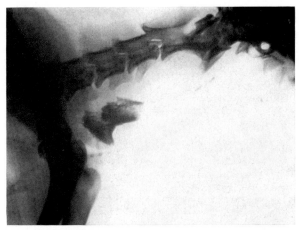

Fig. 297. A foreign body (a bone) in the cervical portion of the oesophagus.

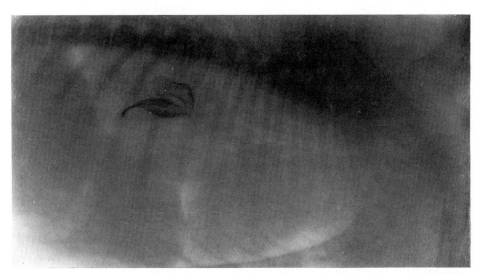

Fig. 298. Foreign body (bone) in the oesophagus.

Treatment is mechanical removal of the foreign body from the oesophagus. We introduce a modified Stadtler's ball (bullet) extractor and extract the foreign body through the mouth.

Technique of Extraction of a Foreign Body from the Oesophagus. The patient is anaesthetised. A Stadtler's ball extractor lengthened to 60 or 90 cms is introduced in 2 or 3 stages, as described on p. 271. The extraction must be done with screen control. The foreign body is seized and by slight rotation its spatial extent is determined. Now one tries to place the foreign body so that its smallest diameter comes to lie transversely to the direction of the oesophagus. By careful manipulation one can sometimes turn it a little, or free the sharp points on the foreign body embedded in the mucosa, by manipulation of the jaws of the forceps. When the foreign body is in the correct position for the application of forceps, it is grasped and extracted by vibratory movements. By such movements it is possible to make the elastic mucosa of the oesophagus glide over the inequalities of the foreign body like a rubber band, so that it does not become fixed again and does not damage the mucosa. In the isthmus of the oesophagus, the foreign body offers marked resistance because of the narrowness of the isthmus caused by the larynx and vertebral column, and there is the risk that it may slip out of the forceps. If the foreign body remains in the isthmus, one must keep it fixed from the outside, grasp it again and help the extraction with the index finger introduced deep into the mouth.

After-treatment of the patient consists of 2–3 days on a fluid diet followed by 5 days on semi-solids.

Technique of Oesophagotomy. General anaesthesia is induced. The middle third of the neck is shaved on the left side, cleansed with ether and iodised. The incision into the skin is made parallel to and on the left side of the trachea for about 10 cm. A cut is made carefully through the platysma myoides muscle. Now a stomach sound is introduced in order to make the identification of the oesophagus easier. The oesophagus is recognised by its bluish-red colour, and, if there is a stomach sound in position, by increased rigidity. It is incised longitudinally between two pairs of forceps, the incision being long enough to enable the foreign body to be extracted smoothly through the wound. The wound in the oesophagus is closed as follows:

1. Closure of the mucosa with a Schmieden suture.
2. Closure of the muscularis with a continuous suture.
3. Closure of the platysma muscle with button (interrupted) sutures.

Post-operatively the dog is fasted for 2–3 days. Pure water can be given during the following days. The skin sutures are removed after 8 days.

If the foreign body remains in the thoracic part of the oesophagus for several days, perforations occur, and this leads to the entry of organisms into the thoracic cavity and to pleurisy. We incline towards the view that perforation due to a foreign body occurs as the result of pressure necrosis after some days. In these infrequent cases after the failure of attempts at extraction, intrathoracic oesophagotomy must be done.

Stomach and Intestine. Various methods of examination are available. The simplest seems to be palpation. The stomach is examined by deep palpation, the examiner standing behind the dog and putting an open hand flat on each side of the hypochondriac region and carefully bringing the two hands together forwards. In this way the region of the stomach can be vigorously palpated. One can estimate how full it is and any foreign bodies present can be felt. Palpation of the intestine is done bimanually, although in small dogs it may be done with one hand. In this way it will be possible to identify painful conditions in the intestine, evidenced by strong contractions of the abdominal muscles. This symptom should not be considered in isolation, because there are other painless conditions in the abdomen which cause contraction of the abdominal muscles on palpation. It is possible by this method to estimate the contents of the intestine. Normally, it is full of a soft food mass. If there is gas present it has a bubbly consistency usually combined with a splashing sound. If the gut is empty one feels the loops of the intestine as firm, hard strands. If the gut is obstructed by stasis of food (especially after feeding with bones) one feels a thick, irregularly formed strand in the abdomen. Usually, such coprostasis is in the hind gut so that it can be diagnosed by digital examination of the rectum. To identify a foreign body palpation is valuable in so far as it confirms a suspected diagnosis. A negative result of palpation when

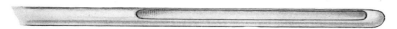

Fig. 299. Instrument for the removal of faeces.

there are other symptoms of a foreign body should not eliminate the possibility of a foreign body. Auscultation of the abdomen may detect peristaltic sounds and may be used in the detection of increased formation of gas in the intestine. Inspection of the gut contents, whether of the vomit or faeces, is also essential. The vomit is examined for variation in the colour of its mucus content (white, yellowish, greenish), for the degree of digestion and for the composition of the broken up food. The faeces are examined for their consistency, colour, admixture with mucus, blood, parasites or foreign bodies, etc. For special microscopic examination faeces are taken with a faeces extractor (Fig. 299) from the rectal ampulla. Aids to diagnosis include X-ray examination, gastroscopy, rectoscopy and examination of the gastric juice.

X-ray examination reveals the presence in the stomach or intestine of radio-opaque objects (bone remains, such foreign bodies as stones, metal, etc.). It shows up accumulations of gas, such as may appear in aerophagy, inanition states and when foreign bodies are present (Fig. 300). If one wishes to visualise distension of a portion of intestine, contrast media are used. We use a thinly-fluid opaque meal to reveal radio-lucent foreign bodies. To estimate intestinal motility on the screen, 125–250 ml are given, and this normally passes through the gut in about 24 hours (Figs. 301, 302). Under normal conditions the opaque meal begins to pass out of the stomach 5–10 minutes after it has been ingested and this process continues for about 3–4 hours. If one is concerned only to show up the mucosa of the stomach (gastritis) the meal is mixed in the proportion of 1 : 1 (contrast and water) and according to the size of the patient ½ a teaspoonful to ½ a table-spoonful is given. To demonstrate inflammatory conditions in the stomach gastro-scopy will also be used in the future. If the hind gut only is of special interest, it can be filled with contrast medium by means of an enema (Fig. 303) and can also be examined with a rectoscope.

To demonstrate the secretion of gastric juice the fasting patient is given a few doses of contrast medium. After a time one can distinguish 3 layers in the stomach. The deepest layer consists of the sedimented contrast medium, the middle layer of contrast medium and gastric juice and the surface layer of air (gas bubbles in the stomach). With some experience one can gain some information about gastric secretion from the thickness of the middle layer. Accurate estimation of the hydrochloric acid content of the gastric juice is performed by giving the fasting patient a substance which stimulates secretion of the acid (alcohol, histamine or caffein). The gastric juice formed is then siphoned off and examined. One first determines by qualitative filtration the free hydrochloric acid with Congo red paper and then estimates the acid quantitatively and also the total acid by titration.

Inflammatory changes in the stomach and intestines in their mildest form are shown clinically by loss of appetite without any specific symptoms. Then follows gastric catarrh in which, in addition to loss of appetite, vomiting and changes in the faeces occur. Finally, a massive inflammation sets in, in which the disturbances

17*

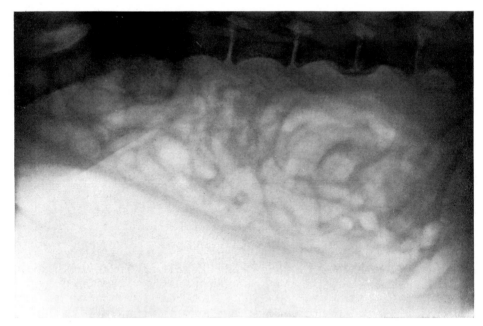

Fig. 300. Aerophagy.

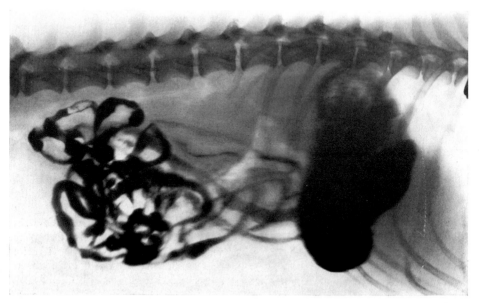

Fig. 301. Contrast demonstration of the stomach and intestinal tract.

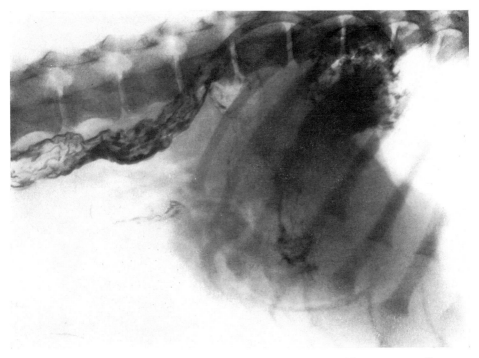

Fig. 302. Demonstration of the intestinal mucosa (jejunum) with contrast medium.

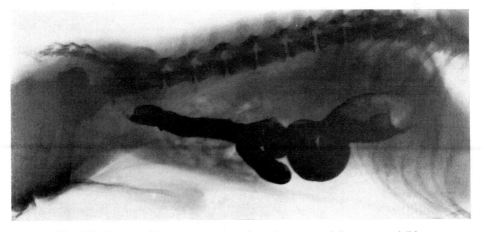

Fig. 303. Enema with opaque meal renders the extent of the rectum visible.

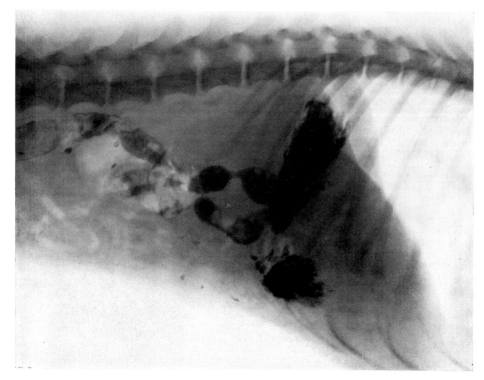

Fig. 304. So-called "dustiness" seen in hypersecretion.

of digestion already indicated occur and also marked changes in the general condition (fever, changes in the pulse rate and quality, etc.).

Gastritis as a clinical entity is rare in the dog. Among marked symptoms caused by the stomach alone we must differentiate **Achylia** (lack of free hydrochloric acid) and **Hyperchlorhydria** (excess of acid) (Fig. 304).

Clinically in gastric achylia or hypochlorhydria there is marked loss of appetite and sometimes vomiting, especially in the morning when the stomach is empty, the vomit consisting only of clear to yellowish frothy mucus. Very often the history indicates that in the morning the patient has eaten grass with definite benefit. The diagnosis can be established by examination of the gastric juice. If there is hyperchlorhydria it will be noted that the patient often vomits after food, the meal being regurgitated in a half-digested state.

Treatment of lack of gastric juice consists of giving a mixture of pepsin and hydrochloric acid:

R.   Dilute hydrochloric acid ⎫ āā   2 parts
      Pepsin   ⎭
      Water   ad 200 parts
      One teaspoonful to two tablespoonful 3 times a day before food.

If there is excess of acid, drugs are given which combine with or neutralise the excess of acid, such as magnesium trisilicate or aluminium hydroxide.

Vomiting (vomitus, emesis) is a symptom, not a disease. Only by careful consideration of the whole clinical picture is it possible to define the aetiology of vomiting. Immediate specific treatment is therefore difficult and one should try to ascertain whether the vomiting is purely a protective mechanism rejecting noxious substances which have been ingested, or whether it is an indication of disease. The consensus of opinion is that vomiting is caused either by direct stimulation of the vomiting centre via the blood, or by cerebral or spinal stimulation of this centre, or it is a case of the so-called reflex vomiting due to peripheral stimulation of the autonomic nervous system. In the dog most cases must be ascribed to reflex vomiting. This occurs in various diseases of the gastro-intestinal tract, the liver, the diaphragm, the serous membranes, etc. In these reflex processes the phenomenon of reflex facilitation is often very evident. Repeated stimulations one after another lower the threshold of excitation so that the slightest stimulus which would normally be subliminal causes the vomiting act.

Clinically vomiting begins with signs of restlessness. The patient makes fruitless movements of chewing, swallowing and gulping. There is marked secretion of saliva. Very often the position of a saw-horse is assumed in order to vomit with the pressure of the abdominal muscles. Vomiting occurs either only once or frequent vomits occur one after another.

The physiological processes concerned are as follows: the moment there is nausea the fundus of the stomach is relaxed, the peristaltic movements of the pyloric antrum are inhibited, the pylorus closes and the fundus is filled with the stomach contents. This causes opening of the cardiac orifice, and by the pressure of the abdominal muscles and cramplike contractions of the diaphragm, the food mass enters the oesophagus. During this time the pyloric antrum remains contracted. Finally, the food that has been for a while in the oesophagus is carried forward by expiration with a closed glottis.

There are also cases which cannot be described as vomiting but must be interpreted as regurgitation. This occurs especially when there is complete obstruction of the oesophagus by a foreign body. The food is usually rejected immediately the swallowing act is completed and without apparent difficulty, although there may be choking movements. The ejection of the food swallowed usually occurs by the peristaltic wave being retarded by the obstructing foreign body and apparently becoming antiperistaltic.

In achloraemia, uncontrollable vomiting (hyperemesis) occurs. Repeated vomiting continuing for a day or perhaps for days is always serious. Examination of the vomit may sometimes provide important clues to the kind of illness present. So-called faecal vomit (the vomit is most markedly undigested or digested and has a faecal odour) suggests that the site of the disease is in the deeper parts of the digestive tract.

In the treatment of vomiting an exhaustive history and a most careful examination of the patient are necessary in order to determine the primary disease condition (Ileus, uraemia, etc.), and then to treat this specifically. In mild forms of vomiting, administration of warm camomile tea by the owner may give relief. Treatment with "Peremesin" (up to 4 tablets several times a day) often gives good results. "Anesthesin" powder (soluble only in alcoholic media) may also be pre-

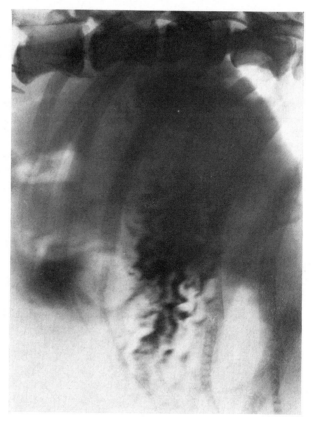

Fig. 305. Marked formation of folds in the stomach in chronic gastritis, revealed by contrast
medium.

scribed. Washing the intestine out with lukewarm enemas is always to be
recommended. Large doses (given intravenously) of Vitamin C and calcium
are helpful. If there is no response to these medications, promazine or chlor-
promazine can be given subcutaneously. The injection may be repeated after
2 hours if necessary. Another drug which works well is opium, in the form of the
tincture in a dose of 5–10 drops twice a day.

Hyperemesis due to achloraemia is treated with frequent intravenous administration of 10 % saline solution (4–12 ml per dose).

Dilatation of the stomach is seen in the dog only in a chronic form due mainly
to faulty feeding of the animal as a pup. At weaning very often excessive quantities
of food are offered, leading to sudden enlargement of the stomach and subsequent
chronic dilatation and its sequelae (achylia, gastroenteritis, malnutrition, etc.)
(Fig. 305).

Dilatation of the stomach may also result when foreign bodies (stones or metal
balls) remain for a long time in the stomach. Prolonged loading of the stomach

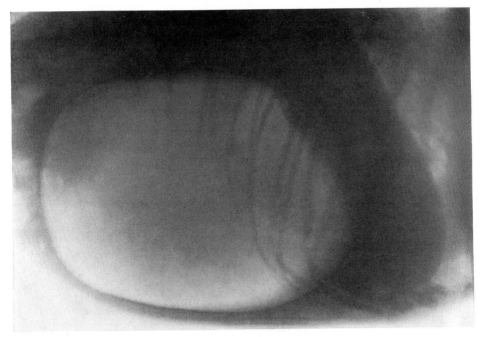

Fig. 306. Torsion of the stomach in a Setter.

may slowly cause dilatation. According to the literature, diverticula of the stomach may also be caused in this way.

Torsion of the stomach is relatively rare. In our experience it occurs only in the larger breeds of dogs (Setter, German Shepherd, St. Bernard, Great Dane). There may be familial or hereditary factors involved in the aetiology.

Clinically the condition is recognised by the acute onset of fermentation and flatulence. Torsion occurs mostly in stomachs that are only partially filled. Probably the torsion occurs from the right side forwards to the left by a downward movement. The cardia and pylorus are twisted through 180° and this causes the clinical symptoms. The animal can take food and swallow it, but immediately vomits. The constriction of the cardia and pylorus not only interrupts the digestive tract, but also obstructs the blood vessels supplying the stomach and thus secretion and absorption cease. There is an enormous formation of gas in the stomach and the viscus becomes grossly distended (Fig. 306). The ribs are expanded outwards by the distended stomach and the epigastric region is tightly stretched, giving a tympanic note on percussion. The patient is very distressed and to lessen the feeling of pressure tries in vain to vomit the stomach contents. Palpation of the abdomen always reveals a marked enlargement of the spleen due to congestion. With such a clear picture of the disease X-ray examination is superfluous.

Treatment is immediate operation in an attempt to restore the position of the stomach. Delay results in disturbance of the nervous control (stimulation of the

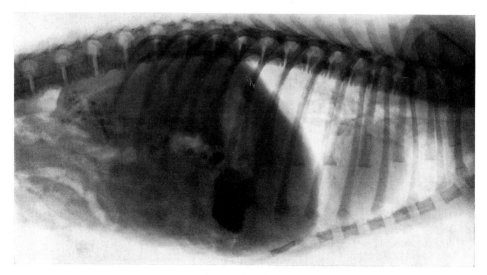

Fig. 307. A foreign body (a stone) in the intestine of a Poodle 10 weeks old.

vagus) because of venous stasis, and this may result in the death of the patient even after a successful operation. The secondary stasis in the spleen disappears immediately after the operation.

Technique of the Operation for the Rectification of Torsion of the Stomach. After extensive shaving and disinfection of the abdominal wall general anaesthesia is induced. After opening the abdomen along the linea alba, the distended stomach bulges tensely into the wound. Very often it is impossible to pass a hand between the stomach and the abdominal wall to the pylorus and so it is useful to make a flap incision on one side into the costal arch. The stomach cannot be returned to its normal position in its distended state so the gas must be relieved by puncture. A purse-string suture is inserted carefully into the thin stomach wall and a wide bore hypodermic needle is inserted in the centre of the suture, thus releasing the gas. After closing the suture 1 or 2 Lembert sutures are put in for added safety. When it is empty the stomach is replaced by drawing it in the direction of the diaphragm and then towards the vertebral column. When the bilateral constriction of the cardia and pylorus has been eliminated there is immediate relief of the signs of obstruction, provided that there has been no permanent damage to the blood vessels. To make sure that the obstruction has been removed, an assistant passes a sound into the stomach. Finally, the spleen is displaced to the left side so that a possible torsion of the spleen is also eliminated. The laparotomy wound is closed in the manner described on p. 281.

After-treatment consists of a mild fast for 2–3 days, glucose being given by the mouth. The owner should not allow his dog to jump, jumping down from a height being especially dangerous.

Ileus ventriculi and also **tumours** are rare and can be diagnosed only by accurate X-ray examination.

Foreign Bodies may be found in the stomach of the dog when indigestible objects are swallowed in games or retrieving. Usually, they are stones, or balls made of various materials such as metal, glass, wood, etc. Unusual objects (wrist-watches,

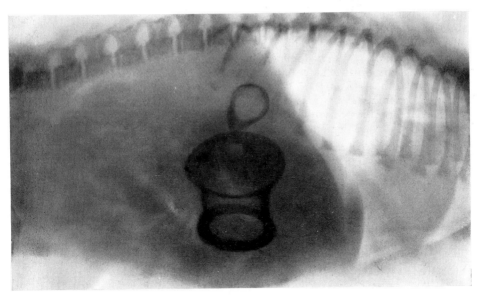

Fig. 308. Foreign bodies (rubber comforters) in the stomach of a Terrier puppy.

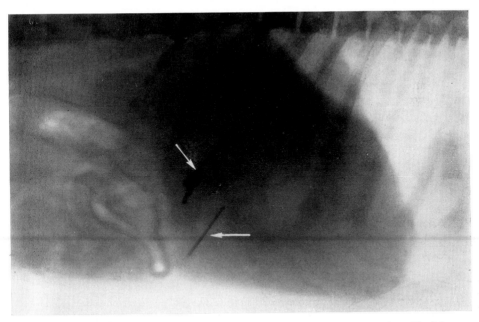

Fig. 309. Foreign bodies (safety pin and sewing needle) in the stomach of an Airedale.

children's comforters, safety pins, etc.) may also be swallowed by dogs (Figs. 307, 308, 309).

The clinical picture may be obscure. Usually, the suspicion that a foreign body is present arises from the history that the dog has been seen to swallow an object with which it often played, or that such an object is missing. Very often the dog is brought in with signs of gastritis. It often vomits a greenish-yellow mucus, its appetite is poor and sometimes it is apathetic. A foreign body in the stomach may be discovered accidentally by a general X-ray examination.

Diagnosis is by X-ray examination. Palpation of the stomach is possible only in lean dogs, because in well-nourished dogs the empty stomach does not reach the ventral abdominal wall and the liver is interposed between the stomach and the abdominal wall. By palpation one can only diagnose with certainty very large and relatively heavy foreign bodies, which, by virtue of their weight, drag the stomach to the floor of the abdomen.

Treatment. When there is a large foreign body in the stomach, delay is contra-indicated, because, if the foreign body passes on into the intestine, dangerous obstruction usually occurs. To remove the foreign body from the stomach four possible methods are available. The conservative method is to give emetics, giving the patient bulky food and then apomorphine hydrochloride (2–3 mg subcutaneously). This method can be helped by allowing the patient to keep its hindquarters raised. The second conservative method consists in giving the patient a pressure enema in such quantity that the fluid traverses the whole alimentary tract and is then vomited. With this method also it is recommended that the hindquarters be raised. These conservative methods may be successful but they are nevertheless uncertain.

The third possibility is the surgical one of gastrostomy, by which the foreign body is extracted through an opening into the stomach. A fourth method is available which we call a surgical-conservative method. By this method a suitable instrument is introduced into the stomach through the mouth; the foreign body is seized and extracted by this route. The method is surgical in so far as an extractor is used and the patient is under anaesthesia or analgesia, and it is conservative because no incision of tissue occurs. For this purpose we use Stadtler's ball extractor elongated to 60 or 90 cm.

Technique of Gastrostomy. After shaving and disinfecting the field of operation in the linea alba, the patient is fully anaesthetised and fixed lying on its back. The laparotomy incision is made into the linea alba in the region of the umbilicus, and it should be made as far as possible from the xiphoid process, so that if necessary the stomach can be drawn out of the wound. After division of the peritoneum the retroumbilical pad of fat must be divided. In order to achieve good approximation of the peritoneal layers when the wound is being closed later, it is recommended that the fatty tissue be immediately separated from the peritoneum (otherwise there is a risk of wound breakdown). The stomach is palpated with two fingers inserted into the wound or, in big breeds of dogs, with the whole hand. Heavy foreign bodies (stones, metal balls, etc.) lie in the depths (near the vertebral column) and light ones (rubber balls, pieces of wood) float in the gastric contents. If needles are sought for, the stomach must be palpated with 3 fingers. When located the foreign body is moved together with the stomach wall into the laparotomy wound and is lightly pinched off with a Doyen's intestinal clamp, so that the foreign body lies loosely in this pinched off sac. The gastrostomy incision should be made in a region poorly supplied with blood vessels, the vascular division between the larger and smaller curvature being the most suitable site. To prevent escape of gastric fluid into the abdomen when the stomach is opened,

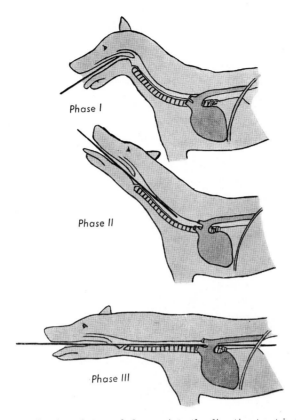

Phase I

Phase II

Phase III

Fig. 310. Introduction of stomach forceps into the digestive tract in 3 phases.

the clamped off portion is carefully brought out through the abdominal incision. The operator stretches the stomach wall over the foreign body with two fingers of one hand and divides it with a scalpel. The gastric mucosa is better opened with scissors after perforation with the knife. The foreign body can then be removed with dressing forceps. The wound is closed with 3 rows of sutures. First the mucosa is closed with a Schmieden suture, using a straight needle with a spring-eye. The suture is inserted from within outwards through both edges of the wound in turn (Fig. 335) so that the edges of the wound are respectively invaginated leaving a plaited pattern on completion of the suture. The second line of sutures includes the muscularis and serous coat and constitutes a running Schmieden suture. Finally, a third row of single sutures is inserted in the form of Lembert's invagination suture (Fig. 331). When the wound has been closed, the exposed portion of the stomach is cleaned and replaced in the abdomen. The intestinal clamp is removed as soon as possible after putting in the first Schmieden suture to avoid damage to the vessels of the stomach wall. The abdominal wound is closed in the manner described on p. 281.

Technique of the Conservative-Surgical Method. General anaesthesia is induced and the patient fixed on its side on the X-ray table. One assistant holds the head and another the animal itself. After inserting a suitable gag, the lubricated forceps is introduced under screen control through the gag in three stages into the digestive tract (Fig. 310). We direct the forceps first into the pharynx (stage 1) (Fig. 311). Then the assistant holding the head and neck stretches the head

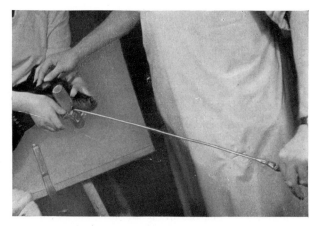

Fig. 311. Introduction of the stomach forceps through the mouth up to the pharynx.

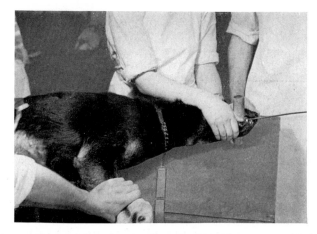

Fig. 312. The stomach forceps is introduced as far as the thoracic aperture with the head stretched
back.

back and the forceps can then slip further in as far as the thoracic opening (Fig. 312). The head
and neck are now lowered but still kept extended until the forceps has passed into the oesophagus and reach the stomach (Fig. 313) (third stage). It is not always easy to grasp the foreign
body. In order to seize it firmly the forceps should be pushed into the fundus with jaws extended.
This can be difficult if one tries to move the forceps; it is better if the assistant moves the head
and neck of the patient so that the forceps can be passively led on to the foreign body (Fig. 314).
It is advisable for the operator to grasp the foreign body through the abdominal wall with his
free hand, fixing it so that it can be gripped firmly with the forceps (Figs. 315, 316). With porous
foreign bodies or those that have a rough surface, the gastric mucosa often shows a tendency
to adhere firmly to the foreign body. In these cases under fluoroscopy one sees a clear zone
between the foreign body and the arm of the forceps. The foreign body can be shelled out of

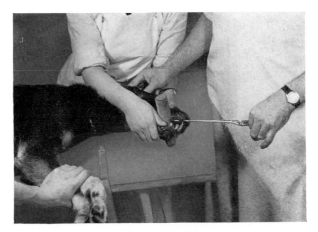

Fig. 313. With the head and neck stretched back the stomach forceps can be slid into the stomach.

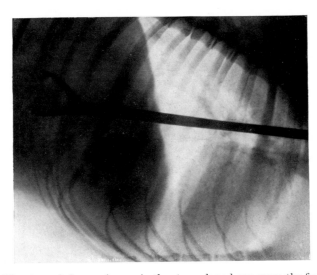

Fig. 314. The stomach forceps is now in the stomach and can grasp the foreign body.

the mucosa by opening and shutting the forceps. If this does not succeed the patient should be given some dilute contrast medium and this releases the foreign body from the mucosa. In cases in which it is not clear whether the foreign body still remains in the stomach or is in the first part of the intestine, it can be located by giving dilute contrast medium (Fig. 317). In the Stadtler ball extractor, the forceps arm, the mid-piece and the handle are firmly soldered together to form a straight whole, and the operator feels every small inequality of the foreign body despite a forceps length of 90 cm. When a stony or metal foreign body is touched a crepitation, similar to that felt in fractures, can be felt in the handle. This is a useful guide but it is not recommended that extraction be undertaken without control on the screen.

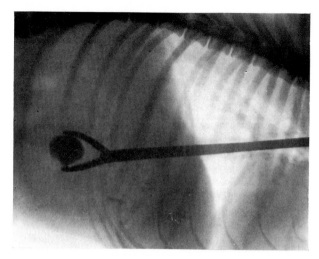

Fig. 315. The foreign body has been grasped.

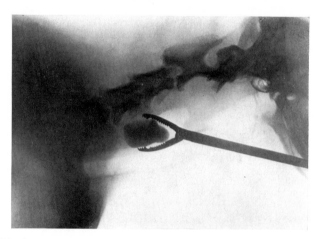

Fig. 316. Extraction of the foreign body through the oesophagus.

In dogs which have two foreign bodies or even one in the stomach and one in the intestine, the one in the stomach is extracted first followed by laparotomy (Fig. 318). This operation is simpler and quicker, because in the first place the laparotomy incision can be a half to two-thirds smaller and, in the second place, gastrotomy is omitted.

Extraction of the foreign body through the oesophagus is done by the same vibratory movements as those used in extraction of foreign bodies from the oesophagus described on p. 257.

After-treatment consists of fasting for 3 days during which the patient should take only a little water. For the next 5 days it is given only soft food. An antibiotic

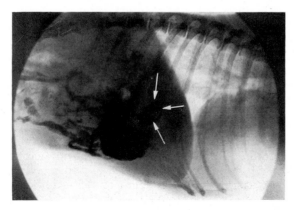

Fig. 317. A radiolucent foreign body in the stomach, which was made visible by the introduction of contrast medium.

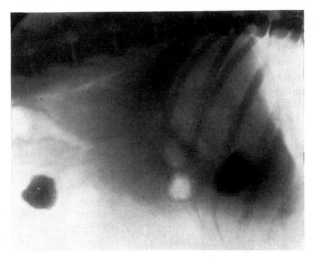

Fig. 318. Two foreign bodies in the stomach and intestine. The stone in the stomach was removed with forceps and the one in the intestine by enterostomy.

should be given only if the temperature rises above 39.5 °C. If the foreign body has been removed by the conservative-surgical method no after-treatment appears to be necessary.

Stenosis and Spasm of the Pylorus are rare. Stenosis of the pylorus is congenital and leads to hypertrophy of the circular muscle layer in the region of the pylorus. This is an instance, as it is in idiopathic spasm of the pylorus, of dysfunction of the vegetative nervous system. The hypertrophy of the circular muscle layer leads to reduction of the lumen of the pylorus and thus to various clinical symptoms.

18   Christoph, Diseases of Dogs

The history usually reveals that the puppies, soon after weaning, have shown constant, persistent vomiting (in pyloric stenosis) or inconstant, intermittent vomiting (in pylorospasm) immediately, or soon after taking food. In spite of a good appetite the nutritional and general conditions of the animals deteriorate. The clinical picture may be extremely variable, because all grades of the disease may occur from complete closure of the pylorus to slight spasms. The patients lag behind their age group in development and nutritional state. Usually there is dehydration due to the continued vomiting. X-ray examination with contrast medium is necessary to establish a diagnosis with certainty. The pylorus is markedly narrow, cordlike and longer than normal. If stenosis is present there is no change after doses of "TEAB" (see p. 254), or of an antispasmodic whereas spasm will be relieved by these drugs. Radiologically enlargement of the stomach is evident in every case. In the early stages of the condition there is marked peristalsis which later gives way to atony. The time required to empty the stomach is always increased (longer than 10 minutes).

Treatment of pylorospasm is conservative. Either "TEAB" (see p. 254) or an antispasmodic such as atropine derivatives, tricyclamol, etc., is given, the treatment being continued for a considerable time. In addition, attempts are made to improve the patient's general condition. The diet should be easily digestible, not too bulky, and given in frequent small quantities during the day. Possibly short-wave or microwave treatment is given. If this treatment gives no results after a certain time, surgery should be recommended.

Technique of the Operation. The patient is fully anaesthetised. The smallest possible laparotomy incision is made in the xiphoid region and the pyloric part of the stomach is drawn out of the wound. The laparotomy wound is covered with swabs and cloths. The operator holds the pylorus with the thumb and index finger and an incision is made through the serous coat of the hardened, hypertrophied pylorus. An assistant spreads apart the edges of the wound and the muscularis is incised until the mucosa is exposed. The mucosa must not be perforated. The longitudinal incision must be made so that the mucosa prolapses like a hernia over the whole length of the stenosis. Before the pylorus is put back into the abdomen, all haemorrhage must be controlled. To avoid adhesion to other abdominal organs, omentoplasty (see p. 283) may be performed. The laparotomy wound is closed in the usual way.

After-treatment is restricted to the care of the laparotomy wound and the improvement of the patient's general condition. If the mucosa has been accidentally perforated and closed with sutures, a 3-day fast should be ordered.

The classification of diseases of the gastro-intestinal tract has already been given (p. 258). It is not always easy to separate these exactly from one another, especially when there is a transition of one disease into another. Although a predominantly gastric disease expresses itself clinically in frequent yawning, retching, eructations, or in vomiting, usually, but not invariably, related to taking food, the symptoms of a disease chiefly of the intestine are rather different. In intestinal disease there is almost always diarrhoea, the consistency of the faeces is altered, they are pulpy or watery, sometimes frothy (fermentation) or contain blood. The anal region is soiled. One result of severe diarrhoea may be tenesmus and this may cause prolapse of the rectum. Peristalsis of the intestine is almost always increased and splashing sounds may be heard on auscultation of the abdomen. If there is catarrhal inflammation of the duodenum, obstructive jaundice may occur. High temperatures are sometimes observed only in infectious diseases (distemper, leptospirosis, etc.).

If the enteritis is chronic the patient's nutritional condition markedly deteriorates (cachexia), the skin loses its suppleness (hidebound) and the coat is dull and unkempt.

The causes of intestinal inflammation, when not due to infectious disease, are mostly bad feeding or eating indigestible substances. In addition one must consider parasites and diseases of other organs which can lead to secondary inflammation of the intestines.

Treatment. First, especially in acute catarrh, food is withheld for 1–2 days, only a little tea being given. For the succeeding days small quantities of oat gruel and minced raw meat are allowed. Milk, sugar and fats are contra-indicated. At the beginning of the treatment emptying of the gastro-intestinal tract with a purgative should be considered, castor oil (1–3 tablespoonsful) being best for this purpose. If the disease is localised in the rectum, dihydroxyanthra quinone (0.15–3.0 g) is given, and flushing out the intestine is recommended. In addition to medicinal charcoal in adequate dosage in the form of a powder or tablets, other drugs which are absorbent, or antibacterial, or inhibit fermentation are used. Tannin albuminate (3–6 tablets) or opium may be prescribed. Silver nitrate pills have a good astringent effect.

In chronic intestinal catarrh, the diet must be carefully controlled in addition to the treatments described above. Small quantities of food are offered frequently during the day. Bones are contra-indicated. Good results have followed the administration of a concentrated decoction of oak bark several times daily. If one thinks it advisable to employ chemotherapy, sulphonamides such as phthalyl-sulphathiazole may be given in a dose of 0.1 g/kg bodyweight daily. The antibiotics streptomycin, neomycin and frumycetin may be given orally.

Obstipation of the intestine (coprostasis) occurs relatively often as a result of taking too large quantities of food, but it is not always caused by a faulty or unbalanced diet. In old male dogs it may be due to prostatic hypertrophy, the hypertrophied prostate narrowing the intestine so that the faeces are obstructed (Fig. 444). The diameter of the pelvis may have been narrowed as the result of fractures (Fig. 495) and this may produce obstruction to the faeces. In such patients obstipation is avoided by regulation of the diet (giving fats). Constipation is also to be expected if stenoses occur as the result of operations. After enterotomy narrowing of the gut may result from the suture technique. If, during the following months, the patient is fed on indigestible food, obstructions occur anterior to the suture site causing dilatation of this part of the intestine (Fig. 319). Portions of food remain in the dilated part of the intestine and ultimately obstipation results.

In badly cared for young dogs the so-called "false obstipation" may be seen, due to matting together of the hairs around the anus so that the animal cannot pass faeces. Removal of the matted hair quickly relieves the apparent obstruction.

Clinically there is a slightly distended abdomen and the patient frequently prepares to pass faeces without result. If the obstipation has existed for only a short time, bimanual palpation causes the patient to contract the abdominal muscles as an expression of pain. Later the abdomen is relaxed, so that the obstructed mass can be felt as a firm, thick cord. X-ray examination reveals the obstruction, which chiefly contains bones (Fig. 320).

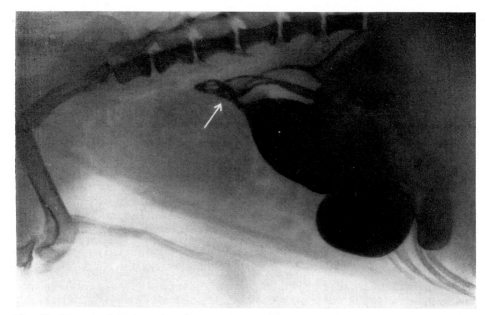

Fig. 319. Stenosis of the intestine after enterostomy. The dog was not restricted in diet following operation so that the food was dammed up in part of the cicatrix and this led to a repetition of the symptoms of ileus.

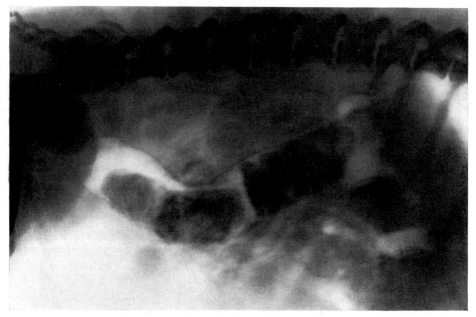

Fig. 320. Coprostasis.

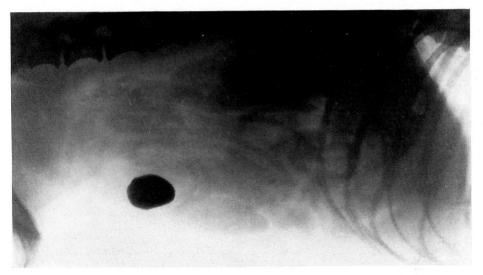

Fig. 321. Foreign body (slag stone) in the intestine of a Pomeranian.

Treatment is by pressure enemas of 100–250 ml of paraffin oil as mentioned earlier. As purgatives, castor oil and dihydroxyanthraquinone are used. If these methods do not succeed, with the patient under epidural anaesthesia, Stadtler's ball extractor is introduced through the rectum, in order to break up the bony material in the rectum. It is advisable to relieve the obstipation gradually over several days in order not to overstrain the patient. Removal of the impacted mass by enterostomy should only be attempted if the measures outlined are unsuccessful.

If a fairly large foreign body has passed from the stomach into the intestine and caused **Ileus** (Intestinal obstruction) very pronounced symptoms may be evident. The most striking clinical signs are summarised by the expression "foreign body triad" and consist of:

1. Loss of appetite
2. Vomiting
3. Cessation of defaecation.

In addition, there may be apathy. Sometimes the patients seek out cool places and adopt the "praying attitude", going down on the forelimbs with hindquarters raised, in order to reduce pressure on the abdominal wall. Palpation shows that the musculature up to the beginning of the ileus is very painful and tense. If the ileus has existed for some time, i. e. 1½ to 3 days, the musculature is relaxed. At this time the abdomen may be successfully palpated and the foreign body detected manually. If X-rays are available the diagnosis can be readily confirmed (Figs. 321 and 322). Foreign bodies which are permeable to X-rays (fruit stones, nuts, wood, leather, fabrics, artificial gut (sausage casing), glass, rubber, etc.) also occur in the intestine. When there is complete obstruction, gas, secretion and food

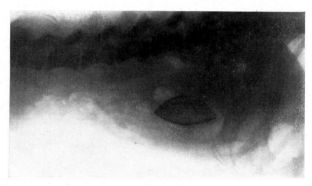

Fig. 322. Compressed ball in intestine.

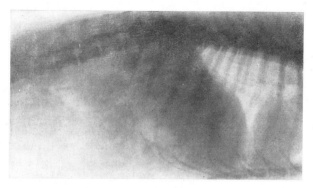

Fig. 323. Large collection of gas in the small intestine; no foreign body can be detected.

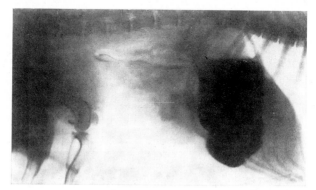

Fig. 324. Barium meal, 30 minutes after administration. The contrast medium is beginning to pass from the stomach into the intestine. In the stomach sedimentation of the contrast medium is already beginning.

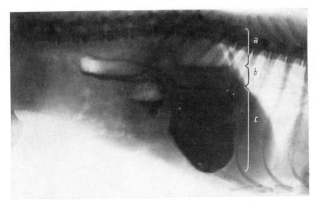

Fig. 325. Barium meal 45 minutes after administration. The contrast medium is passing out of the stomach into the intestine and has already sedimented in the stomach. (a) gas bubble; (b) gastric juice with contrast medium in it; (c) sedimented contrast medium.

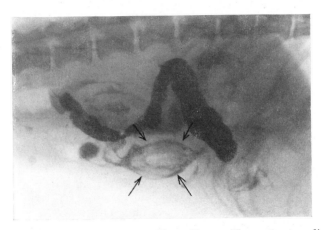

Fig. 326. A foreign body (peach stone) permeable to X-rays. The contrast medium has become deposited in thin streaks over the foreign body, rendering it visible.

collect in the early stage in the section of the intestine anterior to the obstruction. When the ileus is of longer standing a more or less well marked paralysis of the gut appears. X-ray examination reveals collections of gas where it is not normally present, namely in the small intestine (Fig. 323). As a rule, gas in the small intestine shows as a number of individual pockets of gas, whilst gas in the large intestine more or less collects together. When there is gas in the small intestine one must consider the differential diagnosis between aerophagy, fermentation dyspepsia, and atrophy of the mucosa of the small intestine due to severe inanition. These diseases may be eliminated by giving a contrast medium by the mouth to show there is no obstruction. If there is an obturation ileus caused by a foreign body

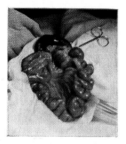

Fig. 327. Ileus due to swallowing string, the knotted end of which had remained in the stomach and peristalsis had caused the small intestine to string itself on the foreign body like a strand of beads. Ultimately intussusception of the small intestine occurred (at the back of the picture).

permeable to X-rays, the contrast medium does not pass as far as the foreign body, but remains in the first loops of the intestine creating a typical picture (Fig. 324). Gas collects at the uppermost point of the small intestine loop. Usually this is limited by a horizontal line over a mobile fluid shadow, this, in turn, being delineated against the darker shadow of the contrast medium (Fig. 325).

Foreign body ileus due to swallowing string or pieces of fabric is rare. Peristalsis causes a large part of the small intestine to wrap itself round the foreign body. Palpation reveals a firm cord giving rise to a suspicion of intussusception (Fig. 327).

Treatment. Conservative methods such as giving paraffin oil by the mouth and rectum may be tried. Purgatives should be given only if there are no obvious signs of an ileus, or if X-rays have shown that the spatial extent of the foreign body in the intestine will not lead to obstruction, or if it can be determined with certainty that the foreign body lies in the colon. If there are marked symptoms of ileus one should not delay surgical interference. It is of no consequence what part of the intestine contains the foreign body, because we can digitally palpate the whole alimentary canal through a laparotomy incision in the linea alba.

Technique of Laparotomy in the Linea alba. To prepare for the operation the skin in the region of the proposed abdominal incision is shaved and cleansed with the utmost care, the hair around the shaved area being well moistened and combed aside. The anaesthetic is selected according to the extent of the operation to be done. In most cases lumbo-sacral epidural anaesthesia is used for the abdominal region. Finally, the patient is tied down on its back. An undocked tail must also be fixed to the operation table and in male dogs the prepuce is clamped with a Doyen's ovarian forceps. The operation field is cleansed and defatted with ether and iodised, the aim being to apply a protective layer on the incompletely aseptic skin and also to dry it off completely. The surgical team scrub up with soap and hot water containing a strong solution of antiseptic, washing the hands and forearms for about 10 minutes. The mechanical cleansing reduces the bacterial infection of the skin which is augmented by a final wash in 1 % solution of sublimate. Meanwhile the instruments required are sterilised for 15 minutes in a steam steriliser. The scalpels and scissors are put for 30 minutes in synthetic n-propyl alcohol as steam sterilisation blunts them. The instruments are put on the instrument table only when the patient and surgeons are ready.

The surgeon and his assistants spread the surgical drapes concertina-wise over the patient in such a way that the slit in the drape lies over the linea alba. The drape measures 85 × 95 cm. In the middle, parallel to its longer side, an incision 30 cm long is made. The skin at the caudal angle of the slit in the drape is clamped off near the symphysis and its cranial angle near the sternum (according to the size of the patient). In male dogs the incision is ended in front of the prepuce. Now the outer skin is divided with the scalpel for about 5–8 cm over the linea alba. The edges of the skin wound and of the borders of the slit in the drape are brought together with two clamps each. The two clamps on the towels at the caudal and cranial angles of the slit in the towel are moved back to the cranial and caudal angles of the wound. The wound is thus completely

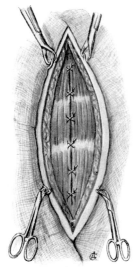

Fig. 328. Closure of the laparotomy wound with Sultan's diagonal suture.

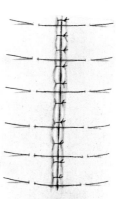

Fig. 329. Relaxation stitches inserted over the skin suture.

uncovered. The surgeon cuts first through the subcutaneous fat and, if the linea alba has been directly incised, through the connective tissue of the sheath of the rectus muscle. If the incision is beside the linea alba (paramedian) first the layer of the outer rectus sheath and the inner layer of the rectus sheath must be divided. Any bleeding is controlled with Pean's forceps. The peritoneum now appears and is grasped by the surgeon and assistants with forceps and an incision about 1 cm long is made in it. Finally, the peritoneum is fixed with one peritoneal clamp on the left side and one on the right. The wound is carefully enlarged with blunt-ended scissors, under the guidance of the index finger of the free hand to protect the underlying viscera. At each wound angle the peritoneum is again fixed with a peritoneal clamp. The retro-umbilical fat is cut off short with the greatest care and the wound is covered with strips of sterile gauze.

Closure of the laparotomy wound is done with Sultan's diagonal suture. This suture includes all the layers of the abdominal wall (peritoneum, inner layer of the rectus sheath, the rectus abdominalis muscle and the outer layer and its sheath). Care should be taken not to leave it too loose or to tie it off too tightly. The suture material may be silk, nylon or catgut (Fig. 328). Instead of the Sultan's diagonal suture each layer (peritoneum, muscle and fascia) of a paramedian incision may be closed separately with interrupted stitches or a continuous suture. If fatty tissue is included in the suture of the peritoneum it may lead to a hernia through the scar. After removal of the lateral clamps on the cloths the skin is closed with stitches tied off, the assistant making a ridge under each stitch with two forceps. These stitches are iodised. In male dogs which cannot have a bandage, because it would become soiled with urine, a relaxation suture is inserted. In bitches this is done only if there is some discrepancy between the circumference of the chest and abdomen so that the bandage tends to slip (Fig. 329). In such cases a strip bandage (Fig. 71) may be applied. In the relaxation suture 2–6 stitches are put in widely separated from the wound. The ends of the stitches are grasped on the one hand by an assistant and on the other by the surgeon. Now a strip of gauze is pulled through from the caudal end over the skin sutures and under the relaxation stitches to the cranial end which is drawn under the stitches. This is removed on the 3rd day after the operation and the skin stitches are removed on the 6th to the 8th day according to circumstances.

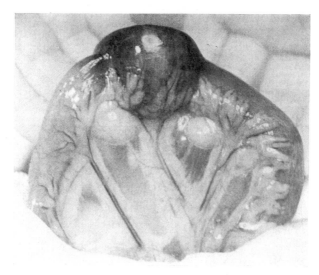

Fig. 330. A foreign body (a stone) in the intestine of a dog brought out through the abdominal incision.

Sometimes a few days after the operation, wound dehiscence occurs. This may be due to variable absorbability of the catgut used, to poor technique in putting in the suture, or to an individual idiosyncracy of the dog's tissues.

Clinically there is prolapse of the omentum or in severe cases of the intestinal loops. Commencement of the breakdown is indicated by a marked, watery and odourless flow of secretion (peritoneal fluid) from the wound. Careful palpation of the wound confirms the diagnosis.

Treatment consists of immediate repetition of the operation (under anaesthesia). The wound area is carefully cleaned up and any sutures still remaining are removed. Prolapsed abdominal contents are cleansed and irrigated with warm physiological saline and replaced in the abdomen. The edges of the wound are scraped with a sharp spoon and re-sutured. As a prophylactic against peritonitis, it is recommended that a sufficient quantity of an antibiotic be instilled into the abdominal cavity and, in addition to this, a sterile gauze drain about 2 m long is put into the abdominal cavity. This drain is removed during the next 4 days. The second closure of the wound after such breakdown usually heals by primary intention.

Technique of Enterostomy. Lumbo-sacral epidural anaesthesia is used. Laparotomy is performed as described above (p. 280), the incision into the abdominal wall being kept as small as possible. It should be large enough to allow two fingers to be easily inserted into the abdominal cavity. The omentum is deflected cranially with the index finger. If the intestine can be freely palpated with the finger, the foreign body is sought. Usually, because of its weight, it lies deep in the abdomen. The part of the intestine containing the foreign body is brought with the bent finger to the wound and, as far as is possible, a piece of normal intestine is drawn through the wound. By means of a light pull on the intestine and with the help of the index finger, the foreign body is brought forward (Fig. 330). If the foreign body cannot be found in this way it is necessary to pull out a piece of intestine and, if it is a normal portion, to reflect it cranially. If it is distended and altered

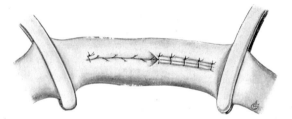

Fig. 331. Lembert's seromuscular suture with a Schmieden suture under it.

intestine, it is drawn out caudally until the foreign body appears. If the diagnosis has been made only by palpation it is essential to palpate the whole alimentary canal in this way in order to find a possible second foreign body which has escaped palpation. The part of the intestine containing the foreign body is brought out of the wound and the remainder of the intestine replaced. The contents of the exteriorised intestine are massaged cranially and caudally until about 5–7 cm on each side of the foreign body are empty and an intestinal clamp is lightly applied. If it is impossible to massage the foreign body into a healthy part of the gut, one should at least try to displace it cranially, because there the changes in the gut have abated somewhat relatively to those at the site of the foreign body. An assistant holds the gut with the index fingers and thumbs of both hands, the abdominal cavity is protected by swabs and the surgeon cuts down parallel to the gut on to the foreign body. The incision must be long enough to enable the foreign body to be extracted without force. It is extracted with Pean's forceps by pressure on the insertion of the mesentery, and removed wrapped in sterile swabs. The gut is closed with a Schmieden suture after the intestine and its mucosa have been cleaned as much as possible. Schmieden's suture is a continuous one and is inserted with a straight needle taking in the whole wall of the gut from the mucosa, i.e., from the lumen of the gut outwards (Fig. 335). This suture brings together the edges of the incision and at the same time invaginates them so that serous membrane is apposed to serous membrane. When the gut incision has been closed, the intestinal clamps are immediately removed and the intestine is lightly compressed on both sides of the incision by assistants. The closed wound is cleansed with physiological saline. The surgeon washes his hands again and with fresh instruments inserts over the Schmieden suture a Lembert's seromuscular suture (Fig. 331). An omentoplasty is applied to the gut wound and is fixed cranially and caudally with a situation suture. The gut is replaced in the abdomen and the intestinal loops are covered with omentum, the omentum previously reflected cranially being pulled back with the index finger. The laparotomy incision is closed in the manner described on p. 281. Before the last suture is tied off, a large quantity of physiological saline is put into the abdominal cavity with a glass funnel, in order to compensate for the loss of fluid and salt.

After-treatment consists of fasting for 3 days, during which time the patient is given drinking water containing a high percentage of glucose. The purpose of this is to convert the toxic products of putrefaction in the gut, indol and skatol, into harmless glucuronic acid. If there is no defaecation during the days after the operation, a cautiously increased intake soon brings about the desired result. Support of the circulation during the post-operative period is obviously necessary. As a result of the stenosis produced in the intestine, the patient is put on a diet (no bones, no sinewy meat) for 6–9 months after the operation. After this time the stenosis has become adjusted, so that a normal diet can be given.

One often reads in the literature that when there are marked changes in the intestine caused by obturation ileus, resection of a limited section of the intestine should be done. In our clinic, procedures of this kind have always had poor results. If one remembers the pathological and physiological processes which go on in the obturated intestine, these poor results are easily explained, since the whole afferent section of the intestine is altered, so that one must do a resection immediately behind the pylorus. The pathological and physiological changes caused by obturation ileus on the intestine have still not been fully investigated. The obturated intestine at first shows only local superficial changes as the blood supply is not markedly impaired, and these are completely reversible if the obstruction is relieved without delay. In the early stages of obturation they are restricted to slight changes at the site of the obturation itself: slight oedema indicates an inflammatory reaction chiefly in the subserous tissue. The serous coat tends to lose its shiny gloss and after a short time the pathological changes may be very marked. General stimulation of the local nerves causes much increased peristalsis and this soon results in hypertrophy. Accumulations of gas and fluid act as stimuli anterior to the site of obstruction, as also do the increasingly obstructed intestinal contents and there are always toxic and bacterial stimuli. Likewise, hyperaemia can be noted behind the stoppage. Further, as the result of dilatation of the blood vessels and consequent slowing of the blood flow, severe venous stasis ensues which gives the intestinal loops a cyanotic colour. The marked excess of blood damages the nerves of the blood vessels so that complete paralysis of the vessels occurs. This is critical for the fate of the section of the intestine concerned, because intestinal musculature responds to the failure of the arterial blood supply by loss of peristaltic power and gradual complete paralysis. Meanwhile, the marked accumulation of gas and fluid in the intestine, which previously acted as an additional stimulant to increased muscular activity, now acts as a motor relaxant of the obturated part of the intestine. Most of the fluid in the small intestine is derived from a greatly increased secretion of intestinal juice by the stimulated mucosa of the intestine and the large digestive glands. This causes abundant transudation into the lumen of the intestine which is accentuated by the damaging effect of marked dilatation and persistent hyperaemia. On the other hand, absorption in the section of the intestine is markedly reduced or even suspended from the beginning of the stoppage. This interference with compensating absorption leads to a dangerous lack of water in the body, but in the intestine itself to a persistent increase of its contents. The congestion and irritative effect of the gut contents quickly extends to the whole intestine, so that the normal absorptive mechanism of the gut is soon markedly upset. There is constant interaction of marked stasis – circulatory disorders – decreased absorption – marked stimulation of the intestinal wall by decomposition products – increases of the motor and secretory functions. Simultaneously, the decomposition of the gut contents in front of the stoppage involves the development of quantities of gas, the amount of which depends on the relationship between the formation of gas and its absorption and to a small extent on the "gas circulation" and the expulsion of gas through the rectum. The rapid accumulation of gas in obturation ileus may be understood if one remembers that normally 9/10ths of the gases in the intestine are eliminated by the lungs after absorption into the blood. Thus the breakdown of the circulation in the intestinal blood vessels causes distension of the gut, whilst on the other hand tympanites damages the blood vessels by reduction of absorption and so leads to circulatory failure. The overdistension of the gut wall by gas must have

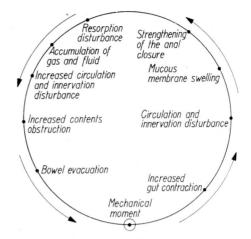

Fig. 332. The vicious circle in Ileus.

a damaging and paralysing effect on the nervous apparatus of the musculature. Many authors consider that the distension of the gut wall due to stasis of the gas and gut contents is the direct cause of all the pathological-physiological symptoms of stoppage of the gut.

Finally, toxic effects produce severe changes in the obturated part of the intestine. Toxic substances may arise as residual products of chemo-physical, fermentative and bacterial decomposition of the intestinal contents or as metabolic products of luxuriant bacterial growth. Since release per rectum is impossible, a favourable prerequisite for the development of a bacterial flora exists, which brings about decomposition of fluids that are most readily broken down. Protein decomposition and carbohydrate fermentation take place on the one hand, and on the other, new products are formed by the bacteria which with their metabolic products accentuate each other. The transudate affords a specially favourable medium for the bacteria, and is at first sero-haemorrhagic and odourless, but becomes foul, stinking and eventually purulent after bacterial decomposition. These toxic products also first stimulate and then tend to paralyse the peristalsis of the gut. The toxic substances attack the mucosa and the damaged gut wall, causing thrombosis which exposes the affected area of mucosa to necrosis.

All these changes may have occurred in a few hours. The stimuli may vary in severity, they abate after the intestinal reactions occur, and to a certain extent there is compensation of the intestinal dysfunction for a varying period of time.

The statements hitherto made about the processes in the occluded intestine relate to acute stoppage of the small intestine and are more typical of its physiological-pathological changes and reaction than obstruction of the large intestine. In the dog in large intestine obstruction the main finding is disturbance of defaecation in the form of coprostasis (Fig. 312). All the phenomena which we encounter as violent reactions in the small intestine occur only slowly by transference to the large intestine. The damage to the gut wall is significantly less severe than that in the small intestine, because the large intestine is not so sensitive and is more resistant to inflammatory change. The schema (Fig. 332) of the vicious circle established in ileus summarises the complex interacting processes in the obturated intestine. In the loops of the intestine, below the obstruction, there is a gradual

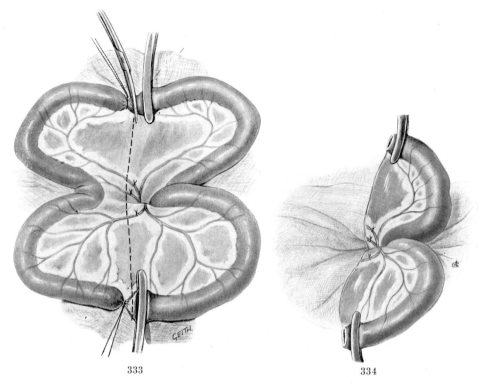

Fig. 333. The part of the gut to be resected is isolated and may be excised.

Fig. 334. The part of the gut to be resected is excised.

emptying and then by loss of tone and turgor, a slow collapse and finally complete stoppage of the intestinal function. In spite of the enormous engorgement of the mesenteric blood vessels these parts of the intestine are only poorly supplied with blood and look pale. After the removal of the obstruction, the intestine below the block is immediately capable of receiving material and quickly recovers its full function, so the inertia must be ascribed to the lack of intestinal contents and their stimulation of the gut wall. Absorption and an increased secretion in the afferent portion of the gut have been observed and it is concluded that these changes are the result of a general body response and extension into the gut far removed from the actual site of obstruction. Obturation ileus has a toxic effect on the whole organism which may become intensified quite rapidly and cause death. This toxic effect is manifested in circulatory dysfunction, respiratory disabilities, etc., and also reflex effects and anaemic changes in the brain leading to exhaustion and failure of the vital brain centres, primarily the vasomotor centre. As a result of the engorgement of the mesenteric blood vessels there is a very much weaker peripheral blood supply. The marked dehydration of the body, which develops as a result of the increased intestinal secretion and simultaneous

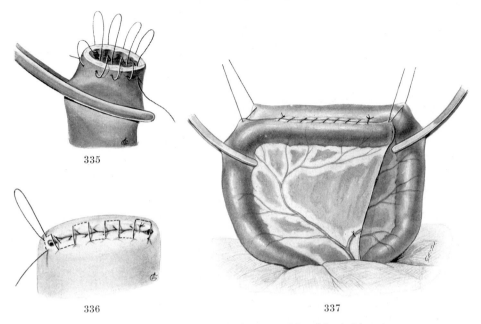

335

336

337

Fig. 335. Closure of the intestinal stump with a Schmieden suture.

Fig. 336. Blendinger's seromuscular suture.

Fig. 337. The posterior seromuscular suture as the first suture in making the anastomosis.

decline of absorption and also possibly persistent vomiting, leads to increased viscosity of the blood, a fall in the blood pressure and decreased secretion of urine.

Intussusception of the Intestine is rare, and occurs mainly in puppies heavily infected with worms. By the time the animal is presented it is often too late for effective treatment. In severe gastroenteritis intussusception occurs as a result of increased peristalsis, the enteritis of distemper being especially liable to cause the invagination. On palpation one finds in the abdomen a fleshy, cylindrical and movable strand. If the invagination is in the rectum it may be possible to detect it digitally per rectum. Sometimes the intussusception proceeds so far that the invaginated bowel protrudes from the anus.

Treatment consists of trying to correct the invagination manually. Laparotomy is performed (see p. 280) and an attempt is made to massage the afferent part of intestine from the efferent part. The invaginated part of the intestine is tremendously swollen as a result of venous stasis (Fig. 327). The portion of intestine into which invagination has occurred is grasped at the end of the invagination and gentle traction is applied to the afferent bowel in an attempt to draw out the invaginated section. Complications appear at the point where the intestine was invaginated, particularly if there are considerable adhesions to the mesentery. As the intestine is very friable, as a result of venous stasis, we perform enterectomy with a laterolateral anastomosis. End-to-end and the side-to-end anastomoses are not suitable for the dog.

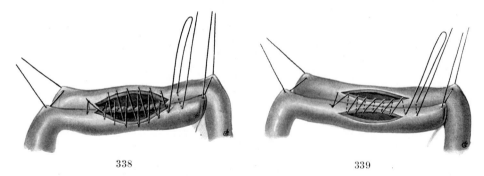

338   339

Fig. 338. Closing the posterior wound edges with a continuous suture as the second suture in making the anastomosis.

Fig. 339. Closure of the anterior wound edges with a Schmieden suture as the third suture in making the anastomosis.

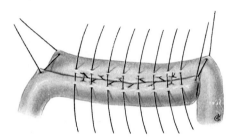

Fig. 340. The anterior seromuscular Lembert suture as the fourth suture in making the anastomosis.

Technique of Enterectomy with Latero-lateral Anastomosis. After laparotomy (see p. 280) the portion of intestine to be resected is withdrawn from the abdomen. The surgeon now ties off the affected part of the gut with catgut loops and fixes the respective ends of the loops with artery forceps. The mesenteric blood vessels leading to the part of the gut to be resected are also tied off with catgut. After massaging away the gut contents, an intestinal clamp is applied to the gut remaining in the body at about 3 cm from the catgut loop (Fig. 333). Now the isolated part of the gut can be removed with scissors. In order that gut contents shall not contaminate the abdominal cavity, swabs are placed under and over the sites of the incisions. The mesentery is cut off as short as possible. The mesenteric vessels are divided distally to the ligatures (Fig. 334). The two stumps are closed with a Schmieden suture (Fig. 335) and a Blendinger seromuscular suture is added (Fig. 336). The intestinal clamps can now be removed and reapplied at about 7–12 cm (according to the size of the patient) from the ends of the stumps, after repeated swabbing out of the contents from the stumps. The freed portions of the gut are placed isoperistaltically at a distance of 5–10 cm from each other and secured with fixation sutures. The continuous suture to be inserted should be about 3–6 cm long (Fig. 337). Both parts of the gut are now incised for about 2–4 cm parallel to one another and the posterior edges of the wound are closed with a continuous deep suture (mucosa, muscularis, and serous coat) (Fig. 338). The anterior edges of the wound are brought together with a Schmieden suture (Fig. 339). The intestinal clamps are

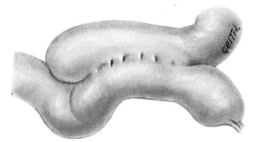

Fig. 341. Specimen of a gut anastomosis 26 days after the operation.

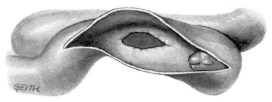

Fig. 342. View of the actual anastomosis 26 days after the operation.

removed and the anastomosis washed with physiological saline. During the operation, the whole section of the gut must be irrigated with physiological saline to guard against drying. An anterior Lembert's button (interrupted) suture is inserted over the Schmieden suture (Fig. 340). After the fixation sutures have been removed, an extensive omentoplasty is applied and the rejoined intestine is replaced in the abdomen. A suture to unite the mesentery does not seem to be essential. The abdominal wound is closed in the manner described on p. 281.

After-treatment is similar to that described on p. 283. If it has been possible to correct the invagination manually, the gut must be rendered quiescent with opium preparations in order to prevent a second invagination.

According to some workers isoperistaltic anastomosis in man should slowly compensate itself in time, the ends of the stumps showing atrophy due to inactivity, so that the gut recovers it former shape. Probably some years are required for this process. It had not yet occurred in a postmortem preparation of ours that was 197 days old (Fig. 343). In our experiments suture ridges were interesting. Investigations of these have shown that these ridges did not project into the intestinal lumen and that whilst the slight stenosis at the site of the operation persisted, the suture ridges were completely extroverted. This is the rationale behind the directions on p. 283 to keep a dog on a diet for 6–9 months after enterectomy, because after this time one can presume that the stenosis caused by the operation will have been eliminated. The specimen in Fig. 341 shows on the 26th day some elevations at the site of the suture which are sutures encapsulated in the tissues. This shows that even after 26 days there is a tendency of the introverted ridge to flatten itself out as a result of the powerful pressure in the intestinal tube. In Fig. 342, a view of the actual anastomosis, no trace of this can be seen. In Fig. 343 the anastomosis has been in existence for 197 days. Here it is evident that the wound edges invaginated when the anastomosis was made are again

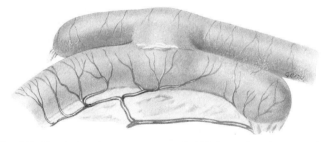

Fig. 343. Specimen of a gut anastomosis 197 days after the operation.

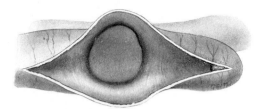

Fig. 344. View of the actual anastomosis 197 days after the operation.

completely restored. Figure 344 confirms this. There is also no sloughing of the wound ridge into the gut lumen.

Figure 345 shows the histological structure 4 days after Schmieden and Lembert sutures. It can be seen that the "Perlon" thread lies in the tissue with almost no reaction round it. The connective tissue in the deeper layers of the mucosa extends into the depth of the invagination ridge and curves round at its tip. There is leucocytic infiltration in the base of the ridge near the "Perlon" thread and in the immediate neighbourhood of the reflection of the mucosa. In addition, round cell infiltrations, partly interspersed with eosinophil cells, lie round the circumference of the central necrosis indicated at (e). From these the cell accumulation extends in the direction of (b). At (d) the tissue seems to be little damaged. The nuclei of the connective tissue fibres do not take up stain and show commencing necrobiosis. The original sectioning lay at (b) in the direction of (e). Evidently, the histological section has been made so that it includes the area in which the edges of the mucosa are fully in contact after the Schmieden suture was inserted. Here we see healing by primary intention.

Figure 346 shows a histological section of the anterior suture of a latero-lateral anastomosis. The suture ridge has not been shed into the gut lumen, but, after absorption of the central necrosis, the blood supply was restricted by insertion of the suture and the insufficient blood supply associated with it, the mucosa was drawn apart in approximately the original position. Scar formation with considerable cell infiltration is seen macroscopically at (a) as a contraction and the mucosa is seen to be richly infiltrated with cells at its base around the former section. Regeneration of the circular muscles (c) has not yet occurred. The suture was inserted along a line from (a) to (b).

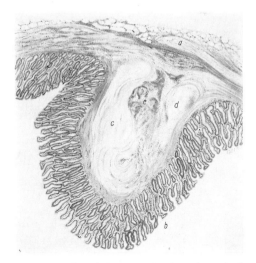

Fig. 345. Histological section of a Schmieden and Lembert intestinal suture 4 days after the operation.

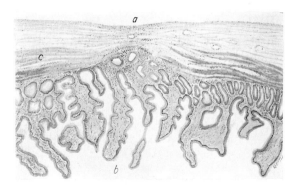

Fig. 346. Histological section of the anterior suture of a latero-lateral anastomosis after 197 days.

In **Prolapse of the Rectum** it is necessary to distinguish between **Prolapse of the Anus** and **Prolapse of the Rectum**. Sometimes there may be an intussusception at the same time as prolapse of the rectum. The cause of such prolapses may be due on the one hand to weakness of the sphincter, and on the other to enteritis, or severe constipation causing tenesmus.

Clinically if only the terminal part is prolapsed (prolapse of the anus), a rounded bluish-red protrusion appears at the anus. In other cases a cylindrical sausage of the same colour protrudes (Fig. 347). The mucosa can always be identified on the surface of the protrusion. If the condition has existed for some time, the surface looks stretched and shiny and in some cases one finds ulcer-like patches and necrosis. Defaecation, if not impossible, is made difficult in all cases.

19*

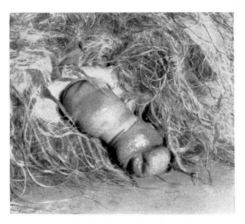

Fig. 347. Prolapse of the rectum.

Treatment may be given in various ways. The simplest method is to replace the prolapsed intestine by pressure with moist cold compresses under epidural anaesthesia. A purse-string suture is then inserted at the anus and the intestine rendered quiescent with opium preparations. The suture is removed after 4–5 days. During this time the knots should be undone twice a day to allow defaecation and very little, easily digestible food is given.

If this is not successful, rectopaxy may be performed. A laparotomy incision is made in the lower third of the abdomen and the rectum is drawn cranially until the prolapse is eliminated. The rectum is fixed to the abdominal wall with sero-muscular sutures after scarification of the peritoneum at the point of attachment in order to produce a quicker adhesion. We have had little success with this method. Resection of the rectum is the most reliable technique and we prefer the following method. The patient is tied down on its side under epidural anaesthesia (Fig. 32). A gauze tampon is inserted in the rectum. A piece of the prolapsed intestine is pulled out of the anus so that the resection can be done on as much healthy intestine as possible. The external intestinal wall is divided and sutured to the internal wall with closely placed sutures. The blood vessels of the mesocolon are ligatured separately, otherwise haemorrhage into the abdominal cavity may occur.

Another method is to insert a cruciform stitch with a straight needle. The prolapsed gut is stitched as near as possible to the point of eversion and then the prolapsed gut is removed at some distance from the suture. The gut is thus fixed at 4 points and may now be joined up with closely placed sutures.

After-treatment consists of a fast for 3 days and on succeeding days as little food as possible is given.

Inflammation of the Anal Sac often occurs in the dog. These sacs lie on both sides of the anus and in defaecation passively empty their secretion into the faeces. If the regular evacuation of this secretion no longer occurs because of soft faeces, the retained secretion becomes inspissated and inflammation results.

Clinically this condition is shown by licking of the anus, clamping down of the tail, sudden sitting down and the so-called tobogganing. The itching or pain at the anus causes the patient to rub the anus on the ground, the hind limbs being brought forward between the forelimbs and then the hinder parts are dragged along the ground. Palpation of the anal sacs with a finger introduced into the anus reveals taut distension of both sacs. If the condition exists for a long time, one of the anal sacs may rupture and a fistula develops, the opening of which constantly enlarges.

Treatment in mild cases consists of frequent manual emptying of sacs. The index finger is introduced into the anus and the sac is carefully emptied by pressure from the outside with the thumb, resulting in a stinking grey to yellowish, pasty secretion appearing from the anal opening. If the inflammation is severe the anal sac should be filled with antibiotic solution. In advanced or recurrent cases destruction of the glandular tissue must be attempted. This may be accomplished by instillations of iodine, the instillations being given initially 3 times daily at 3-day intervals, using Lugol's solution, and later once a week using tincture of iodine. In order to fill the anal sacs the patient is placed on its side and the tail pulled forwards over the back so that the anal orifice protrudes. One can now distinguish laterally two small openings about 2–3 mm, anterior to the skin–mucosal junction, which are the orifices of the anal sacs. A fine blunt ended cannula is carefully introduced into these and the sacs are filled with the solution.

If fistulation occurs the sacs are irrigated with antibiotics or tincture of iodine through the fistula opening. At this time one should aim for the production of a soft stool and the frequency of defaecation should be limited by scanty feeding to reduce irritation in the inflamed area. The tail may be drawn to one side by a bandage attached to the collar to allow better ventilation of the anal region.

If these conservative methods are not successful extirpation of the anal sacs must be considered.

Technique of Extirpation of the Anal Sacs. After shaving, cleansing and disinfection of the anal region the patient is restrained on its side (Fig. 32) or on its abdomen under epidural anaesthesia. The dog should be starved for 24 hours before the operation and the rectum emptied by an enema. A blunt sound is introduced to the bottom of each sac and the outer skin is firmly grasped, either by an assistant or with Pean's forceps. A longitudinal incision is made into the skin and the anal sac is carefully dissected out. In doing this, special care must be taken to preserve the external anal sphincter and the levator ani muscles as damage to them may lead to incontinence of faeces. The whole of the anal sac is extirpated and removed at its outlet. The wound is then closed by skin suture. If the wall of the anal sac is damaged by a fistula the operation is made more difficult, because this involves the most careful and complete removal of the glandular tissue.

After-treatment is chiefly directed to protecting the wound area from injury. This involves fasting for 3 days and then scanty feeding. The tail is held to one side with a bandage to the collar. An Elizabethan collar will prevent the patient from licking or gnawing at the wound. Itching occurring as healing begins can be reduced by the application of 5% benzocaine ointment.

Diseases of the Circumanal Glands cause a r ng-shaped swelling round the anus. The surface is tuberculated and single or multiple fistulae may occur giving a grater-like appearance. There is marked pain.

Treatment is by moist camomile compresses and local antibiotic treatment. If there are marked fistulae, attempts may be made to destroy these by electrosurgery. It is especially valuable to rest the affected area as already described under inflammation of the anal sac.

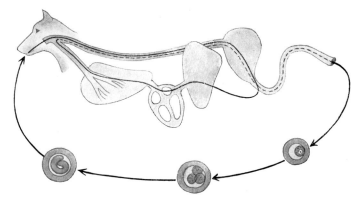

Fig. 348. The life cycle of the ascarid worm *(Toxocara canis)*.

Endoparasites of the digestive canal are of some importance in the dog and include ascariasis, taeniasis, ankylostomiasis and coccidiosis. Usually, we find *Toxocara canis*, but also *Toxascaris leonina*. These ascarids are predominantly inhabitants of the small intestine. They lay considerable numbers of eggs in batches and these pass out with the faeces. A single negative examination for the eggs does not therefore indicate that the host is free from these parasites. It is best to examine the morning faeces microscopically on several successive days to be sure that no ascarids are present. If the eggs of *Toxocara canis* pass out in the faeces they become embryonated in days or weeks and are then infective. If they are swallowed by a host, the larva is set free in the intestine, bores through the gut wall and thus gets into the blood or lymph stream. It migrates to the alveoli of the lung and there breaks out of the capillaries into the bronchi and migrates up to the trachea, from which it is coughed up and swallowed to become sexually mature in the intestine (Fig. 348). As the larva enters the bloodstream, infection of the foetus during pregnancy may occur. *Toxascaris leonina* does not go through this migration through the bloodstream.

Clinically infection occurs by licking or ingesting objects fouled by the faeces. If the host harbours only isolated ascarids, there are no clinical symptoms. Evidence of disease occurs only with heavy infections, especially in young dogs, and these may ultimately cause death. At first the dogs are less active, they are quickly tired by play, the mucosae are pale, and the hair is rough and lustreless. In spite of good feeding emaciation or cachexia occur. Very often the faeces are pulpy and food containing worms may be vomited. Sometimes the gut is completely packed with ascarids and this may be palpated very readily. A distended or "pot-bellied" appearance of the abdomen may be a marked feature. The metabolic products of the ascarids appear to have a neurotropic effect and this causes paralysis of the hind limbs, cramps, circling movements, hysteria, etc. Such patients often have a garlicky odour to the breath. Diagnosis is made by the presence of ascarid eggs in the faeces or vomit. The clinical symptoms described may be confirmed by the results of palpation. X-rays with a contrast medium show the contrast medium in thin threads in the gut.

Fig. 349. *Echinococcus granulosus.*

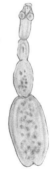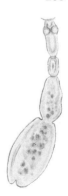

Treatment is by administration of oil of chenopodium. We use the following routine. The patient is starved for 12–18 hours. We give one drop for each month of life 3 times at intervals of 1 hour, with a maximum of 3 drops for small breeds and 5 drops for large breeds. Half an hour after the last dose the dog is given a good teaspoonful of castor oil. The effect may then occur up to 4 hours later. Chenopodium oil cannot be kept very long and soon loses some of its vermicidal properties, and for this reason rather higher doses can be given. If a litter of young dogs is infected with worms, the mother is also treated. In view of the life cycle of *Toxocara canis* a repetition of the treatment after about 14 days is recommended.

Piperazine derivatives are also used as a vermifuge for ascarids. The dose is a single peroral dose of 100 mg per kg bodyweight. It is not essential to starve the dog, no side effects are to be expected, and the dose may be repeated after 14 days.

Special attention should be given to hygienic measures in order to reduce the possibility of re-infection to a minimum. The bedding and kennels must be thoroughly disinfected with boiling soda solution. Normal disinfectants cannot destroy the thick-shelled ascarid eggs. The houses, runs, feeding bowls, etc., may be burned off with a blowlamp.

Household remedies are garlic and carrots. For about a week one gives puppies a daily teaspoonful of a mixture of about $^2/_3$ of carrot juice to $^1/_3$ of cloves of garlic. This is done mainly where microscopic confirmation of diagnosis has not been made, as specific worm treatment being somewhat damaging to the young animal is only justified when worms are actually present.

Taeniasis is mostly seen in the adult dog, less often in young ones. As various species of tapeworms (and partly subspecies) occur in the dog, the following table by SCHULZE (Monatshft. Vet. Med. 7, 128, 1952) gives a synopsis of them. It gives their various names and most striking characteristics and intermediate hosts.

The clinical picture in light infections may pass unnoticed as little damage is caused to the host. Heavy infections cause inflammation of the gut, intussusception and cachexia, a rough and lustreless coat and nervous disorders. In light infections the liver is also involved, suffering prolonged injury from the toxic effects of the metabolic products of the worms and rendering the dog more susceptible to intercurrent disease. So far as hygiene is concerned, tapeworm infection of the dog is important in many ways, not only in relation to transmission of *Echinococcus granulosus* (Fig. 349), which is a rare but serious condition in man, but also as a source of infection of pigs, sheep, goats, etc., with *cysticerci*, which reduce the state of health of these animals and their slaughter-house value.

Treatment. Before treatment the animals should be fasted for 12–18 hours. We give arecoline hydrobromide 2 mg per kg body weight by the mouth. It is important to dose according to body weight. Because of the unpleasant taste of the drug it can be mixed with syrup. Many dogs vomit a few minutes after dosing and for this the treatment described on p. 263 is used. After the dose of arecoline has been given the owner is sent out into the open to exercise his dog for 20–30 minutes. Then a high enema of lukewarm water is given, even if a result has already been achieved. It should be pointed out that self-prepared 1 % solutions of arecoline lose a good deal of their taenicidal activity after about 4 weeks and should therefore be kept in ampoules at the required concentration.

Arecoline acetarsol is a combination of arecoline with an organic arsenical compound. It is supplied conveniently in tablets of 0.024 g and 0.15 g, the dose being 6 mg/kg of body weight. If used correctly this works just as reliably as arecoline solution. Dogs with affections of the heart and kidneys may collapse after doses of arecoline. The owner should be warned of this possibility before dosing, especially with sensitive breeds. For dogs liable to collapse, we give the dose in fractions 2–3 times at intervals of 10 minutes. If the patient is brought back into the consulting room in a state of collapse, we give 2–3 mg of apomorphine hydrochloride subcutaneously. The apomorphine is not an antidote against arecoline poisoning as are atropine and scopolamine, but by its emetic effect it produces a rapid mechanical removal of the arecoline from the stomach and therefore decreased absorption. After the apomorphine the affected dog is given a respiratory stimulant in order to produce better breathing. In severe cases manual heart massage and a careful washing out with an enema of lukewarm water are recommended.

In recent years the taeniacides Dichlorophen, Niclosamide (100 mg/kg about 12 hours after a light meal) and Bunamidine hydrochloride (20–40 mg/kg on an empty stomach) have been found more effective.

Infection may also occur by the larvae penetrating the intact skin.

Ancylostomiasis is caused in the dog by *Ancylostoma caninum*, and *Uncinaria stenocephala*. The life cycle of these hookworms begins with the expulsion of their eggs in the faeces. They develop into larvae in a damp environment and are infective after two ecdyses. If these infective larvae are swallowed by a host, they enter the circulation and pass via the lungs to the gut where they attach themselves to the mucosa feeding on the epithelium and sucking blood. As a moist environment is the most favourable one for their development the disease occurs only in dogs whose quarters are damp. The clinical picture is not clearly defined. Very often hookworm infection is accidentally discovered by examination of the faeces. The most prominent symptom is cachexia, and anaemia may occur.

Treatment. Carbon tetrachloride (0.3–0.4 ml per kg body weight) may be used or tetrachlorethylene (0.2–0.3 ml per kg body weight) or oil of chenopodium. As it is mostly a question of adult dogs, chenopodium oil may be given in doses rather higher than those stated on p. 295.

The most effective treatment is by Bephenium compounds at a dose rate of 20 mg/kg of one of the salts or Thenivin in a dose of 200–250 mg/kg twice daily.

Specific name	Characteristics	Intermediate Host	Length	Other points
Diphyllobothrium latum Tapeworm with grooves on its head	Segments broader than long or quadratic	Lower crustacea Fish (pike, perch, etc.)	2.9 m	Also occurs in man, cats, fox, etc.
Dipylidium caninum Tapeworm like a pumpkin seed	Segments shaped like pumpkin seeds, rose-coloured	Dog flea Dog louse	10–40 cm	Very common, also occurs in man, cat and fox
Taenia pisiformis *Taenia serrata* Serrated tapeworm	Segments broader than long, posterior end of them looks rather broader than the anterior end, the edges therefore look rather serrated	Hare, rabbit	60–100 cm	Especially infects hunting (sporting) dogs after feeding on the entrails of rabbits containing the *cysticerci* which are mostly grape-shaped
Taenia hydatidgena *Taenia marginata* The milled-edged tapeworm	Posterior border of each segment contained as an enveloping cuff over the anterior border of the next segment	Pig, Sheep (*Cysticercus tenuicollis*)	1.5–3 m	Especially in dogs fed on slaughterhouse scraps from home-slaughtering
Taenia multiceps *Taenia coenurus* *Polycephalus multiceps* (Blister worm)	Segments shaped like pumpkin seeds. White and mostly 2.3 mm longer than those of *Dipylidium caninum*	Sheep, cattle (*Coenurus cerebralis*)	40 cm	Especially in sheep dogs
Mesocestoides lineatus Unarmed tapeworm	Segments reddish, like a sack standing on end	Insects feeding on faeces (?) Infection of the dog mostly by ingestion of the young tapeworms in mice, rats, lizards and the hen	30–50 cm	Also occurs in the fox, marten, mink and cats, etc.
Echinococcus granulosus The tapeworm with 3 segments	Very small only 3–4 segments	Various mammals, man (!)	2.5–5 mm	Very dangerous for man, but rare

Piperazine hydrate also has a good effect. Two doses at an interval of a few days must be given. To dislodge these obstinate parasites, the dose may be increased to 150–170 mg per kg body weight under careful supervision.

Coccidiosis also occurs in the dog but its biology will not be considered in detail. The most typical symptom is intractable diarrhoea which may persist for months. The results of infection are cachexia, a coat of poor quality and possibly also anaemia.

Treatment is with the sulphadimethoxine at the rate of 50 mg/kg daily. Special attention should be paid to hygienic measures to prevent re-infection.

7. Diseases of the abdomen and peritoneum

Strictly speaking, this section is outside the adopted classification, because the abdomen does not represent an organ. Abdominal ascites, tumours, injuries and peritonitis will be described.

The methods of examination of the abdomen are palpation, percussion, auscultation, and laparoscopy. Laparoscopy is a valuable diagnostic aid in our opinion which has only recently been introduced for diagnosis in the dog. Diagnosis of liver diseases especially may be improved by this technique.

Ascites abdominalis is always of secondary origin. Usually, there is venous congestion such as occurs in progressive heart failure, from pressure of tumours on the large vessels, or from pathological changes in the liver or kidneys. A change in the composition of the blood (Hydraemia) may result from severe intestinal disturbances and ascites abdominalis may follow this. Infectious diseases (tuberculosis, streptotrichosis, etc.) may be primary affections in abdominal ascites. Finally, the malformation of the blood vessels described on p. 234 which may cause a dropsical condition should be remembered.

In assessing the clinical picture an attempt should always be made to determine the primary disease so that the appropriate therapeutic measures can be taken. The most striking feature is the enlargement of the abdomen (Fig. 350).

To detect a suspected abnormal collection of fluid in the abdomen, one tries to induce waves in the abdominal contents. To do this the investigator stands behind the patient, puts one hand flat on the lateral wall of the abdomen and taps quickly, with two fingers of the hand flexed at the wrist, on the opposite abdominal wall. The wave movement thus caused is transmitted uniformly so that it is detected by the hand laid flat on the abdomen. By percussion the upper border of the fluid can be detected only with difficulty, because the loops of intestine which are mostly lighter rise up and obscure the horizontal limit of the fluid. It is possible to demonstrate it by X-rays (Figs. 352 and 353).

Diaphragmatic respiration is markedly hindered by the increased pressure in the abdomen, so that the patient shows a marked costal type of breathing. In abdominal ascites there is usually no rise of body temperature.

Treatment is directed initially towards the primary lesion. If there is a heart condition, appropriate treatment is given. In kidney diseases, we must try to bring about diuresis and dietetic measures are prescribed. If the transudate is not diminished in this way or if the quantity of fluid present is so great that a situation

Fig. 350. Abdominal ascites in a Fox terrier.

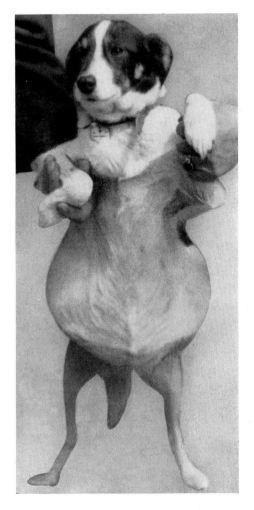

threatening life develops, the fluid is removed by puncture. Quantities of 8–12 litres can be removed by this method. Care should be taken to remove the fluid slowly because rapid changes in the pressure conditions in the abdomen may cause failure of the circulation (flooding of the large vessels with blood). The fluid drawn off may be serous, haemorrhagic or chylous (milky). A chylous transudate indicates a high fat content, whilst a pseudochylous one is chiefly composed of albumin (globulin). The two may be differentiated by shaking up with ether: the chylous transudate is clear, whilst the pseudochylous one remains milky.

Paracentesis is performed with a trochar of suitable size with the patient lying on its side, the puncture site being between the navel and the symphysis pubis, about 2 finger-breadths away from the linea alba. Local anaesthesia is not usually necessary. The site of the puncture is shaved and iodised. The trochar and the blunt-ended sound, which must be introduced through the trochar, are boiled. The trochar is taken up in the hand and the depth to which it is to be inserted is marked with the thumb. It is then quickly thrust into the abdominal cavity with moderate pressure and when the trochar is drawn out the cannula allows the transudate to flow out. If the fluid appears to be escaping too rapidly (when there is marked distension) the outflow is interrupted for a while, so that the body can adapt itself to the altered pressure conditions in the abdomen. Measures to support the circulatory system (see p. 230) may be necessary during the paracentesis. When the intra-abdominal fluid has been greatly reduced, parts of the omentum may be drawn into and obstruct the cannula. If this occurs a sterile blunt-ended sound should be introduced far enough to free the opening of the cannula. The operation is terminated by removal of the cannula. To do this the trochar is again introduced and then quickly pulled out together with the cannula.

In paracentesis, proteins are removed from the body. It is often necessary to repeat the puncture and a second puncture within 8 days must be interpreted as

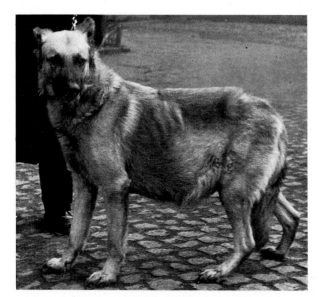

Fig. 351. Abdominal ascites.

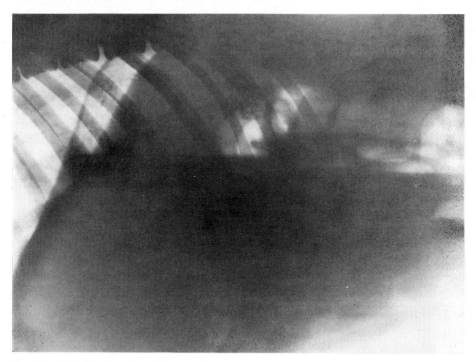

Fig. 352. Abdominal ascites. The air-filled intestinal loops have imposed themselves over the
level of the fluid.

Fig. 353. Abdominal ascites. Demonstration of the horizontal level of fluid in the abdominal cavity was possible only by means of a pneumoperitoneum. The patient was held with forequarters raised and standing on the hind legs (see Fig. 246).

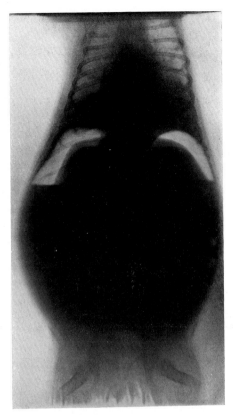

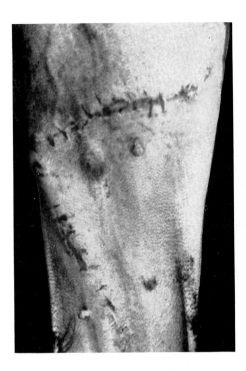

Fig. 354. Scar after flap incision.

prognostically unfavourable. Removal of proteins may lead to emaciation of the patient, so amino acid mixtures should be given for a considerable period. A suitable preparation is methionine.

Tumours are often encountered in the abdomen and mostly arise from an organ (liver, ovary, etc.). Tumours developing free in the abdomen are rare and are chiefly teratomas.

The clinical picture is of a general malaise with a normal temperature. Poor appetite causes cachexia. A striking feature is the increase in the circumference of the abdomen. Usually bimanual palpation reveals a more or less spherical structure in the abdomen. Tumours which arise from the liver are exceptional in relation to therapeutic measures and are considered in more detail on p. 320.

Teratomas can be diagnosed with certainty by X-rays because of the structures within them.

Treatment is essentially surgical in nature. If a very large tumour has been discovered by clinical examination, it is recommended that the technique of

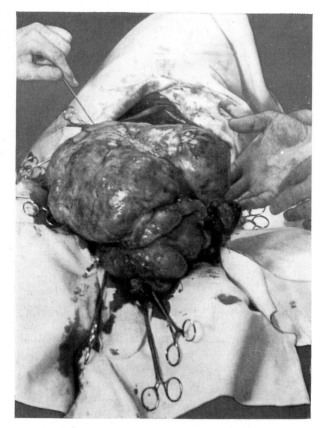

Fig. 355. A very large teratoma of the abdominal cavity.

laparotomy described on p. 280 should be modified, so that the incision is made as a flap incision not in the mid line (Fig. 354). In the removal of a tumour lying free in the abdomen, special attention should be given to ligature of all blood vessels supplying it (Fig. 355).

Injuries of the abdominal cavity are to be expected especially after accidents and bites. If there is an open penetrating wound with protrusion of the abdominal viscera, these are replaced with surgical precautions, possible injuries to organs (e.g. the intestine) are repaired, and the wound is closed. As regards infection the remarks about peritonitis (p. 303) are to be borne in mind.

Injuries of the abdomen that are covered (ventral hernia) are described on p. 306. Gunshot injuries are seen quite frequently (Fig. 356). One can deduce whether viscera are injured or not from the direction of the entry and exit wounds, or from the shot still present in the body. In our experience, in doubtful cases which cannot be resolved by X-rays, the owner should be advised that an exploratory laparotomy be performed. Very often the intestine is penetrated in several places, so that resection of it is unavoidable.

Fig. 356. A wound from an abdominal shot injury. The intestine was penetrated several times. 31 cm of the intestine were resected and recovery followed.

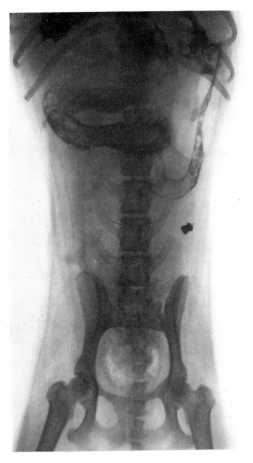

Peritonitis is inflammation of the peritoneum caused by infection with bacteria of various kinds. Paracentesis and laparotomy may lead to inflammation of the peritoneum and also peritonitis may commence in an organ necessitating laparotomy (foreign body in the intestine, perforating placental ulcer, etc.). The peritoneum has extraordinary powers of absorption, so that although the inflammation may be only localised initially it may become generalised.

Clinical picture. In acute peritonitis there is usually generalised illness with a high temperature. The abdomen is tucked up and painful to palpation. Because of the pain the patient moves cautiously. Urination and defaecation may cease. Very often there is vomiting associated with retching. Respiration is superficial and chiefly costal in character. The mucosae are a dirty red colour. The pulse is quickened, small and feeble, sometimes wiry or threadlike. On paracentesis a cloudy, serous, purulent or sanguineous fluid containing fibrinous flocculi is obtained. Increase in the size of the abdomen occurs only in chronic peritonitis. This leads to weakening of the abdominal muscles which are no longer painful to palpation. The patient is completely apathetic and lethargic. Peritonitis is rarely the primary disease. It is mostly associated with the diseases of the abdominal organs already mentioned and often occurs following abdominal surgery. It is important, therefore, that one should pay particular attention to the condition of the peritoneum in every laparotomy performed on patients with a high temperature. When inflammation is beginning, the peritoneum is very reddened, lustreless and sometimes no longer transparent. There may be fibrinous deposits on the organs and collections of fluid in the abdominal cavity.

Treatment. Prophylactically, a gauze drain should be inserted into any abdominal cavity liable to peritonitis. We use sterile, selvedged, gauze bandage (4 m long) and this is inserted into the abdomen leaving a short portion protruding through the caudal angle of the laparotomy wound. The protruding portion is soaked in antibiotic solution. The purpose of this strip is to act like a wick to extract the fluid collecting in the abdomen. The drain is gradually removed during the next 4 days (1 m daily). If there are fibrin flocculi in the abdomen, as many as possible are removed by washing out with physiological saline before closure of the abdominal wound.

Instillation of tetracycline suspension (about 10 mg per kg body weight) into the body cavity is recommended. In addition, when there is peritonitis it is essential to institute effective systemic antibiotic treatment as soon as possible.

8. Hernias

The hernia most often seen in the dog is umbilical hernia, and this is not a true hernia as it is only a prolapse of the preperitoneal fatty tissue or of the omentum emerging from a round opening in the navel. It is difficult to decide what part faulty ligature or cutting of the umbilical cord or hereditary predisposition play in the aetiology of the condition. Very often, puppies with umbilical hernia are brought to the veterinarian after fruitless attempts have been made to correct the hernia with strips of white rubber plaster or penny pieces. Treatment with irritant ointments is just as foolish and has the disadvantage that it leads to accumulations of scar tissue which complicate a later operation.

Technique of the Operation for Umbilical Hernia. According to the extent of the umbilical hernia, it must be decided whether the operation should be done under antiseptic or aseptic conditions. If there is only a small extrusion of fat it may be done antiseptically. On the other hand, if there is a considerable extrusion, aseptic precautions are recommended because of the possibility of injuring the filmy inner hernial sac. The field of operation is shaved, cleansed and iodised, and after a local injection the patient is tied down on its back (Fig. 29). An incision is made over the umbilical area parallel to the long axis of the body and the outer skin is carefully dissected from the inner hernial sac, freezing the sac up to the hernial ring. It is now severed at its tip with a Pean's forceps and slowly twisted off. The contents of the hernia are replaced in the abdominal cavity. The hernial sac is now tied off with a transfixing catgut suture. Before it is removed it is carefully opened to confirm that it is empty. If it contains no abnormal contents it is excised at up to 3 mm from the ligature. A Sultan diagonal suture (Fig. 328) allows the stump to disappear. The skin is brought together with sutures and a relaxation suture is inserted (see p. 281). This suture is removed after 3 days and the skin sutures are removed after 8 days. If there is a bigger extrusion (more than 2 fingers broad) the internal hernial sac must be cut off at the hernial ring and both layers of the peritoneum must be closed together.

Inguinal hernia is extrusion of the abdominal viscera through the inguinal canal (Fig. 357). Usually, the viscera appear through the ostium vaginale in the processus vaginalis so that this latter constitutes the peritoneal hernial sac. It is possible, however, that the viscera appear beside the ostium through a separate peritoneal sac, although this form is very rare.

Inguinal hernias are most often seen in bitches, in which the processus vaginalis is in the form of a small sac, normally containing a little fat which is distributed in the round ligament of the uterus. This is the reason for the relatively frequent occurrence of these inguinal herniae which are congenital or acquired. In the operation one must pay particular attention to tumours of the caudal mammae so that a hernia of this kind is not cut away under the impression that it is a tumour.

Fig. 357. Inguinal hernia.

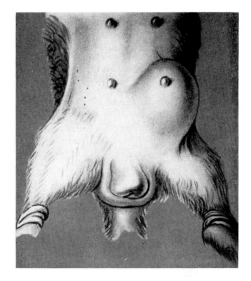

The clinical picture is of a hernial protrusion of variable size and which may have a sausage-like shape in the inguinal region. If this protrusion is replaceable the hernial opening (inguinal canal) will admit 1 or 2 fingers. The contents of the hernia may be omentum, gut, uterus or bladder. Sometimes there is a small portion of herniated omentum in which the fat increases so much that the hernia is irreducible. Similarly the pregnant uterus may enter the hernia with resultant incarceration in the sac.

Treatment is entirely surgical.

Technique of the Operation for Inguinal Hernia. Epidural anaesthesia is induced and the animal restrained on its back. An incision is made obliquely over the hernial protrusion and the fatty tissue is carefully incised until one reaches the hernial sac formed by the peritoneum. The hernial sac is dissected free as far as the inguinal ring. The dissection should always be done from the cranial to the caudal end. Special care must be taken not to injure the external pudendal artery and vein which emerge from the inguinal ring at the caudal end of the hernia. The contents of the hernia are replaced by stroking them along the hernial sac and by twisting, and the sac is tied off near the outer inguinal ring and removed. If omental adhesions are present, the hernial sac is opened, the omentum tied off and the stump of it replaced and the sac is then ligatured and cut away. The inguinal ring is closed with a Sultan's diagonal (catgut) suture. The suture sites lie in the external oblique abdominal muscle and in Poupart's ligament, so that suturing involves some risk of damaging the femoral artery and vein. The sutures should always proceed therefore from Poupart's ligament, i.e., from the lateral aspect, to the external oblique muscle. Finally the skin is sutured.

In male dogs inguinal hernia is relatively rare. When it occurs there is a hernial protrusion the size of a nut or child's fist. If the abdominal contents pass down into the depth of it, it is known as a scrotal hernia. Incarceration of the intestine within the hernia leads to the symptoms of acute ileus. An inguinal hernia of small dimensions may easily be confused with ectopic testis. In scrotal hernia the scrotum is enlarged. By palpation the pouch of the widened tunica vaginalis and soft masses (gut or omentum) inside it can be felt.

Treatment is by surgical removal of the hernial protrusion.

Technique of the Operation for Scrotal Hernia. The patient is prepared as described above. After freeing the hernial protrusion and reduction of the abdominal viscera, the spermatic cord is tied over the tunica vaginalis with catgut, removed and the inguinal ring is closed with a purse-string suture. If the testes are retained the inguinal ring is narrowed by a purse-string suture inserted through Poupart's ligament and the external oblique muscle and tied just tight enough to ensure blood supply to the testis. It is not very easy to estimate the correct size of opening to be left and inexperienced surgeons would be well advised to forego the preservation of the testes and complete the operation by complete closure of the inguinal ring. If the spermatic cord is sufficiently adherent to the hernial sac that it cannot be freed without risk to the future nourishment of the testes, castration should be performed.

In traumatic inguinal hernia, attention must be given to the hernia contents. Sometimes there are injuries to the intestine, etc., which require special care, resecting, etc.

Interstitial inguinal hernia should really be classed among the abdominal herniae because it emerges beside the tunica vaginalis, so that the peritoneum is usually ruptured and an inner hernial sac is absent, the contents of the hernia being subcutaneous beside the tunica vaginalis.

Ventral hernia may occur at different places on the abdominal wall. Excluding the herniae which arise from protrusions of abdominal contents through preformed openings (e.g. the inguinal canal), abdominal hernias occur mostly as the result of accidents or bites (Fig. 358) involving trauma due to blunt objects.

Clinical picture. As the skin remains intact, but the musculature is damaged, the viscera bulge out together with the peritoneum (inner hernial sac). Often the peritoneum is also damaged so that the viscera come to lie directly under the skin (subcutaneous prolapse). If this occurs, an inner hernial sac is formed after a time out of connective tissue, once the acute symptoms have subsided. On palpation of a ventral hernia a soft, superficial, cap-shaped protrusion is felt, which is sharply circumscribed. After reduction a distinct opening is felt in the abdominal wall. If the trauma has gone deep, it is possible that the abdominal muscles have been damaged at different places (an oblique hernia canal). The viscera in such cases very quickly adhere to the muscles, the contents of the hernia cannot be replaced and the opening of the hernia cannot be determined. It may be in the middle of the protrusion or at its border, so that special care is needed in the operation.

Treatment. In early cases judicious measures may bring about spontaneous resolution (traumas in the flank region). After accidents in a few specially selected cases (where there is no strangulation or damage to internal organs) conservative treatment may be adopted. Tight bandages are not suitable because they do not hold well. Forsell's percutaneous tamponade is preferable. The contents of the hernia are reduced and a tampon is put over it. The size and form of this tampon are decided by the circumference of the hernia ring. Several stitches are put into the skin fold lateral to this ring and these are tied over the tampon so that it is strongly pressed down on to the hernia. If there is a circular hernia ring, a purse-string suture may be inserted which presses firmly on to the tampon. The tamponade is removed after 10–14 days. If abdominal organs are also injured or if strangulation occurs, surgical treatment is essential. When the upper abdomen is involved, general anaesthesia is usually employed, otherwise epidural or local anaesthesia may suffice. The patient is prepared as described on p. 280, the contents of the hernia are replaced, and the individual layers of the muscles closed with catgut sutures. This can be done in every early case of abdominal hernia, but, if the hernia has existed for several days, the musculature is infiltrated by reactionary inflammatory processes and is so friable that the sutures tear out. In these cases the operation should only be undertaken 3–4 weeks after the accident, conservative methods being used in the meantime. The operation is performed through a skin incision. The panniculus is divided and the hernial sac is dissected out up to the hernia ring, where the hernial sac can be tied off and excised. As there are very often adhesions

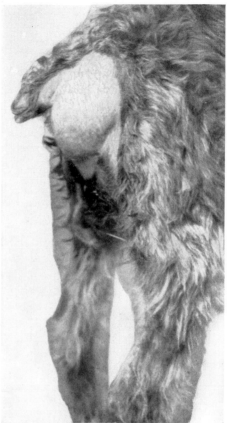

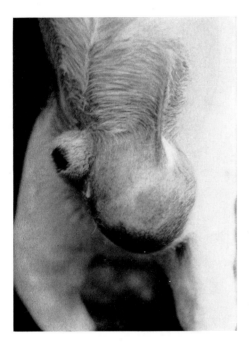

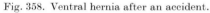

Fig. 358. Ventral hernia after an accident.   Fig. 359. Perineal hernia.

of the viscera to the hernia sac, it is recommended that the sac should be opened up. The adhesions are freed, the viscera are replaced and the hernial sac is removed at the hernia ring. The opening is closed with a Sultan diagonal suture.

Perineal hernia. This is extrusion of viscera through the pelvic cavity into the perineal region (Fig. 359). Usually, it is unilateral, rarely bilateral. The contents of the hernia may be intestine or bladder. Perineal hernia occurs quite often in old dogs. There is no inner hernia sac, but the contents of the hernia reach the perineum between the lateral and ventral walls of the pelvis and the rectum. The levator ani and coccygeus muscles are partially atrophied and partly stretched to their maximal extent. The cause of perineal hernia is tenesmus due to prostatic hypertrophy, chronic constipation, etc.

The clinical picture is chiefly of a soft, reducible swelling in the perineum beside the anus. At the affected site the muscle is very atrophied and one can introduce some fingers, if not the whole fist, into the hernial opening. If the bladder is

20*

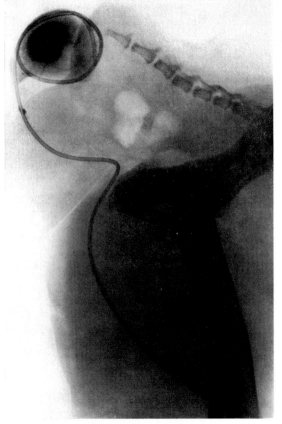

Fig. 360. Perineal hernia with prolapse of the bladder. The catheter shows the course of the urethra. The bladder is full of contrast medium.

Fig. 361. Perineal hernia with incarceration of the urinary bladder shown by contrast medium.

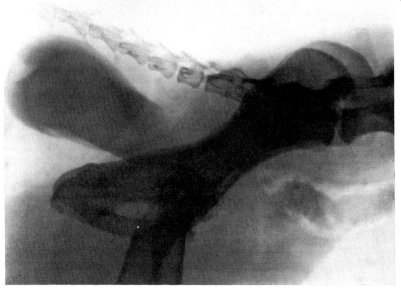

retroflexed, an elastic catheter introduced into it may be palpable in the hernial sac (Fig. 360). In such cases there are difficulties of micturition because there is a kink at the neck of the bladder. By the continuous flow of urine out of the ureters the perineal hernia is progressively enlarged (Fig. 361). Often accompanying the hernia there is a diverticulum of the hind gut which has prolapsed into the hernia. In most cases this is a loop of hind gut which only appears to be a diverticulum (Fig. 362). In differential diagnosis one must consider a periproctal abscess, which is distinguished from perineal hernia by signs of inflammation. Accurate diagnosis is important because the treatment of these two conditions is fundamentally different. A periproctal abscess must be opened whereas this could prove disastrous in perineal hernia.

Treatment should be directed initially to achieving regular and soft stools.

Technique of the Operation for Perineal Hernia. The patient must be starved for 48 hours and the hind gut must be emptied by a high enema. The operation should be done as far as possible under aseptic conditions. Epidural anaesthesia is employed. The field of operation is shaved, cleansed and iodised and the patient is tied down in the manner described on p. 30. A swab is inserted into the relaxed anal opening and the anus is closed with a purse-string suture (Fig. 363). The pelvis may be raised in order to keep the replaced hernial contents away from the hernia. The skin is incised and the contents of the hernia are freed (Figs. 364 and 365). Now the hernia

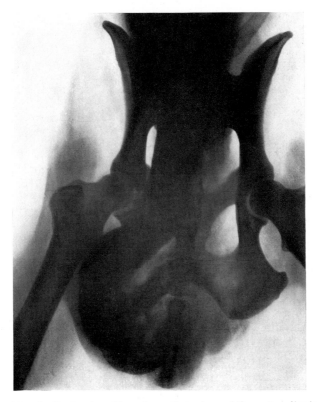

Fig. 362. Perineal hernia. Contrast medium shows that a loop of the rectum lies in the hernial sac.

opening is closed using small, fully-curved needles to insert deep catgut sutures. In doing this the external sphincter of the anus, the external levator ani and the sacrotuberal ligament are brought together by closely-placed sutures (Figs. 366, 367, 368, 369). The tissues are extremely friable (atrophy and deposition of fat) so that a large number of sutures should be inserted. Several layers of sutures should be put in over one another. The operation ends with suture of the skin incision.

After-treatment is chiefly regulation of the feeding. If relapses occur one should consider whether a vesicopexy (of the bladder) or rectopexy (of the rectum) would not give a better result (see p. 292).

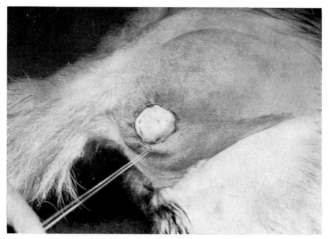

Fig. 363. Operation for perineal hernia. Insertion of a swab in the rectum and closure of the anus with a purse-string suture.

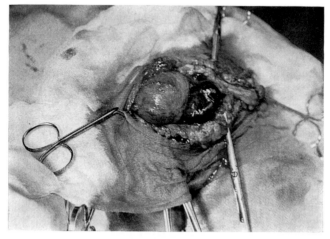

Fig. 364. Operation for perineal hernia. After a skin incision the contents of the hernia consisting of bladder and omentum are shown.

Diaphragmatic hernias. In these we must distinguish between actual diaphragmatic hernias and traumatic rupture of the diaphragm. Diaphragmatic hernia is chiefly congenital and is shown by the fact that the organs prolapsed into the thorax have a covering of peritoneum. In traumatic rupture of the diaphragm there is a prolapse of a large proportion of the abdominal organs (liver, stomach, intestine, omentum) into the thorax.

Clinical picture. Diaphragmatic hernias cause no symptoms or troubles and are mostly found accidentally by X-ray examination of the alimentary tract. On

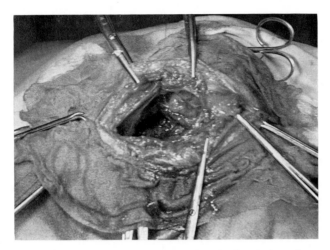

Fig. 365. Operation for perineal hernia. The contents of the hernia have been replaced in the abdomen.

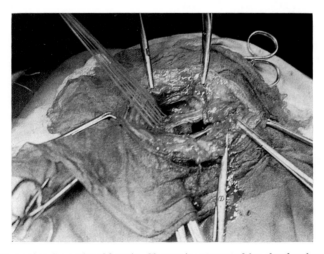

Fig. 366. Operation for perineal hernia. Closure is attempted by closely placed stitches.

the other hand, traumatic rupture of the diaphragm with prolapse of the viscera into the thorax may cause the most pronounced clinical symptoms. The history is one of sudden dyspnoea after an accident, or dog fight, or after more than usually severe physical stress. The patient's respiration is markedly costal, the ribs are maximally expanded and the abdomen is contracted. In addition to shortness of breath there are local symptoms depending on the kind and number of the viscera prolapsed into the thorax. In prolapse of the liver or spleen, or in the presence of fluid, there may be dulling of the percussion note. If the stomach and intestine have prolapsed, the percussion note is tympanitic. There are no respiratory sounds in the region of the prolapsed organs, whilst on the other side auscultation may

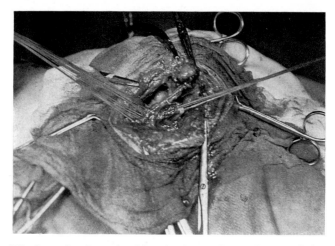

Fig. 367. Operation for perineal hernia. A second row of sutures is inserted.

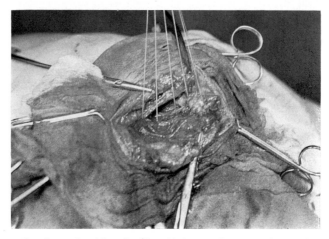

Fig. 368. Operation for perineal hernia. The third row of sutures almost closes the wound.

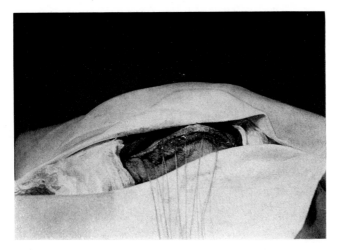

Fig. 369. Operation for perineal hernia. The subcutaneous tissue is also closed by the suture.

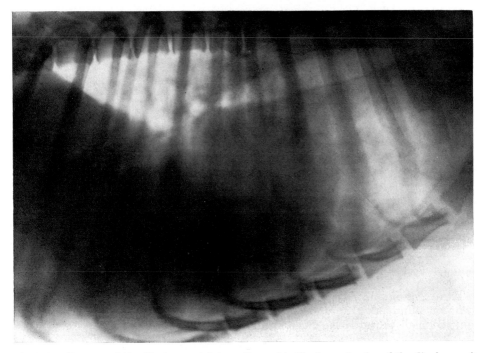

Fig. 370a. Rupture of the diaphragm (plain radiograph). The lower border of the diaphragm is
obscured in the lower half.

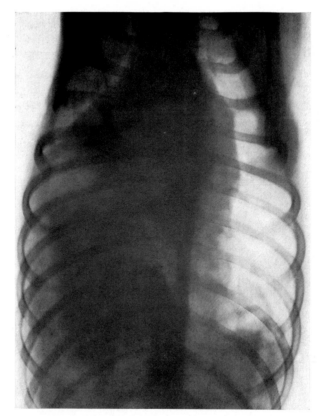

Fig. 370 b. The same patient radiographed dorso-ventrally. The left half of the thorax is full of
"masses" whilst the right half is still full of air.

show these to be increased. On auscultation peristaltic sounds may occur which
are not synchronous with respiration. By palpation of the abdomen it is sometimes
possible to feel the organs drawn into the thorax. X-ray examination gives an
especially clear picture when the intestine is shown up by contrast medium (Figs.
370 a–d). If there is torsion of the stomach or intestine, their distension may result
in dangerous dyspnoea. Constriction of the spleen leads to rapid congestion and
this, by limiting the thoracic region, causes serious dyspnoea. Sometimes also
constriction of a lobe of the liver may occur with resultant hydrothorax or abdominal ascites.

Treatment of a diaphragmatic hernia should be expectant if there are no clinical
symptoms. In traumatic rupture of the diaphragm on the other hand, an attempt
must be made to repair the defect in the diaphragm.

Technique of the Operation for Traumatic Rupture of the Diaphragm. The operation field in the
epigastric region is shaved, cleansed and iodised. In order to be able to control the respiration
of the patient intubation is necessary. The patient is tied down on its back and the abdomen is

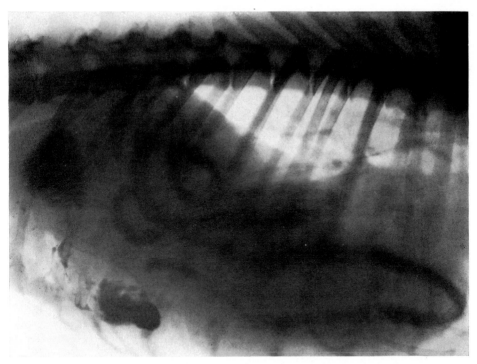

Fig. 370c. The same patient; the intestinal loops have been made visible by contrast medium.

opened with a lateral incision 2–3 finger-breadths from the costal arch. One is tempted to make the incision directly at the costal arch in order to give access to the lesion, but this incision has produced complications in post-operative healing so caution is advisable. If one cannot manage with a lateral incision, a median incision in the linea alba should also be made (flap incision). At the moment when the peritoneum is divided, controlled respiration must be started. After opening the abdomen the viscera prolapsed into the thorax are replaced, special care being given to the replacement of the liver, which is often very friable and may rupture with dangerous haemorrhage.

Single silk sutures are inserted close together in the deepest parts of the rupture of the diaphragm and these are continued along the tear. Before the last stitch is tied off, the lungs must be maximally expanded with the respirator, so that no atmospheric air remains in the pleural cavity. Before the abdominal wound is closed (see p. 281) the tightness of the diaphragmatic sutures is re-checked. If no muscle relaxants have been given, spontaneous respiration will commence immediately after the operation.

Mesenteric hernia is extremely rare. It occurs by the passage of a loop of the small intestine or the colon through a split in the mesentery.

The clinical picture is very variable. The symptoms resemble those of ileus but are disappointing radiologically because the gas distension is not so typical. Contrast medium is sometimes able to pass into the intestine because the displaced

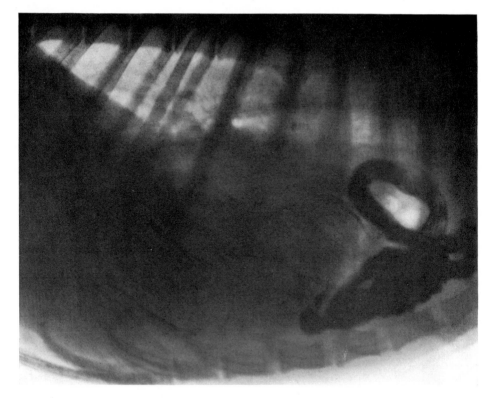

Fig. 370d. The same patient; the contrast medium has passed into the anterior part of the thorax.

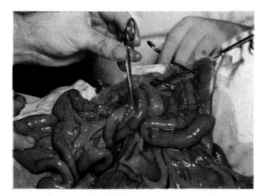

Fig. 371. Mesenteric hernia. The artery forceps shows the point of entrance of the section of
the gut drawn to the left.

intestine is not strangulated. On palpation a soft mass is felt in the abdomen. The mesenteric hernia shown in Fig. 371 was discovered only after two exploratory laparotomies. During preparation for the first exploratory laparotomy the intestine had replaced itself and an opening in the mesentery was not suspected. Three weeks later the same symptoms appeared and a second laparotomy revealed the condition shown in Fig. 371.

Treatment is by laparotomy with replacement of the intestine and closure of the opening in the mesentery.

9. Diseases of the liver and pancreas

It is very difficult to carry out a clinical investigation of the liver in the dog. Palpation is only possible where the patient is emaciated or where there is a great increase in the size of the organ. To perform palpation, the clinician stands behind the patient and, introducing the finger tips under the costal arch, tries to approximate the two hands. In this way one can appreciate alterations in the size of the liver and changes in its surface. By radiography it is possible to determine the cranial border of the liver by estimating the position of the diaphragm (it is high up when the liver is enlarged), and its caudal limit, after administering a contrast medium (the outlined stomach restricts the shadow of the liver posteriorly). Radiographic examination may be facilitated by the induction of pneumo-peritoneum (the introduction of air into the abdomen) as by this technique all the abdominal organs are better delineated, and in this way it is sometimes possible to visualise individual lobes of the liver (Figs. 372 and 373). Visual inspection of the liver can be performed by the technique of laparoscopy. A laparoscope is introduced into the abdominal cavity and a direct inspection of the liver can then be made through the instrument. Unfortunately, however, functional disorders of this large and important gland cannot be assessed by these methods and therefore various functional tests are employed. The estimation of serum bilirubin, SGPT, and alkaline phosphatase and the bromsulphalein retention tests are of great value as a means of estimating liver damage.

The pancreas is not accessible to ordinary clinical investigational methods.

As the liver is such a difficult organ to investigate, one looks for evidence of disordered function in the secondary changes which appear in the body. In the first place these are often revealed in disorders of the digestive organs. Colour changes occur in the tissues, the urine and the faeces. If the detoxicating activity of the liver is reduced there may be disorders of the central nervous system. Bile salts may accumulate in the body fluids. As the liver is an extremely vascular organ, where there are widespread pathological changes there may be stasis of blood which affects the whole body. In this respect dropsical conditions are especially common. Liver disease (cirrhosis, chronic congestion, neoplasia) was incriminated as the cause of ascites in 68 out of 91 cases by one worker.

Icterus (jaundice) is a condition which is specially related to liver disease and is polymorphic in nature. Obstructions to the outflow of bile from the liver lead to obstructive and absorptive icterus. Haemolytic icterus occurs when there is excessive breakdown of red blood cells with a consequent excessive supply of haemo-

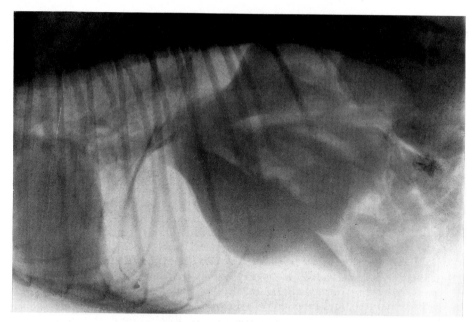

Fig. 372. Demonstration of the liver by means of a pneumoperitoneum. The diaphragm is a narrow strip dividing the abdomen from the thorax (latero-lateral irradiation).

globin for the formation of bile. Where there is severe disease of the liver itself, retention icterus occurs. Clinically these three forms are only rarely seen as separate entities, usually various combinations of them occurring. The most striking symptom is the yellow coloration of the skin and mucosae, which can be most easily seen in the sclerotic of the eyes. The urine usually has a rich content of bile and is therefore brown, or even dark green. In obstructive icterus the bile is prevented from entering the intestine and therefore the faeces are pale, grey, and resemble cement, and peristalsis is somewhat diminished. As the bile is also essential for the proper digestion of fats, there may be a so-called fatty stool, which has the consistency of clay, is grey in colour and has a rancid odour. In haemolytic icterus there is often a marked enlargement of the spleen, the serum may be cherry red in colour because of its increased haemoglobin content, and the faeces are rather dark in colour because of the increased outflow of bile. The accumulation of bile acids in the blood produces autointoxication which is shown by lassitude, haemorrhages into the skin and mucosae, pruritus, bradycardia and bradypnoea.

Treatment must be aimed at rectifying the underlying cause of the icterus where known. In most cases the aetiology is obscure, so that treatment must be symptomatic and mainly directed towards removal of the bile acids from the body. An attempt should be made to regulate peristalsis by the use of neutral salts. Cholagogues, which increase the amount of bile, and chloretics, which stimulate bile secretion, may be used. We prescribe Carlsbad salts and bile salt preparations. Drugs which increase the excretion of urine (diuretics) also increase the removal

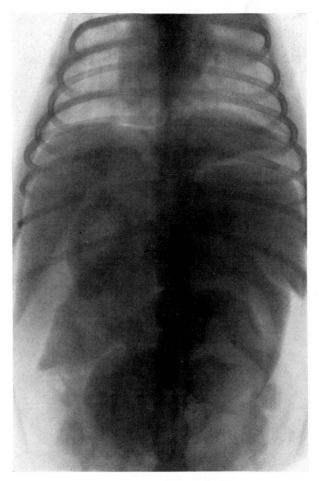

Fig. 373. Demonstration of the liver by means of a pneumoperitoneum (dorso-ventral irradiation).

of bile. To reduce the amount of fat in the intestine, reduction in the fat and albumin intake is necessary. Where fat digestion is impaired, choline preparations may be prescribed. It is essential to ensure effective defaecation and to this end laxatives may be required.

Chronic interstitial inflammation of the liver (cirrhosis of the liver). In this condition there is an inflammatory process in the liver which results in the formation of excess connective tissue. This new connective tissue contrasts over a period of time with resultant pressure atrophy of the liver cells and a hardening of the organ. The disease is a chronic process and is seen more often in the older dog.

Clinical signs are not very characteristic, the earliest often being the development of ascites. It may be possible to appreciate the irregularities on the liver surface by palpation, or radiography may reveal the increase in size of the organ. Liver function tests are necessary to assess the functional ability of the affected organ.

As diagnosis is so difficult, it is always advisable to bear in mind the possibility of liver damage and to try to protect the liver in all cases of severe disease, especially in the older dog. In foreign body ileus, for example, indol and skatol are absorbed and will damage the hepatocytes if they are not protected. Protection can best be afforded by increasing the storage of glycogen in the liver cells by the intravenous injection of 5–10 m*l* of 40 % glucose, or fructose. The amino acid preparations which have a lipotropic action, such as methionine and cysteine, also have a protective action on the liver. The vitamin B complex plus vitamin C may be given in high dosage. In dropsical conditions, liver hydrolysates, which are especially rich in amino acids, the B complex vitamins and especially in the purine bases such as adenine, may be administered. The use of the glucocorticoids (see p. 466) may be effective.

Neoplasia. New growths in the liver may be primary or secondary by metastasis. Unlike the condition in man, carcinoma of the canine liver is not associated with cirrhosis. Primary carcinomata are more common than secondary growths, and the bile duct cells more frequently involved than the liver cells.

The clinical picture may be very variable. If the neoplastic foci are extensive there may be production of ascites. If the tumours are small they are usually symptomless, but may possibly be detectable on palpation in a lean animal. The larger growths produce digestive upsets, seen mainly as loss of appetite and vomiting. If food is given forcibly it is usually regurgitated. Some of the larger tumours may be detected on radiography with contrast medium (Fig. 374). Sometimes in older bitches it is extremely difficult to differentiate between a liver neoplasm and one involving the ovary, and a laparotomy may be required before a definite diagnosis can be made.

Treatment can only be by surgical removal and is not often successful. The poor results are due to the fact that the dog is often moribund when presented for examination, and the difficulty of effective haemostasis in the friable liver tissue. Where the patient's condition warrants surgical intervention the possibility of successful surgery can only be assessed by an exploratory laparotomy.

Liver Fluke (Metorchis conjunctus). JORDAN & ASHBY (J. Amer. vet. med. Ass. **131**, 239–240, 1957) found more than 100 flukes in a 4-year-old bitch which had been destroyed because of ascites. In addition to cirrhosis of the liver, there was proliferation of the bile ducts, acute nephritis and myocardial degeneration. The animal was thought to have been infected by eating raw fish.

Pancreatic Diseases, Diabetes mellitus. In this condition large amounts of sugar are excreted in the urine due to a deficiency of insulin production by the Islets of Langerhans. It is comparatively rare in the dog. Bitches are more frequently affected than dogs and there appears to be a breed predisposition in the Dachshund and the Miniature Poodle. The onset of the condition in the bitch often appears to be associated with the end of oestrus. There is an aggravation of the diabetic condition during and soon after oestrus, the increase in blood sugar often leading to diabetic crises. This association with oestrus seems to indicate that there is some connection between the control of sugar metabolism and the hormonal control of the oestrus cycle.

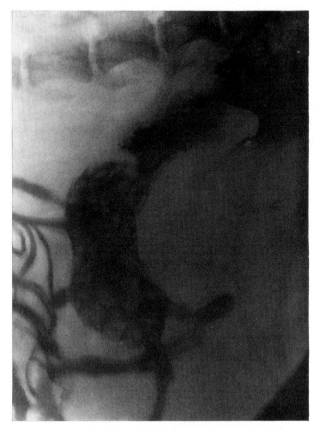

Fig. 374. Diagnosis of a liver tumour by contrast medium. The stomach has been displaced caudally by the tumour.

Clinically the patients are emaciated and cachectic (Figs. 375a and 375b), the normal blood sugar content of about 100 mg per cent is increased, the renal threshold is exceeded and so sugar is excreted in the urine. As a result of this disordered sugar metabolism, acid breakdown products appear, composed of excess of protein and fat. This acidosis (β-oxybutyric acid, acetic acid and acetone) produces auto-intoxication and leads to diabetic coma. Polydipsia and polyuria are always present, leading to a heavy burden being placed on the kidneys. The urine is almost colourless and watery with a little sediment, but because of its high sugar content it has a high specific gravity. The passage of large quantities of urine of a high specific gravity, therefore, should raise suspicions of Diabetes mellitus. The high sugar content leads to the precipitation of very small crystals, which adhere to the hair of the prepuce or the vulva, causing the hairs to stick together. Diagnosis should only be based on repeated findings of increased blood and urine sugar, because glycosuria may occur in other diseases, e.g. alimentary

21 Christoph, Diseases of Dogs

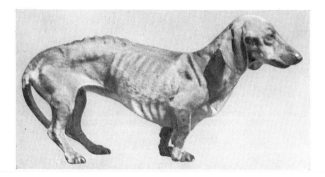

Fig. 375a. Marked cachexia in Diabetes mellitus.

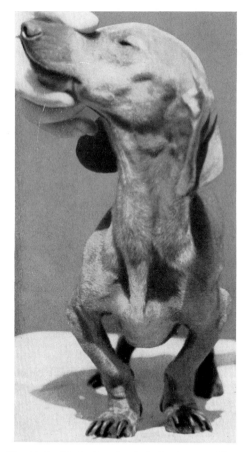

Fig. 375b. Marked cachexia in Diabetes mellitus.

conditions, or infectious diseases such as rabies. Diabetic patients tend to have a lower resistance to skin infections and thus one may see eczema, acne, or furunculosis. In advanced cases central opacities of the lens occur, and this may lead to complete blindness (diabetic cataract). The dog shows general weakness, with loss of vigour, cramps and loss of consciousness, leading progressively to coma and death.

Prognosis should be guarded, as the life expectation of diabetic dogs is not very high. Most of the cases recorded died within the first six months of diagnosis being made. Only a third lived longer than one year, three lived more than two years and two more than three years.

Treatment is difficult in the dog. Carbohydrates should be restricted, or even eliminated from the diet, which should also be rich in fats and protein. Insulin is given as replacement therapy and acts by reducing the release of sugar from the liver and muscle reserves, stimulating the utilisation of glucose and acting as an antagonist to the diabetogenic hormone of the pituitary gland. The amount of insulin to be given must be worked out in each individual case by monitoring the blood and urine sugar content. Speaking generally, about 8 to 24 units, according to the size of the patient, are injected subcutaneously. Usually the higher the blood sugar value and the more marked the glycosuria, the more insulin is required, e.g. where there is 270–300 mg per cent of sugar, 40–60 units of insulin a day may be required. The daily dose is divided into two injections and given after food in the morning and in the afternoon. It is essential to allow at least four hours between the two doses, otherwise a cumulative effect may occur. The second daily dose should be given not later than 5 p.m. because the blood sugar usually falls towards evening. Zinc protamine insulin may be used and this persists for 24 hours. As a practical measure it is recommended that the dog should be given just enough insulin to bring the thirst to normal proportions. Successful control of the diabetes is shown by increasing body weight with subsequent maintenance of a constant body weight. Over-dosage leads to hypoglycaemic shock, with cramps and loss of consciousness. In this event the dog will need to be given large intravenous doses of glucose immediately. Acidosis, where it exists, should be treated by the administration of sodium bicarbonate.

Pancreopathies (other disease of the pancreas) are often secondary to other conditions. The exocrine portion of the pancreas produces enzymes and other secretions and must possess great adaptability in its qualitative and quantitative response, according to whether carbohydrates, proteins, or fats are included in the diet. Where there is liver disease, or if the intestine is damaged, the pancreas will always be affected.

Acute pancreatic diseases are usually very quickly fatal. SINGLETON and RHODES (Vet. Rec. **69**, 110–111, 1957) reported a case of acute pancreatic necrosis following a duodenal abscess in a 7-year-old Labrador, which died within 12 days after vomiting and showing marked epigastric pain. The abscess was near the papilla of VATER, and this led to obstruction of the outflow of bile which then refluxed into the pancreas through the duct of WIRSUNG.

Pancreatic atrophy is not uncommon in the dog and results in defective secretion of amylase, lipase and trypsin. Clinical signs of this condition are digestive upsets and emaciation. Some workers are of the opinion that in many cases the condition is preceded by liver damage by the virus of C.V.H. The most effective treatment

21*

is feeding raw pancreas, the choline content of which helps to prevent degeneration of the liver. Injection of methionine is also said to be beneficial. Pancreatin may also be used with success.

Chronic disease of the pancreas was not recognised until fairly recently. Disease of the exocrine portion of the organ leads to digestive difficulties. The dog is ravenous for food, but remains emaciated and there may be coprophagia. Fermentation in the intestine leads to unpleasant flatulence and the faeces are often altered, the so-called fatty stool being characteristic of the condition. Faeces are soft, grey or milky, often greasy, foul smelling and poorly digested. In some cases the liver is so badly damaged that icterus occurs and dropsical conditions are often seen in association with pancreatic disease. Again pancreatin will often prove effective.

Tumours of the pancreas, by damaging the exocrine portions of the gland, tend to produce the clinical syndrome of chronic disease.

10. Diseases of the urinary system

In the investigation of renal disease it is necessary to combine the clinical examination with various laboratory tests, in order to assess the functional efficiency of the kidneys. Palpation of the kidneys is only possible in lean animals, and in such cases it may be possible to detect abnormalities in their size, or irregularities on their surface. Where there is a painful condition, careful palpation will produce contraction of the muscles of the loins and the abdominal wall, the animal evincing pain and possibly snapping at the clinician. Palpation of the bladder is easier and is done with one hand to estimate the degree of distension and the thickness of the wall. Abnormal contents of the bladder, e.g. stones or tumours, may be detected in this way. In the smaller breeds palpation may be done with both hands, one hand pressing the bladder away from the abdominal wall into the pelvis, while the index finger of the other hand is inserted into the rectum and the bladder palpated with the tip of the finger. By this technique it is possible to estimate the strength of the bladder wall quite well.

Urine analysis is of great diagnostic value in the investigation of renal disease. The urine may be collected during micturition or with a catheter, the latter method being more useful, as there is then less risk of contamination with the vaginal or preputial secretions. To catheterise the bitch we use a vaginascope with a slotted safety-glass speculum. With the animal in a standing position the speculum is inserted with the slot dorsal in position. The handle is then turned through 180° so that the opening of the urethra appears beneath the slot in the speculum. The metal catheter can now be inserted under direct visual control (Fig. 376). Soiling of the vaginascope handle by spontaneous voiding of urine is prevented by the fact that the handle is held vertically and dorsally. The speculum is withdrawn and the urine collected in a glass flask (Fig. 377). If necessary a hypodermic syringe may be attached to the catheter and a sterile sample withdrawn, irrigation of the bladder performed, or urine withdrawn without exerting any pressure on the abdomen (Fig. 378). In the male dog a flexible catheter containing a metal stylus is used. The dog is restrained on its side with the hindlegs

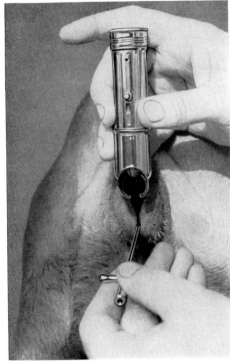

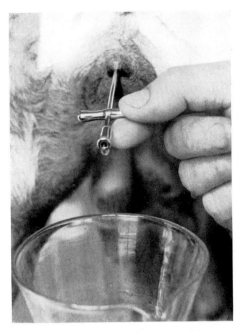

Fig. 376. Insertion of a metal catheter in a bitch.   Fig. 377. Collecting urine from a bitch.

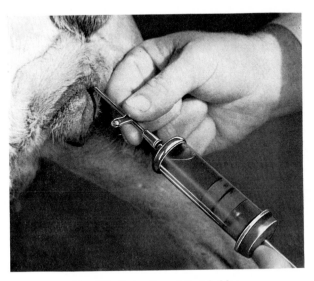

Fig. 378. Irrigation of the bladder.

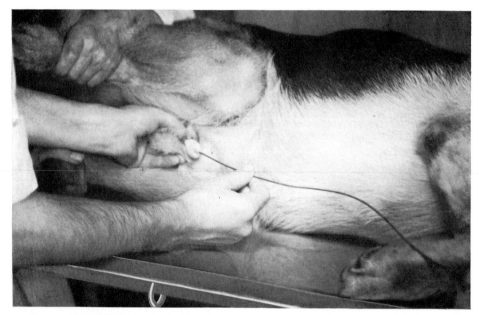

Fig. 379. Catheterisation of the male dog.

flexed. The penis is exposed and retained by digital pressure on the sheath, the catheter being introduced into the urethra with the other hand (Fig. 379). The stylus is then held stationary whilst the catheter is advanced into the bladder. Urine will now flow out through the catheter or may be withdrawn with the aid of a syringe as in the bitch.

A normal dog passes urine 1–3 times in the course of 24 hours, the amount passed varying according to the size of the dog between 40–2,000 ml. According to WITZIGMANN ("Studies of the urine of domesticated animals", Hannover 1940), normal urine has the following characteristics:

Colour – bright or amber yellow, clear and watery.
Viscosity – low (Frictional index 1.10–1.20).
Odour – broth-like or garlicky.
Specific gravity – 1035 (Range 1020–1050).
Osmotic pressure lowering of freezing point – 0.385–3.280 °C.
Reaction – acid, pH 6.7.
Optical rotation – greater when fed on meat than when fed on bread.
Albumin – trace.
Sugar – negative.
Urobilin – 6.2–32.4 mg daily (there may be 30–40 % variation in same dog). 0.22–
    1.61 mg per litre.
Indican – 2.9–30.0 mg per litre.
Acetone bodies – 1–4 mg per litre.
Urocanic acid – found only twice.

Creatinine – 0.70–1.87 mg per litre.

Urea – 1.5–6.0 carbon: nitrogen ratio.

Urinary index – 0.94–1.29.

Iron – 1 mg daily.

Phosphorus – on a meat diet 92 % of the phosphorus intake appears in the urine.

Allantoin – positive.

Sulphates, thiosulphuric acid – the sediments of these are of great importance in the assessment of renal disease but they are so variable that a normal amount cannot be defined.

Kidney Function Tests.

Kidney function tests fall into two main groups:

a) those which assess the ability to excrete and to cope with the administration of known amounts of substances, which may be either normal or foreign to the body,

b) those methods in which the blood level of substances excreted in the urine is estimated.

None of the first group can be recommended for use under conditions of general practice. In the second group the most important are the assessment of the blood levels of urea, urea nitrogen and their fractions, and the products of intestinal putrefaction. We prefer to use the blood urea nitrogen (BUN), whilst other workers estimate blood urea. The latter test has some advantages in that it shows defective kidney function earlier and more markedly, as urea nitrogen is increased almost exclusively by increase in urea, and it is an easier and quicker test to perform. The main disadvantage lies in the fact that it is not so accurate, as the urea is not quantitatively broken down and because intermediate creatine, creatinine, purine, amino acids and other metabolic products take part in the reaction.

Estimation of the blood urea nitrogen will shed light on the protein metabolism of the body and also the functional capacity of the chief excretory organs, the kidneys. Increase in BUN is always seen in organic disease of the kidneys, as inflammatory and degenerative processes increase the excretion of the breakdown products of protein metabolism. Obviously increased BUN will also result from increased protein breakdown in feverish conditions, or after haemorrhage into the gastro-intestinal tract, disorders of intermediate metabolism, disorders of vitamin or hormone content, etc. SCHEFFLER (Thesis. Leipzig, 1954) gives the normal value of blood urea nitrogen as between 13–43 mg% with a mean of 28.8 $\pm$ 1.5mg%. If this value is altered by an increased breakdown of protein, it is advisable to carry out a xanthoprotein test, as retention of putrefactive intestinal products in the blood will lead to serious impairment of renal function. According to HELD (Thesis. Leipzig, 1952) the normal range of xanthoprotein is 39.4–62.9 mg%, with a mean of 47.7 mg%. There is often a significant relationship between BUN and the sodium chloride balance of the body. When there is a fall in the chloride level there is a slow increase in the BUN, and conversely parenteral administration of sodium chloride leads to a sudden fall in BUN. In the first instance the increase in BUN precedes the loss of chloride. The normal value of blood chloride according to SCHEFFLER (Thesis. Leipzig, 1954) lies about 430.9 mg%; we regard values

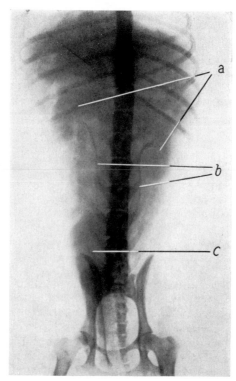

Fig. 380. Intravenous urography. (a) kidneys; (b) ureters; (c) urinary bladder, all shown well by the contrast medium.

between 500–600 mg% as being normal. The sodium chloride balance is closely related to the secretion of gastric juice. Where there is frequent vomiting there is a loss of chloride in the gastric juice which is expelled. Enteritis may also cause a hypochloraemia due to disordered chloride absorption and also loss of chloride in the diarrhoeic faeces. The clinical syndrome of chloride deficiency may present certain similarities with uraemia, but as there is no true renal disease it is classed as a pseudo-uraemia. Nevertheless if the condition persists for any length of time renal dysfunction will occur with an increase in BUN, due to the fact that the kidneys cannot function efficiently where there is a low blood chloride level. Where normal urine secretion takes place the serum chloride level must also be normal.

Two radiographic techniques may be employed in the diagnosis of renal diseases, viz. Intravenous Urography and Pneumoperitoneum.

Intravenous Urography (LORENZ, Thesis. Leipzig, 1955). This technique is used when there are suspicions that the pelvises of the kidneys are structurally altered (Fig. 380). It can also be used to assess the functional efficiency of the organ, as the excretion of the contrast medium is delayed when the kidneys are severely damaged by disease.

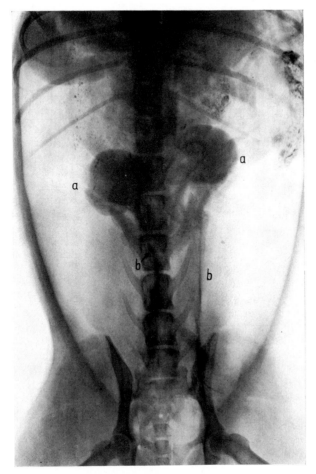

Fig. 381. Demonstration of the kidneys (a) and ureters (b) with the aid of a pneumoretroperitoneum with the pelvis elevated.

Pneumoperitoneum, Pneumoretroperitoneum (SCHWILLE, Thesis. Leipzig, 1958). In this technique air or oxygen is pumped into either the abdominal cavity or the retroperitoneal connective tissues (Fig. 381). The air, being radiolucent, outlines the organs and it is thus possible to gain a fairly accurate picture of the kidneys and ureters, and of any structural changes due to enlargement or contraction.

The bladder can be outlined radiographically by the technique of retrograde filling with a contrast medium or with air. This method is useful for the demonstration of neoplasms within the lumen, increased thickness of the bladder walls, or inflammatory changes in the mucosa. Cystic calculi may be detected by plain radiography depending on their composition. Calcium and phosphorus stones are densely radio-opaque, but cysteine stones may produce no shadow and thus be overlooked. Oxalate stones may sometimes be recognised by their notched borders. Where it is suspected that rupture of the bladder has occurred a pneumocystogram should be attempted. If the bladder is ruptured, then the air will pass into the abdominal cavity and the organ will not be outlined.

Nephritis, often of a severe nature, is a common disease in the dog. The condition is caused by blood-borne irritants in the majority of cases, including toxins, the micro-organisms of infectious disease (distemper, C.V.H., leptospirosis, etc.) and metabolic products such as indol and skatol from intestinal fermentation. Poisons in the form of mercurial preparations, turpentine, creosote, cantharides, tar, squills, etc. may also have a direct irritant action on the kidneys.

Clinical classification of canine kidney disease is difficult as a pathological classification cannot be applied *in vivo*. The pathological processes cannot be accurately demarcated from each other and tend to merge into a continuous process. Nevertheless it is possible to distinguish Renal Insufficiency, Acute and Chronic Nephritis and Uraemia.

Renal Insufficiency. The early signs of this condition often pass unnoticed by the owner, and only after it has been in existence for some time is the dog presented with a history of loss of appetite, increased thirst (polydipsia) allied to normal amounts of urine. The aetiology of renal insufficiency is often to be found in cardiac dysfunction resulting in restriction of the normal blood supply to the kidneys. The process of concentration of urine by the kidneys may also be disturbed. The volume of urine is increased (polyuria), it is pale and watery in appearance and the specific gravity is low. Urine volume may be decreased (oliguria) where there are disorders of filtration or reabsorption. In this case the urine is darker in colour and the specific gravity is raised. In severe cases the production of urine may cease completely (anuria). In renal insufficiency palpation of the kidneys is not very rewarding, the BUN and serum chloride levels remain within normal limits.

Treatment. Prime consideration should be given to improving cardiac output and where possible specific treatment of the heart condition should be instituted (see p. 230). The diet should include mainly carbohydrates, gruel, fruit, and vegetables, whilst meat, cheese, gravies, spices and salt should be severely restricted or withheld altogether. Boiled sugar water or tea should be offered in place of the normal drinking water, and every 3–4 days a thirst day is established on which only fruit is given as a source of fluid. Diuresis may be stimulated by tea sweetened with saccharine, or with one of the saline diuretics.

Intravenous injection of 40 % glucose solution is also recommended to regulate the output of urine, and diuresis can also be maintained by the use of drugs which increase cardiac output (digitalis, strophanthin, etc.). The metabolic rate of the dog is diminished by keeping it at rest as much as possible, so that excretion by the kidney can be reduced. Warm poultices, diathermy or microwave therapy of the kidney region should assist in promoting an increased blood supply to the organs.

Acute Nephritis. Acute nephritis is manifested by loss of appetite, general malaise, vomiting and enteritis. Palpation of the kidney region evokes signs of pain and the dog walks stiffly with its back arched. Micturition may be increased in frequency and is often painful (dysuria). In the early stages of the disease, there is usually oliguria with the passage of a dark coloured urine of high specific gravity. Later the urine becomes more normal in appearance and consistency. The urine may be cloudy due to increased cellular content and large amounts of albumin (up to 2 %) may be found. Albuminuria in itself is not a positive indication of nephritis, as it may occur in persistent pyrexias, overexertion, nervous diseases, etc. Conversely there may be severe kidney damage where the urine contains little or no albumin. Haematuria is a regular feature of acute nephritis and to pinpoint the site of haemorrhage the so-called "3-glass test" is used. The first, middle and final portions of the urine stream are collected into 3 separate glasses. If the final portion is very haemorrhagic this is indicative of renal haemorrhage. The sediment contains small polygonal epithelial cells with large distinct nuclei and many small finely granular or large coarsely granular casts. These casts have been interpreted by BECHER (Nierenkrankheiten Bd. 1, Jena 1944) as denoting degenerative processess. WITZIGMANN (Münch. tierärztl. Wschr. **85**, 313, 1935) associated these casts with acute relapses of nephritis in elderly dogs. Rarely the BUN level is raised, due to the combination of circulatory insufficiency with maintenance of the concentration power of the kidneys.

Treatment. Treatment is similar to that outlined on p. 330. Massive doses of vitamin C (500 mg) and calcium borogluconate (2–5 ml) may be given intravenously. Where there is a bacteriuria, hexamethylene-tetramine may be given. Hexamethylene-tetramine acts by the formation of formaldehyde in an acid urine and it may be necessary to acidify the urine. This may be achieved by the intravenous injection of "Amphotropin" (hexamine camphorate) in a dose of 3.5–5 ml.

Editor's note: This solution is highly irritant if it is injected extravascularly. The acidification can be achieved more easily by the administration of ammonium chloride or 1-methionine.

Hexamethylene-tetramine must not be combined with sulphonamides, as there is a danger of crystallisation in the kidneys. The broad spectrum antibiotics are more effective in clearing a bacteriuria.

Chronic Nephritis. Chronic inflammatory changes may affect the renal parenchyma or the interstitial tissues. The course of the disease is very insidious and the condition may have been in existence for a considerable time before the owner suspects the dog is ill. Polydipsia is a fairly constant symptom and occurs mainly in chronic interstitial nephritis, where it is to be interpreted as a sign of compensatory hyperfunction. It is usually accompanied by polyuria, due to the increased intake of water and to the diuretic action of the retained urea. As there is a gradual loss of chloride there is a corresponding loss of the ability to retain water in the body tissues. This leads to signs of dehydration appearing, especially in the skin which becomes hidebound. The polyuria must be distinguished from the reflex polyuria which one sees in cystitis, consisting of increased frequency of micturition without an actual increase in the volume of urine passed.

Clinically the chronic nephritic dog appears to have a stiff gait, often with an arched back. The conjunctivae are of a pale, rather muddy colour, the coat is staring and lustreless, and there may be areas of alopecia and chronic eczematous changes. In advanced cases acidosis may develop as the formation of ammonia for the maintenance of normal blood pH is reduced, and the fixed blood alkali reserves are exhausted by the free acids. This acidosis may lead to deep breathing, due to a reflex action on the respiratory centre. Auscultation of the heart usually reveals an accentuated second sound, the pulse is hard and tense (bounding), and radiography reveals hypertrophy of the heart, especially the left ventricle.

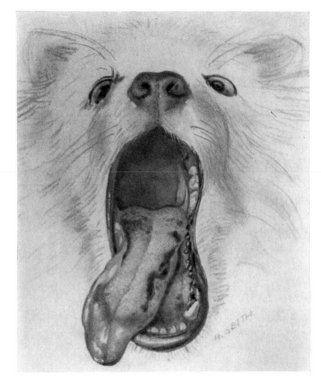

Fig. 382. Necrosis of the edges of the tongue in uraemia.

There is still some controversy as to whether one of the cardinal features of human nephritis, viz. hypertension, occurs in the dog. The circulatory changes described may be due to an irritant action of metabolites retained in the blood on the peripheral blood vessels and on the heart itself. In thin dogs it may be possible to palpate shrunken or irregular kidneys.

A characteristic feature of chronic nephritis is the passage of large amounts of pale urine with a low specific gravity. The kidney's ability to form the normal urinary pigments has been lost and the urine appears very clear and watery. The specific gravity may fall to between 1002–1012, indicating a lack of compensatory ability by the kidney. Damage to the renal epithelium leads to disturbances of reabsorption in the tubules. The excretory substances are washed out by the amount of fluid and the kidney is unable to reabsorb some of the fluid and thus concentrate the urine. In this way the specific gravity may fall until it approaches that of plasma dialysate, where it achieves a sort of balance (isothenuria or hyposthenuria). At this point the filtration capacity of the glomeruli has almost completely disappeared. The albumin content of the urine is very small, often about 1 %, and may be unmeasurable. Cellular constituents are sparse in the sediment but there are usually quite a number of casts present. Hyaline casts are

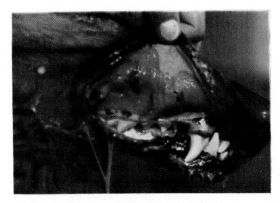

Fig. 383. Uraemia. There are wide, flat erosions on the cheek mucosa and the saliva is viscous and ropey.

characteristic of chronic interstitial nephritis, they are derived from the tubules and are the products of inflammatory changes.

Treatment. Treatment of chronic nephritis is similar to that described on p. 331. In addition, to combat the loss of chloride and the accompanying dehydration, 3–8 ml of 10 % sodium chloride solution are given intravenously.

Uraemia. Uraemia represents the final stage of kidney disease. Clinically it is shown by increasingly marked lassitude which may progress to complete apathy. The skin becomes hidebound, the dog becomes emaciated, and the polydipsia so marked that the animal drinks from puddles and even its own urine. Due to the failure of the kidney to excrete waste products, auto-intoxication occurs and the body tries to excrete through the skin and mucosae, with a resultant urinous smell of the breath (Oral foetor). Ulcers appear in the mouth and on the tongue, breaking down to leave raw areas covered with a greyish-green deposit (Figs. 382, 383). Another sign of uraemia is persistent vomiting, and in the terminal stages blood appears in the vomitus and the faeces. The acidosis of the blood slows and deepens the respirations and in the later stages muscular spasms or convulsions may occur. The dog may become completely anuric, or the small quantity of urine passed shows all the signs of a very severe nephritis. The BUN level increases rapidly and may be of the order of 200 mg %, with a corresponding fall in the blood chloride level (hypochloraemia). The prognosis must be regarded as unfavourable if the chloride continues to fall, as hypochloraemia is a sign that the maintenance of the anionic state of the blood is threatened by the accumulation of the products of protein breakdown. If this continues, death in uraemic coma will occur.

Treatment. Treatment of uraemia is similar to that of renal disease in general. The mouth cavity may be rinsed out with sage tea and the ulcers painted with iodised glycerine (see p. 247). As there is usually some degree of hypothermia, warm packs are recommended. Acidosis may be corrected by the administration of sodium bicarbonate, and charcoal may be given to absorb some of the putre- factive toxins produced in the bowel. It is important to ensure that there is a free flow of urine from the bladder and any obstruction (Calculi), or dysfunction

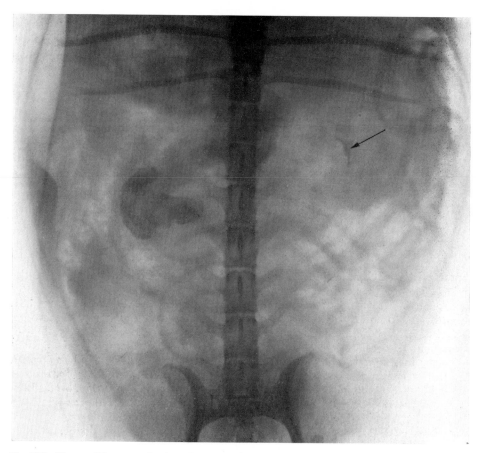

Fig. 384. X-ray of the stones in the pelvis of the kidney in Fig. 385. The arrow points to the right kidney pelvis shown up by intravenous pyelography. In order to show up the kidneys better a pneumoperitoneum was done. As the right kidney was functional the left kidney was removed.

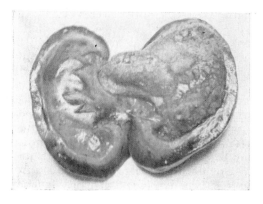

Fig. 385. Stones in the pelvis of the kidney, visible in the radiograph in Fig. 384. The stones were removed by nephrectomy.

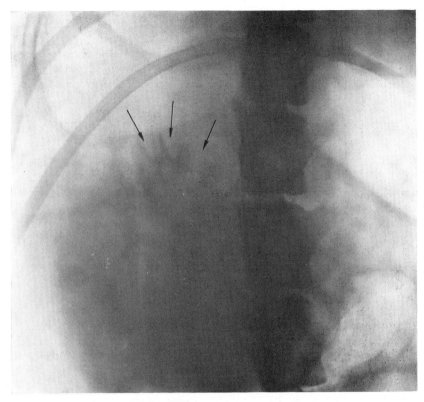

Fig. 386. Tumour of the kidney. By means of a pneumoperitoneum and intravenous pyelography
it was shown that only a small part of the kidney is functional (shown by the arrows).

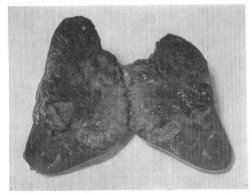

Fig. 387. Kidney tumour (compare the
radiograph in Fig. 386), only the anterior
third of this kidney was still functional.
Postmortem examination showed a
markedly infiltrating adenocarcinoma
partly forming cysts.

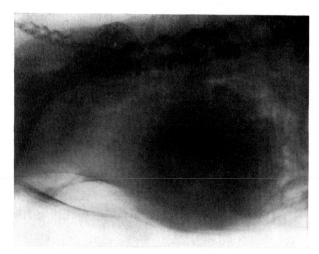

Fig. 388. Enlarged bladder with thick walls in cystitis.

(paralysis of the bladder), must be corrected as soon as possible. Peritoneal dialysis will often reduce the BUN level temporarily.

Renal Calculi (Kidney stones). The formation of stones in the pelvis of the kidney of the dog is extremely rare and is often asymptomatic, such calculi often being discovered on radiography of the abdomen. The stones may be outlined by the use of intravenous pyelography or pneumoretroperitoneum. Calculi producing illness can be removed by nephrotomy, or, if only one kidney is affected, nephrectomy (Figs. 384, 385, 386, 387) may be performed.

Cystitis (Inflammation of the Bladder). Cystitis may be due to three main causes: Haematogenous infection; Ascending infection; Trauma.

Acute Cystitis. In this condition small amounts of urine are passed frequently but the total daily amount passed remains normal. Palpation of the bladder will evoke signs of pain and it may be possible to appreciate some thickening of the wall of the viscus. The urine has an ammoniacal smell due to fermentation within the bladder, it is dark in colour, of increased viscosity or stringy, and usually alkaline or neutral in reaction. Albumin is usually present and the sediment contains triple phosphate crystals and epithelial cells. If the condition persists for any length of time, cells from the deeper layers of the bladder epithelium may appear. Bacteria are to be seen in the sediment in most cases.

Chronic Cystitis. There is a similar clinical picture but the frequent micturition is more marked. There may be general malaise with inappetence, lassitude and sometimes pyrexia. Often the dog will strain for quite long periods but only produce a few drops of urine. Palpation reveals thickening of the bladder wall and any pressure will evoke signs of pain (Fig. 388). Pus and blood may be appreciable macroscopically in the urine. The latter is alkaline in reaction, has an ammoniacal odour and the sediment contains triple phosphate crystals, bacteria, leucocytes and erythrocytes.

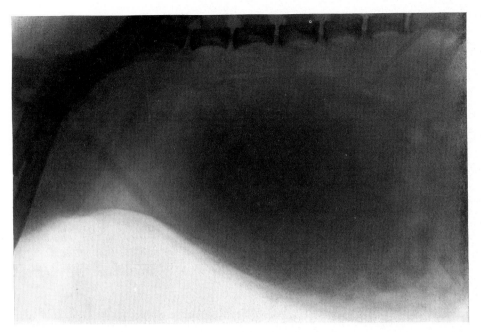

Fig. 389. Retention of urine. The bladder extends up to the costal arch.

Treatment. The patient should be rested as much as possible and the bladder kept warm, by woollen cloths, diathermy, microwave therapy, etc. The bacterial content of the bladder may be reduced by the flushing action of diuretics or the administration of large amounts of fluids (see p. 330). The infection may be treated by the use of hexamethylene-tetramine (see p. 331). The bladder may also be irrigated with solutions of the broad-spectrum antibiotics, or the latter may be administered systemically.

Capillaria plica infection. This helminth parasite occurs in the bladder and may cause marked clinical signs, which may lead to errors in diagnosis. In a case described by OTTEN (Kleintier. Prax. **2**, 114–166, 1957) a purulent vaginal discharge aroused suspicions of pyometra. Exploratory laparotomy revealed only cystitis and urine examination showed the presence of numerous eggs of *C. plica.*

Treatment. In the case reported above, piperazine paste (1 cm/kg bodyweight) was given for 4 days. The bladder was also filled three times with 10 ml piperazine solution to which prontosil had been added. Egg production was diminished but not stopped by this treatment. It has been reported that methyridine is effective in this infection.

Paralysis of the Bladder. Paralysis of the bladder may result from diseases of the spinal cord, the cauda equina, or the peripheral nerves supplying the bladder. Injury to the bladder wall or the sphincter by overdistension may also lead to paralysis. The condition may be manifested by retention or incontinence of urine.

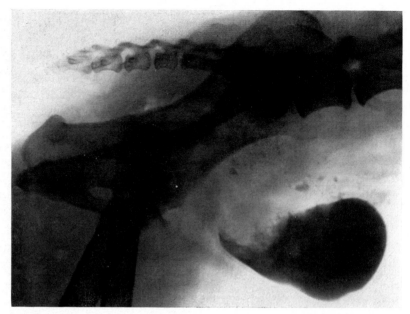

Fig. 390. Neoplastic infiltration of the bladder. Both the ureteral openings are closed by polypoid growths. Resection of the bladder and implantation of the ureter into the rectum were performed but death from uraemia and hydronephrosis occurred after 4 days.

In retention, the bladder is overdistended and can be felt as a large, firm, smooth, spherical swelling in the abdomen (Fig. 389). Careful pressure on the bladder may overcome the resistance to outflow and urine can be expressed.

In incontinence, the bladder is again enlarged but it is only moderately full and of a flabby consistency. The urine spills over after reaching a certain level in the bladder, but the dog does not appear to realise that micturition is occurring and does not adopt the customary stance.

Treatment. This will depend on the aetiology as the condition is seldom a primary one. It is important to prevent infection of the paralysed bladder and the viscus should be emptied as frequently as possible by manual expression or catheterisation. Muscular paralyses are treated by the application of warm packs, diathermy, microwave and infra-red therapy. Nervous paralyses can be treated by injections of strychnine (strychnine nitrate 1% solution, 0.1 mg per kg bodyweight subcutaneously for no more than 4 successive days) or by the use of Faradic stimulation.

Prognosis should always be guarded, but in the case of a muscular paralysis recovery may be expected in a comparatively short time.

Displacement of the Bladder. Displacement of the bladder from its customary position may occur in perineal hernia (see p. 307). In this case the bladder is retroflected into the hernial sac and there is kinking of the neck with resultant obstruction to the flow of urine. Before repairing the hernia it may be necessary to puncture and drain the bladder.

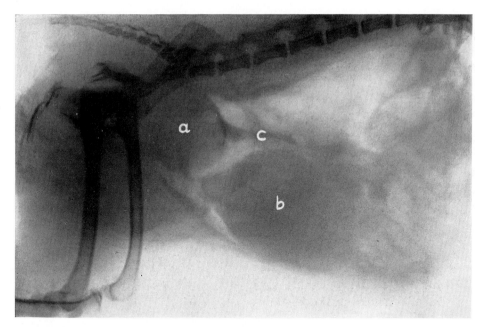

Fig. 391. Tumour between the neck of the bladder and the uterus made visible by a pneumo peritoneum and filling of the bladder with contrast medium. (a) tumour; (b) bladder; (c) uterus.

Neoplasia of the Bladder. Tumours of the bladder are comparatively rare in the dog. The clinical picture is similar to that seen in chronic cystitis, but there may be more haematuria. It may be possible to palpate the tumour within the bladder, but usually there is so much inflammatory thickening of the wall that this may be difficult. Radiography after filling the bladder with contrast medium will more accurately delineate the lesion (Fig. 390). A pneumoperitoneum radiograph will facilitate the differential definition of the site of the tumour growth (Fig. 391).

Treatment. The only treatment is surgical removal. Cystotomy is described on p. 344. It is imperative to completely remove the tumour and where the whole bladder is infiltrated it will be necessary to remove the whole viscus and implant the ureters into the rectum.

Rupture of the Bladder. Rupture of the bladder should always be borne in mind in street accidents. Dogs are usually allowed out on the street to pass urine and even a slight blow may rupture a full bladder. It is important to enquire as to whether the animal has passed urine after the accident. If not a catheter should be passed, as reflex spasm of the sphincter may lead to urinary retention. If no urine can be obtained in this way then air should be pumped in and a radiograph taken (see p. 328).

Rupture of the bladder is to be regarded as a surgical emergency as there is usually severe shock, and peritonitis soon ensues due to contamination of the peritoneum by urine. The technique is similar to that described on p. 305.

Urolithiasis. The formation of calculi in the bladder of the dog is quite common in certain breeds. The calculus forms by a nucleus of cells and renal casts collecting,

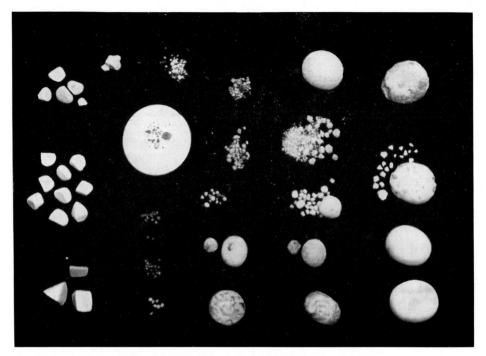

Fig. 392. Various vesical and urethral stones.

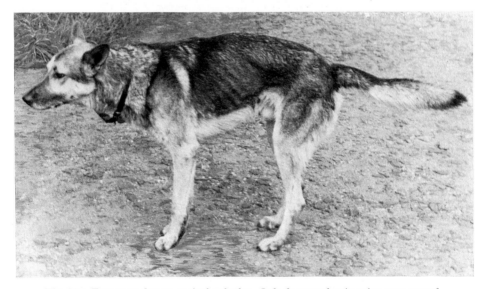

Fig. 393. Tenesmus due to vesical calculus. Only haemorrhagic urine was passed.

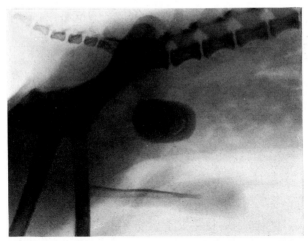

Fig. 394. Vesical calculus with concentric layers in a male terrier. The external layer of the stone consisted chiefly of ammonium urate and calcium phosphate whilst its centre was composed of calcium carbonate and calcium phosphate.

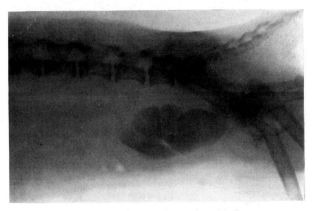

Fig. 395. Vesical calculus in a bitch.

on which salts are deposited. This may occur because there is too high a concentration of salts in the urine, but the part played by the protective colloids is more important. Certain districts seem to have a high incidence of urinary calculi. In the post-war years when the standard of canine nutrition was low, calculi were not often seen, whereas today they are often diagnosed. It would seem, therefore, that the plane of nutrition plays some part in calculi formation in the dog. The calculi themselves are usually composed of phosphates or urates.

The clinical picture is basically the same as that seen in cystitis, but there is usually more tenesmus. After considerable straining efforts the dog manages to pass only a small amount of blood-stained urine (Fig. 393). Sometimes this tenesmus is not seen but there is a greatly increased frequency of micturition. It may be possible to palpate the stones within the bladder. In contradistinction to foreign bodies in the intestine, bladder stones can only be moved to a limited extent and in the direction of the pelvis. In the bitch, catheterisation may reveal the calculus by the grating sensation imparted by contact with the catheter. Usually vesical calculi are easily visible on plain radiography (Figs. 394, 395 and 396).

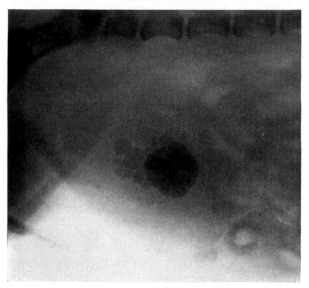

Fig. 396. Vesical calculus (with concentric layers) in a dog.

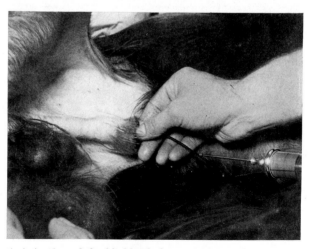

Fig. 397. Antiseptic irrigation of the bladder before cystotomy. A syringe with a blunt-ended needle is attached to an elastic catheter.

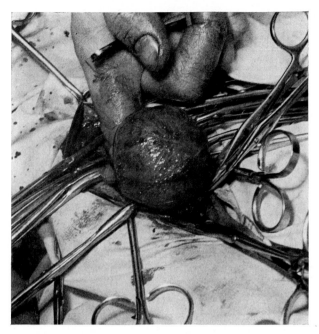

Fig. 398. A very inflamed bladder (cystitis) protruding through the laparotomy wound.

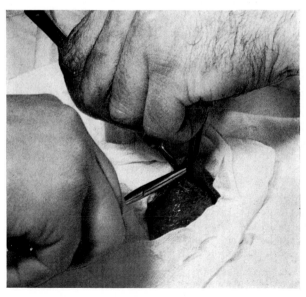

Fig. 399. Cystotomy. The bladder is opened with a scalpel between artery forceps and dressing forceps.

Treatment. No medical treatment is known which can disperse the calculi and the only available treatment is surgical removal.

Technique of Cystotomy. As opening of the bladder breaches surgical asepsis, the bacterial content of the urine must be reduced as much as possible by pre-operative irrigations with antibiotic solutions. A few hours before operation the bladder is filled with a penicillin solution containing 400,000 units, and the catheter is left *in situ* (Fig. 397). The patient is prepared for surgery in the usual way. Anaesthesia is the lumbo-sacral epidural type. The incision is made in the supra-pubic position and should be about 7 cm long. In the case of the male dog, the incision is made alongside the penis. The bladder is brought out through the wound (Fig. 398), and the wound edges are packed off with gauze. The fundus of the bladder is now opened, the size of the incision depending on the size of the stone(s) (Fig. 399). The wound edges are separated by an assistant with forceps and the stones removed with the aid of artery forceps. Small stones may be hidden in the neck of the bladder and so normal saline solution is forced in through the catheter to wash them into view, where they can be removed with a gauze swab. If the pressure through the catheter is insufficient, a blunt-ended cannula is introduced through the bladder incision, and with the aid of a syringe, saline is squirted into the viscus (Fig. 400). When all stones have been removed the bladder wound is closed preferably with a double row of Lembert's sutures. In most cases, however, the bladder wall is too thickened to be invaginated, so Über-reiter's sutures are employed. Closely placed, deep sutures are used to approximate the edges of the wound and between these, to seal the wound completely, more superficial sutures are placed (Fig. 401). Finally the bladder is washed with normal saline, the suture line is covered with omentum, the bladder is replaced in the abdomen and the latter is closed in the usual way. Before actual closure, the abdomen may be irrigated with sterile normal saline or 100–200 mg terramycin.

After-treatment of the wound is routine, but one must attempt to prevent a recurrence of stone formation. To do this it is necessary to know the composition of the calculi removed. If these are composed of triple phosphate, attempts should

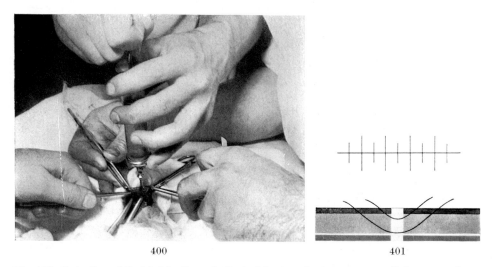

400   401

Fig. 400. Irrigation of the bladder through the incision in order to remove small stones or urinary gravel with the aid of a gauze tampon.

Fig. 401. Suture of the bladder by Überreiter's method.

be made to keep the urine as acid as possible and the diet should be made up of meat, fish, eggs, etc., but containing no milk, fruit or vegetables. There should be a high fluid intake. In the case of urate stones again there should be a high fluid intake and this may include milk.

Lactovegetable, uncooked foods, vegetables, fruit and potatoes should all be included in the diet, but meat and fish are restricted, and cocoa and chocolate forbidden. Oxalate stones call for a reduction in fluid intake and the prohibition of vegetables, tomatoes, fruit, cocoa, chocolate and tea. With cysteine stones a low protein, high carbohydrate diet should be prescribed.

Hyaluronidase has an important prophylactic effect as it acts as a hydrophil colloid, probably preventing the accumulation of crystals by reduction in surface tension. As the viscosity of the urine is decreased, the crystals are more easily flushed out when the bladder is emptied. For the first 3 post-operative days, the dog is given 10 VRE of "Hylase", followed by 3 injections at 2 day intervals and 4 injections at 4 day intervals. After an interval of 8 weeks, 10 further injections are given with a week's interval between each of them. Unfortunately recurrences are frequent despite all prophylactic measures.

Urethral Calculi. Urethral calculi are found almost exclusively in the male dog. Due to the anatomy of the penis, small stones or gravel tend to become wedged in the urethra at the caudal end of the os penis.

The clinical picture is dominated by tenesmus, the dog constantly straining to pass urine, but only a few drops of blood-stained urine emerging. If the obstruction is not so complete, the urine may emerge in a thin stream. The bladder becomes very distended and may be palpated as a firm spherical swelling occupying almost the whole of the abdomen. A catheter passes only a short way along the urethra before encountering resistance, and often the gritty nature of the calculi can be appreciated by the feel of the contact. Radiography may not show up the stones,

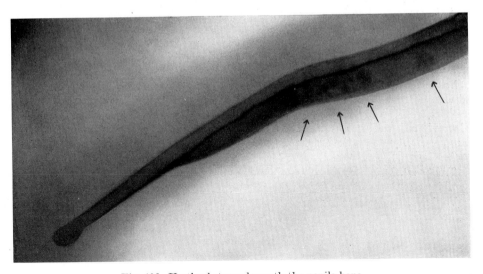

Fig. 402. Urethral stones beneath the penile bone.

either because of the low radio-opacity of the calculi, or due to the fact that they are obscured by the os penis (Fig. 402).

Treatment. In the vast majority of cases urethrotomy will be required. In mild cases an attempt may be made to break up the collection of stones with the metal catheter, plus urethral irrigation. The urethral injection of hyaluronidase may break up the stones by reducing surface tension.

Technique of Urethrotomy. Epidural anaesthesia is induced after the usual surgical preparation of the site. A metal sound is passed as far as the obstruction to indicate the site of operation. The penis is seized between the thumb and forefinger, and the skin of the sheath is stretched and incised along the median raphe. The urethra can now be seen and is incised over the calculi. There is considerable haemorrhage at this point as the urethra is surrounded by muscle. The mucosa is fixed with mosquito forceps and the calculi removed with a small spoon. Gentle pressure on the bladder will wash any remaining stones out through the urethral incision. When the urethra is free and the catheter can be passed easily into the bladder, the urethral mucosa is sutured to the skin wound by small Perlon sutures. The fistula thus created usually heals up within about six months and the urine is then passed in the normal manner (Figs. 452–455).

11. Diseases of the female generative system

Examination of the female sexual organs is limited to visual inspection of the external genitalia, the vagina through a vaginascope, palpation of the abdomen (pregnancy, pyometra, ovarian neoplasia) and radiography. The latter may be used to determine the number of foetuses in the uterus, the presentation of the puppy in dystocia and possibly increase in the size of the uterus in pyometra. Certain haematological techniques (erythrocyte sedimentation rates, differential white cell counts, electrophoresis, etc.) are of value in certain conditions and are discussed in the relevant sections. For vaginoscopy we use the Chiron vaginascope. This instrument has a glass speculum with a bevelled anterior rim to facilitate insertion. It is advisable to lubricate the speculum with paraffin oil or a bland ointment before use. Any changes in the portio or inflammation of the vaginal mucosa can be studied closely by means of the adjustable lens (Fig. 403), and a prolapsed mucosa can be inspected by withdrawing the speculum.

Vaginitis. Inflammation of the vagina appears clinically as a muco-serous discharge from the vulva. Vaginoscopy reveals a reddened and inflamed mucosa with excessive fluid. In the portio (cervix uteri), which remains closed, there is also evidence of inflammation. Vaginitis is relatively rare as a clinical entity and the possibility of cystic hyperplasia (pyometra) of the uterus should be excluded before a diagnosis is made.

Treatment. Irrigation with acridine dye solutions followed by the instillation of antibiotic ointment is probably the most effective treatment.

Vaginal Neoplasia. New growths in the vagina occur mostly as pedunculated tumours in the older bitch. After a time the tumour protrudes from the vulva, and may become excoriated and ulcerated if not removed (Fig. 404). Removal is fairly easy, but as most of the tumours arise from the floor of the vagina, care must be taken not to injure the urethral opening. It is advisable to introduce a catheter into the urethra to protect it during operation. As most of the tumours

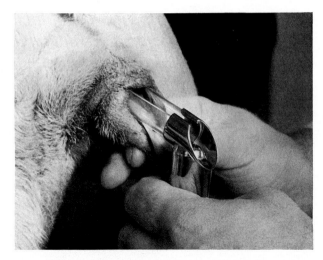

Fig. 403. Vaginoscopy with a slotted speculum.

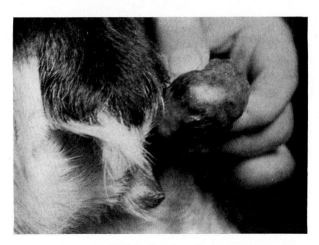

Fig. 404. Pedunculated vaginal tumour.

are pedunculated, they can be removed by placing encircling ligatures around the pedicle under local anaesthesia and then cutting through the stalk.

Condylomata (cauliflower-like growths) are rarely seen in the vagina. Complete extirpation of this type of growth is usually impossible, as they often involve the whole of the vagina up to the cervix. Those protruding through the vulva can usually be removed fairly readily.

BAIER & RÜSSE (Berl. Münch. tierärztl. Wschr. **72**, 355–359, 1959) describe a technique for the removal of deep-seated vaginal tumours. After a medial incision of the perineum, the whole length of the vestibule is opened and the introitus

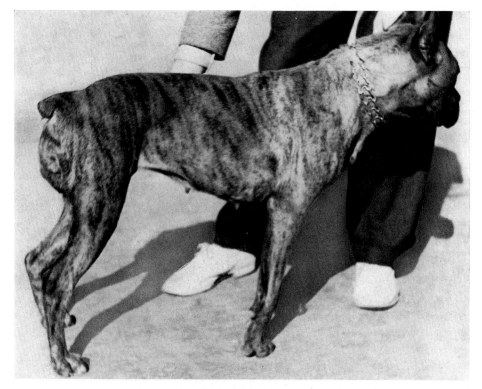

Fig. 405. Vaginal tumour in a Boxer bitch. The tumour was on the dorsal wall of the vagina and
simulated a perineal hernia.

vaginae is freed. The vagina within the pelvis can now be exposed by retroversion.
The incision is closed in three layers, viz. vestibule, subcutaneous tissues and skin.

Hyperplasia of the Vaginal Mucosa. Occurs occasionally in young bitches
(especially Boxers) in the first oestrus and is often confused with prolapse of the
vagina. The hyperplastic mucosa bulges out through the vulva and may be
mistaken for a vaginal polyp (Fig. 406). The condition usually subsides with the
end of the heat period. The hyperplasia tends to recur at each succeeding oestrus
and the mechanical obstruction renders mating impossible. Surgical treatment
should therefore be undertaken to relieve the condition.

Technique of Operation for Vaginal Hyperplasia. Epidural anaesthesia is induced and the
bitch is tied down on her side as shown in Fig. 32. The urethra is protected by the insertion of a
catheter (Fig. 407) and the protruding tissue drawn out with forceps. To diminish the risk of
vaginal stenosis, the hyperplastic mucosa is removed transversely to the course of the vagina. It
is very important to grasp the edges of the wound with clamps, otherwise they will be retracted
into the vagina and may be difficult to relocate (Fig. 408). The withdrawn tissue is carefully
divided with scissors and all bleeding vessels, which are mainly superficial, are clamped and ligated.
Closely placed Perlon sutures are inserted, the ends being left rather long as they have to be
removed after eight days, possibly under anaesthesia (Fig. 409).

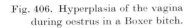

Fig. 406. Hyperplasia of the vagina during oestrus in a Boxer bitch.

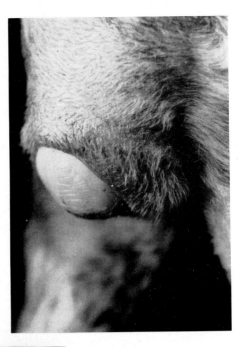

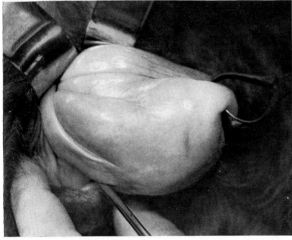

Fig. 407. The hyperplastic tissue withdrawn with tumour forceps and a metal catheter inserted into the urethra.

Normal Pregnancy. Oestrus in the bitch usually occurs twice a year and lasts for about 21 days. The first heat period normally occurs when the bitch is 7–8 months old, but mating is not usually allowed until the 3rd or 4th oestrus. The optimum time for mating is between the 11th–14th day of oestrus when the bitch will most readily accept the dog. At the moment of ejaculation, the bulbus cavernosus of the penis swells to seal off the vagina caudally and effectively "tying" the two partners together for 20–35 minutes. Usually the dog will turn around when tied so that

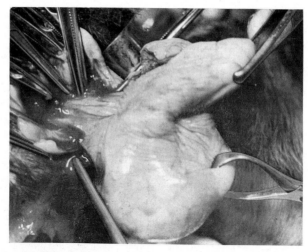

Fig. 408. The tumour is removed with scissors and the edges of the wound are fixed with artery
forceps. In the foreground, the catheter in the urethra.

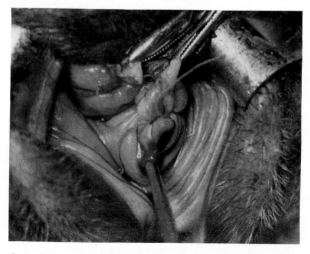

Fig. 409. The edges of the wound are drawn together. Now the catheter may be removed.

the two animals are back to back. During this tied period, the sperms migrate up
to the Fallopian tubes where fertilisation of the ova takes place. On the 11th day
after fertilisation, the fertilised eggs migrate to the uterus and become implanted
in the endometrium. Cyst-like swellings, denoting the sites of development of the
foetuses, develop along the uterine horn about the 19th–21st day of gestation.
About the 40th day, the individual swellings become merged into a general dilata-

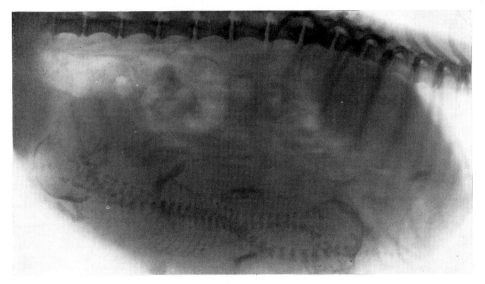

Fig. 410. Pregnancy.

tion of the uterine cornu. The gestation period is on average 62½ days with a range of 56–64 days, and ends with parturition.

The owner usually requires as early a diagnosis of pregnancy as possible. Unfortunately the output of hormones in the urine of the pregnant bitch is very small and BUTSCH (Thesis. Zürich, 1945) found that the Cuboni, the Allen–Doisy and the Ascheim–Zondek tests were of no value in the dog. Palpation and radiography are the only methods of pregnancy diagnosis applicable to the bitch.

Abdominal palpation will permit a diagnosis of pregnancy if carried out between the 21st and 42nd day, as the cyst-like dilatations of the uterus can be appreciated during this period, the 24th–26th day being the optimum time in our experience. At this time the foetuses can be palpated as swellings the size of a hen's egg. It is possible to miss a pregnancy, especially in fat bitches and those of the toy breeds, where the foetuses may be carried under the costal arch. Palpation should always be carefully carried out and not performed after about the 35th day because of the danger of inducing abortion. In the later stages of pregnancy the foetuses can be seen on radiography (Fig. 410).

Normal parturition begins with a fall in body temperature of 1–1½ °C, 12–48 hours before the actual birth. The bitch has made herself a bed, her teats are swollen and the vulva is enlarged and oedematous (Fig. 411). Often the bitch will go off her food for about 24 hours before parturition commences. The cervical plug becomes liquefied and the cervix commences to open. It is important to note these signs of impending parturition, especially when the pregnancy has exceeded the normal length of time. A vaginal examination should be made to determine whether the cervix is open or not, as it may be necessary to use drugs to assist the birth process. Birth commences with labour pains and the darkly coloured amniotic sac bulges through the relaxed cervix into the vagina. The time

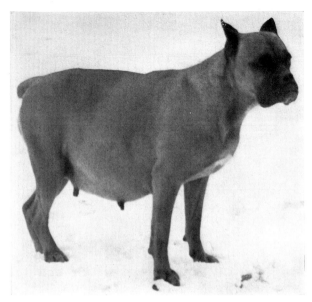

Fig. 411. Advanced pregnancy in a bitch with a well developed milk line.

interval between the birth of one pup and the next should not be allowed to exceed 2 hours. SCHULZE (Mhefte Med. **10**, 533–539, 1955) made a detailed study of labour in multiparous bitches. It appears to be immaterial to the birth process of the bicornuate uterus whether the foetuses are alive or dead, and the same function occurs in abortion. If dead and living pups are present together in the uterus, the living are always expelled before the dead ones. The process of birth is probably initiated by intra-uterine pressure. The puppies are born either head or tail first, and the foetal membranes and the umbilical cord are divided by the bitch. It is believed that the foetal membranes and the placenta contain substances causing labour pains, so the bitch should not be prevented from eating them. Sometimes the bitch bites through the cord in a ragged manner, in which case the owner should ligature the cord about a finger's breadth from the abdominal wall, and cut it off neatly.

The normal puerperium commences with a slight rise of temperature (39.0–39.3 °C). The uterine discharge increases for the first 5–8 days post-partum and then gradually decreases until it has virtually ceased by the 21st day. Involution of the external genitalia occurs during the first week.

Superfoetation (Superfecundation). Breeders often hold the erroneous opinion that once a bitch has been successfully mated she cannot conceive to further services during the same heat period. The birth of pups of obviously different sires indicates that superfecundation can, in fact, occur.

If a bitch is not to be mated during oestrus, one can prevent dogs annoying her by deodorising the oestrual vaginal secretions, and many preparations are available for this purpose. Chlorophyll tablets given orally are said to effectively deodorise the vaginal secretions.

Failure to accept the dog or to conceive may be due to many different factors. Surgical manipulations are somewhat risky due to the small size of the organs involved. BARDENS (North Amer. Vet. **38**, 280–284, 1957) described a technique for curettage of the uterus during oestrus. He performed a laparotomy, opened the uterus at the level of the bifurcation, and curetted the endometrium, finally irrigating the uterine cavities with normal saline. Out of 5 bitches treated in this way, 2 conceived at the next oestrus. We do not perform this operation but prefer to rely on hormonal treatment of sterility. A suitable dose of follicle-stimulating hormone is given on the 5th and 7th days of eostrus and the bitch is mated between the 11th–13th days.

If mesalliance occurs, antiseptic irrigation of the uterus immediately after mating will not prevent conception. It is necessary to give follicle-stimulating hormone to counteract the activity of the corpora lutea and produce a secondary endometrial proliferation and thus prevent implantation. A suitable dose given subcutaneously on the 6th, 8th and 10th days after service is usually effective. Too high a dosage may produce cystic glandular hyperplasia of the uterus (Pyometra). After the injection the signs of oestrus become more marked and it is essential to ensure that further mating does not occur. HEBER (Thesis. Leipzig, 1959) studied the effect of such treatment upon the subsequent fertility of the bitch and found that it was not significantly reduced. The temporary infertility occurring was in the region of 9 %, which does not vary much from expected natural incidence of sterility of unknown origin. An intramuscular injection of oestrogen within 48 hours of mating is equally effective. After the 11th day after mesalliance, implantation can no longer be prevented by hormonal means and it is necessary to resort to surgical intervention. This can be done from the 19th day onwards, as by that time the cyst-like dilatations of the uterus have formed. Laparotomy is performed by midline incision (see p. 280) and a needle of suitable length is inserted into the tip of each cornu and passed through the foetal sacs as far as the bifurcation. The needle is then withdrawn, injecting a little 1 % silver nitrate solution into each foetal sac. Finally the puncture wound in the cornu is closed with a seromuscular suture, and the abdominal wound is repaired. The contents of the foetal sac undergo an aseptic disintegration and resorption, as there seems to be little systemic disturbance to the bitch. After the 40th day of gestation, pregnancy can be interrupted by standard Caesarean techniques, as by this time the uterine cornua are uniformly dilated. If the bitch is not required for future breeding, ovaro-hysterectomy can be performed at any time during the pregnancy (see p. 365).

Abortion. Abortion may be the result of trauma or infection. In the first instance it may be caused by blows, kicks, being squeezed in doors, etc. Usually one or two puppies are expelled and there is no pyrexia. In our experience it is unwise to attempt to produce expulsion of the whole litter. The bitch should be allowed to rest in a quiet room, away from all excitement and the action of the corpora lutea augmented by the intramuscular injection of 5–10 mg progesterone every second day. We have seen bitches which, having aborted one or two foetuses, have carried the remainder to term and delivered a live litter.

Abortion due to infection may be seen as a rare complication of distemper. Usually in such cases there is either spontaneous abortion or the foetuses die and disintegrate, so that at term the bitch presents with a uterus filled with a yellowish-brown creamy fluid in which remnants of the foetuses may be found. *Brucella canis* infection is a fairly common cause of abortion in certain kennels.

Aids to parturition. Various procedures may be employed if parturition is delayed or dystocia occurs. These include; lubrication of the birth canal, increasing labour pains, forceps delivery, episiotomy, embryotomy, Caesarean section and Caesarean hysterectomy.

Lubrication of the birth canal can be achieved by instilling antiseptic lubricants or linseed mucilage into the vagina through a Schimmelbusch syringe.

Increase in uterine contractions may be effected by massage of the abdomen towards the pelvis, by hot compresses on the abdomen, or by the administration of 1–4 tablespoonsful of infusion of cinnamon. Where secondary uterine inertia occurs, oxytocic drugs are employed. The best known of these are extracts of the posterior lobe of the pituitary gland, which are standardised in Voegtlin units (V.E.). As these extracts contain vasopressor and antidiuretic factors, the more sophisticated preparations containing only the oxytocic fraction should be used, otherwise the vasopressor action may cause collapse due to spasms of the coronary circulation. Overdosage may lead to a continuous spasm of the uterine musculature (tetanus uteri) which may eventually cause rupture of the viscus. Four to 15 V.E., according to the size of the bitch, are injected and if there is no response it is unlikely that further doses will be of any value. Ergot (*Secale cornutum*) has an ecbolic action but it is no longer used as the variable content of alkaloids renders its action unreliable. (Editor's note: The more refined preparation of ergot, viz. ergometrine, has a definite, if restricted, use in canine obstetrics.)

There are few indications for the use of forceps delivery in the bitch. If possible traction should not be applied to the puppy's head as there is a danger of fatal injury to the spinal cord and medulla oblongata. It is better to pick up a fold of skin and apply traction through this. There are no ideal whelping forceps and various artery forceps, dressing forceps and even bullet forceps have been used for this purpose. After applying the forceps it is important to ensure that the uterine mucosa has not been caught up in the forceps grip, otherwise serious damage may be caused leading to sepsis (Fig. 412). The birth canal should be well lubricated and the presentation of the foetus determined by digital exploration.

In an anterior presentation it is important to determine whether the head is in the right position for delivery, i.e. the head is within the pelvis or has descended far enough for the nose to be within reach of the finger. It must be possible to push the foetus back within the uterus by repelling the head, otherwise forceps cannot be applied. Care should be taken to ensure that the pup's lower jaw does not catch on the pelvic rim otherwise damage to the mucosa may occur. Under digital control the forceps are applied to the lower jaw and the head is guided into the pelvis by light traction. The index finger is then passed over the shoulder of the foetus and the limb extended on each side. The pup can now be extracted, exerting traction in a backward and downward direction.

In the flexed shoulder position, in which the forelegs are crossed, attempts should be made to correct the presentation with the tip of the finger. If this fails, the skin at the level of the shoulder is grasped with forceps and drawn forwards carrying the forelimb within reach of the finger, which is then used for the correction. If only one limb is presented, careful palpation will reveal whether it is a fore or a hindlimb, often in the latter case the tail is also presented. The hindlimb is

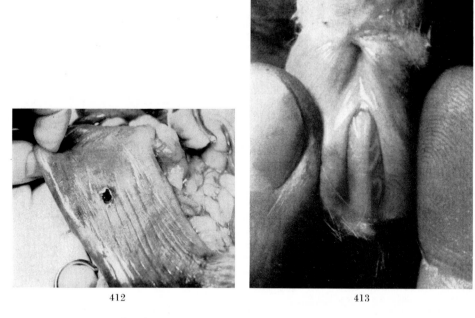

412   413

Fig. 412. Perforation of the uterus due to inexpert use of midwifery forceps.

Fig. 413. Vaginal atresia as a result of healing after a perineal tear during whelping.

grasped at the level of the stifle and fixed with forceps, whilst attempts are made
to find and bring the other leg into the pelvis with the finger. Once this is accomplished delivery is straightforward. Where it is a foreleg alone which is presented
(lateral head position), forceps delivery is not usually possible.

Episiotomy is indicated where there is a narrow vulval opening and should
only be used where this is the only obstacle to delivery and where there is only one
foetus. Long handled scissors are introduced into the vulva and the constriction
is divided under digital control. This procedure should not be performed where
there are several foetuses as oedema of the incised area, with consequent renewed
restriction of the vulval opening, very soon develops.

Embryotomy should be avoided as far as possible, as the extent of the procedure
cannot be assessed at the outset. Cutting or sawing instruments cannot be used
in the bitch and it is necessary to remove portions of the foetus by grasping them
with forceps and pulling them apart. Care must be taken to ensure that portions
of the vaginal mucosa are not included in the jaws of the forceps. Where the head
is presented, but the shoulder is flexed, an incision is made with episiotomy scissors
into the skin of the side of the neck through which are passed artery forceps to
grasp the shoulder blade and draw it with the foreleg out through the wound.

Embryotomy may be indicated where there is a posterior presentation of a dead
and putrefying foetus in which the abdomen is so distended with gas that it is

23*

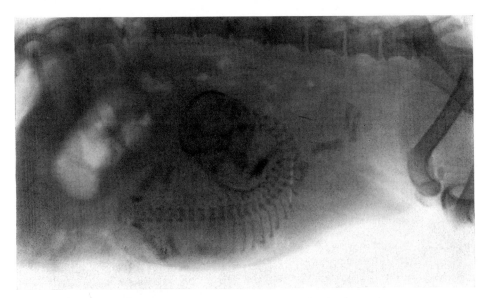

Fig. 414. Lateral head position. A forelimb lies in the vagina.

too big for the birth canal. In this case the abdominal wall is pierced with forceps or scissors and the abdominal and thoracic viscera removed with forceps. The foetus is then so reduced in size that delivery can be effected.

A definite indication for embryotomy is where there is lateral deviation of the head with one foreleg presented (Fig. 414). The presented limb should be withdrawn as far as possible and removed. Through the gap thus created, the ribs, thoracic organs and cervical vertebrae are removed with forceps, again care being taken to avoid injury to the maternal mucosa. In all embryotomy operations it is essential to lubricate the birth canal adequately. We tend to restrict this procedure to a fairly narrow field, as the prime consideration in canine obstetrics must always be the wellbeing of the mother and embryotomy can jeopardise the life of the bitch.

Caesarean Section. Caesarean section, in our experience, is much superior to either forceps delivery or embryotomy for the protection of the life of the mother and the puppies.

Technique of Caesarean Section. The bitch is prepared for surgery in the usual way and secured on her back after the induction of epidural anaesthesia. The abdomen is opened by an incision through the linea alba, the omentum is pushed forwards and the uterine horns delivered in turn through the wound (Fig. 415). If an ecbolic has been given shortly before operation the uterus is usually very contracted and it may be very difficult to bring the organ out through the wound. In such a case rupture of the uterus may occur and it is then essential to perform a hysterectomy. For this reason, Caesarean section should always be delayed until at least 2 hours have elapsed after the last ecbolic injection has been given. If the uterus is undamaged by the manipulations, a longitudinal incision is made in one horn, opposite the attachment of the broad ligament and between the last two placental areas before the bifurcation (Fig. 416). The incision must be of sufficient length to allow passage of the foetus without tearing the wall of the uterus (Fig. 417).

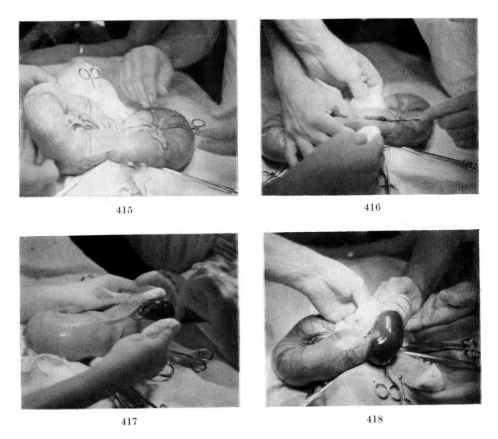

415   416

417   418

Fig. 415. Conservative Caesarean section. The uterus has been brought out through the wound in the abdominal wall.

Fig. 416. Conservative Caesarean section. Incision near the bifurcation between two placental points of attachment or between the bifurcation and the attachment of the first placenta.

Fig. 417. Conservative Caesarean section. The first embryo is extruded.

Fig. 418. Conservative Caesarean section. The first embryo has been completely extruded and can now be seized by an assistant and pulled out.

The cornu is held by assistants on both sides of the commisures of the wound. Where the foetuses are putrefying, the surgeon works them down the cornu through the uterine wall and when they are sufficiently extruded through the incision, they are grasped by an assistant and carefully removed from the operation site complete with membranes and placenta (Fig. 418). When the horn in which the incision has been made has been emptied, the foetuses on the other side are massaged round the bifurcation and out through the incision. If the pups are alive and healthy, the surgeon may introduce two fingers through the incision and deliver the foetuses manually. Where there is any doubt as to whether the foetuses are infected, then the method outlined above should be strictly adhered to.

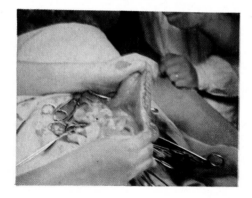

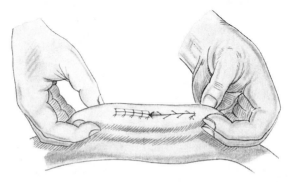

Fig. 419. Conservative Caesarean section. Closure of the incision in the horn of the uterus. The underlying suture is a Schmieden suture and over it is a single Lembert suture.

The puppies are removed from their membranes by an assistant and their umbilical cords tied off. Any mucus should be cleared from the mouth and nose and the pups should be vigorously massaged to stimulate respiration.

It is important to ensure that all the pups have been removed by palpation of each cornu as far as the ovary and the vagina as far as the vulva. The uterus is then closed by a double suture, the deep one being a Schmieden suture and the superficial one a Lembert suture (Fig. 419). The empty uterus soon commences to contract, so to ensure that the sutures are inserted close together, an assistant stretches the incision during suturing. If the uterus fails to contract, 10 V.E. of pituitrin are applied with a sterile swab and this will initiate contraction in most cases. If there is no response then hysterectomy must be considered. A portion of omentum is drawn over the uterine wound and sutured into place to seal off the uterus, and it is then replaced in the abdominal cavity which is closed in the usual way. The bitch should be allowed to suckle the pups as soon as possible.

Caesarean Hysterectomy. This operation is indicated where the uterus shows changes which militate against satisfactory healing, e.g. bluish-green discoloration of the uterine wall, marked friability, rupture, injuries due to previous attempts at forceps delivery, etc. The technique differs from that described later in the chapter in that both horns are brought out through the abdominal incision, clamped off and laid out posteriorly. Each horn is now opened and the contained puppies delivered. Usually a pup is wedged in the body of the uterus and this must be removed before division of the uterine stump can be performed.

Dystocia. Dystocia may be of two main types, a) maternal dystocia and b) foetal dystocia.

a) Maternal dystocia – this may be due to primary or secondary uterine inertia, obstruction due to pelvic deformity, vaginal tumours, or uterine torsion.

Primary uterine inertia occurs when the womb is overloaded and is present from the onset of parturition. The usual signs of approaching labour, e.g. vulval oedema, milk production, etc., are absent. Ecbolic drugs are of little use in this condition and delivery can only be effected by Caesarean section, probably followed by hysterectomy.

Secondary uterine inertia occurs when the uterus is overloaded with a large litter. The uterine contractions are normal at the beginning of labour, but become progressively weaker until they cease before labour has been completed. The bitch should always be allowed to eat the afterbirth as it contains natural ecbolic hormones. Inertia may also result from puppies which are too large or are wrongly presented. Treatment of this condition is by the use of ecbolic agents.

Where the pelvis is too narrow due to healed fractures or rickets (Fig. 494), recourse must be made to Caesarean delivery. If the birth canal is too narrow due to strictures, vulval hypoplasia, etc., episiotomy may be performed, but if the litter is large, Caesarean section may be the method of choice.

In cases of torsion of the uterus, this may be difficult to diagnose as often only one horn is involved, and this cannot be appreciated by vaginoscopy. Often the diagnosis can only be made by exploratory laparotomy. Treatment is by Caesarean delivery and often hysterectomy is necessary as there is damage to the blood supply of the affected horn.

Tumours do not usually cause dystocia unless they have arisen since the bitch was mated. Treatment is surgical removal of the obstructing tumour or Caesarean section.

b) Foetal dystocia – this is due to faulty presentations or positions, or overlarge foetuses.

Among faulty presentations and positions may be mentioned the flexed shoulder position, the lateral head position, transverse presentation and lateroflexion (Fig. 420). These conditions are treated by forceps delivery or embryotomy, bearing in mind that embryotomy should only be undertaken when there is only a single pup, or when the affected pup is the last of the litter. This precaution is necessary as embryotomy is invariably followed by swelling of the soft parts of the birth canal, which may cause dystocia for any remaining puppies.

Transverse presentation may occur by the foetus passing into the other horn rather than into the body of the uterus. Successful correction of the presentation is difficult as the contractions of the two horns exert equal pressure on the foetus. Embryotomy may be tried if it is the last pup, otherwise Caesarean delivery is indicated.

By lateroflexion we mean a posterior presentation in which the hindlegs are flexed so that they lie almost against the thorax. Correction of the position is virtually impossible so that embryotomy should be tried or Caesarean section performed.

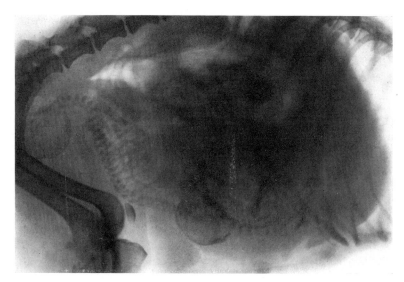

Fig. 420. The radiograph indicates the faulty position (on its back) of the presenting puppy.

Overlarge foetuses mean that the pups are too large to pass through a normally developed pelvis. In multiple pregnancies only one foetus may be too large and in such cases forceps or embryotomy should be used. In some breeds (Bulldogs, Pekingese, Pugs, etc.) where the head is normally large in comparison with the body, one should always anticipate trouble with overlarge foetuses and Caesarean section is often to be recommended. In the dwarf breeds, a single embryo is often overlarge, and where it is important to get a live puppy Caesarean section is preferable to either forceps delivery or embryotomy. We cannot support the theory that the sire is the main factor in determining the size of the foetus. On the contrary, we feel that the dimensions of the bitch have the decisive influence in this matter.

Certain pathological processes in the bitch may cause intrauterine foetal death. Where the contents of the uterus are sterile, mummification will occur, possibly at different stages of development. Often in the course of normal births, mummies of this kind may be expelled along with normal living puppies (Fig. 421). There do not appear to be any characteristic clinical signs in this condition. Sometimes the owner will observe that the abdominal enlargement of the bitch decreases again after a time. Bitches with the entire litter mummified usually show no signs of impending parturition. In spite of the usual drop in body temperature the mucus plug does not dissolve and the os uteris shows no tendency to open. Diagnosis may be made by palpation or radiography. Where there is total mummification of the litter, treatment is by Caesarean section, but where there are live pups normal parturition will usually take place.

On the completion of whelping when there has been dystocia, the bitch should be carefully examined by palpation and radiography, if necessary, to ensure that no puppy is retained in the uterus. Finally we inject a suitable quantity of posterior

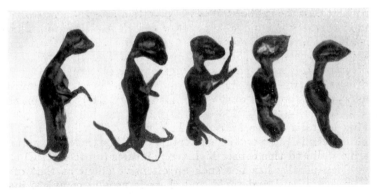

Fig. 421. Mummified, badly developed puppies. Delivered by Caesarean section on the 65th day of pregnancy. (Photograph by the University Dept. of Illustration.)

pituitary extract to stimulate involution of the uterus and promote lactation.

Puerperal Sepsis. Infection of the uterus or vagina in the puerperium is manifested by apathy, inappetence, neglect of the puppies, an offensive purulent discharge, pyrexia (up to 41.0 °C), a rapid, hard pulse and pale conjunctivae.

Treatment is by systemic antibiotic therapy which usually produces a fall in temperature after 24 hours. Supportive treatment should include circulatory stimulants and local antibiotic douches. HARASZTI (Acta Vet. Acad. Sci. hung. **8**, 329–335, 1958) recommended curettage as also did BARDENS (see p. 353), the indications being catarrhal inflammation of the uterus after delivery, or where there was poor involution after abortion.

Usually there is a failure of lactation in puerperal sepsis so it may be necessary to hand rear the puppies. The pups' abdomens must be massaged to stimulate peristalsis and defaecation. Massage of the perineal area will also encourage micturition. Bitch's milk contains 7.5 % of albumin, 8.3 % fats, 280 mg calcium and 240 mg phosphorus per 100 ml of whole milk, but only 3.7 % sugar. BJÖRK, OLSSEN & DYRENDAHL (Nord. Vet. Med. **9**, 285, 1957) propose a mixture which has proved very successful. To 800 ml of whole cow's milk are added 200 g of cream, one egg yolk, 6 g of bone meal and 4 g of citric acid. During the first three weeks of life the pups are fed six times daily with a feeding bottle, no feeds being given during the night. The amount of feed depends upon the age:

Age in days	Amount of feed as percentage of body weight
3	15–20
7	22–25
14	30–32
31	35–40

The mixture is kept in a refrigerator, sufficient for each feed being taken out and used as required. As a feeding bottle we use a pharmacological flask of 100–250 ml. An opening is made in the flask large enough to allow the introduction of a dropper pipette. In the rubber top of the pipette a hole is burned with a red hot needle and in this way it is possible to allow sufficient of the milk mixture to be sucked out. In the process of adapting the puppies to artificial feeding during the first days of life, the bottle should be removed after a few sucks because the physiological processes involved in sucking from the maternal teats are basically different from those when sucking at a rubber teat. There is a certain degree of risk of aspiration of the milk during the initial stages of adaptation to artificial feeding.

Perforating Necrosis of the Placenta. This presents a clinical syndrome very similar to that seen in puerperal sepsis. In this condition there is a partial necrosis of the uterine wall and this causes high temperatures (up to 41.0 °C) and a dirty discharge, which usually has not such an offensive odour as that of puerperal sepsis. The pulse is hard and rapid and there is usually complete inappetence, great thirst, and complete neglect of the puppies. As regards treatment, irrigation of the uterus should not be attempted as this may lead to perforation of the necrotic area and subsequent peritonitis. The bitch may be given high doses of penicillin on the first day as a means of differential diagnosis. If there is not a rapid reduction of the fever in the next twelve hours, as is obtained in puerperal sepsis, it may be presumed that placental necrosis is present. After the pyrexial stage, which usually lasts from two to three days, the temperature drops, becomes subnormal, and death usually follows on the fourth to fifth day. In these cases the patient's life can only be saved by immediate hysterectomy (see page 358). In the uterus one or two necrotic areas are found, which are easily distinguishable from the pressure necrosis of the uterine wall which tends to occur in protracted labour.

Uterine Prolapse. This mishap occurs immediately after whelping. Complete prolapse of both horns of the uterus is rare, as is partial prolapse of one horn or of the uterine body. Treatment of a recent prolapse is by conservative measures. The bitch is anaesthetised and restrained on her side (see Fig. 32). The hindquarters are raised as high as possible by tilting the operating table and the prolapsed organ is treated with cold antiseptic fluids. Replacement is now attempted beginning with one prolapsed horn and returning it as far as the bifurcation with the help of moist cloths. The same procedure is carried out with the second horn if it is prolapsed, and the body of the uterus and vagina is then replaced. During this procedure the bitch is given an injection of 4–10 V.E. of pituitrin, which produces involution of the uterus. Finally the vulva is closed with a mattress suture of "Perlon", which may be removed after 3–5 days. If this method is unsuccessful the uterus must be amputated.

Technique of Amputation of the Prolapsed Uterus. The bitch is prepared in the usual way for laparotomy in the mid line (see page 280). The operation is carried out under epidural anaesthesia and the uterine horns are double ligatured with catgut and "Perlon" in the region of the Fallopian tubes. A second "Perlon" ligature is applied to the tip of the horn and the tissues are divided between them. A long dressing forceps is now introduced into the cornu to seize the tip and evaginate the horn by traction. The same procedure is carried out with the second horn and the laparotomy wound is then closed. Finally an encircling ligature is applied round the prolapsed vagina in front of the urethral opening, secured by a transfixing ligature, and the prolapsed uterus is removed. The stump is then closed by a row of fine sutures and replaced into the pelvis.

Eclampsia in the bitch. This is a condition which tends to occur during or after whelping, in which convulsions occur without true disturbances of consciousness.

The causes of the condition have not been fully elucidated but, bearing in mind the striking results obtained by administration of calcium, it would seem apparent that there is some imbalance in calcium metabolism. It seems probable that a certain hormone and also vitamins play an important part in the aetiology of the condition. Enormous demands are made on the calcium reserves of the bitch during the latter weeks of pregnancy, when the puppies are maturing and the milk supply is being elaborated. Immediately after the last war, when the feeding of pregnant bitches was not very good, eclampsia was regarded as a disease occurring invariably during whelping, whereas now only isolated cases of it are seen. We see it especially in small breeds (Pekingese, Dachshunds, etc.), and have only diagnosed it once in the large breeds. Clinical signs are a rapid rise of temperature (40.5 °C and more), hyperpyrexial convulsions, in which the limbs are stretched out in a tetanic convulsion and there is opisthotonus. Due to contraction of the temporal and facial muscles the eyes tend to protrude (exophthalmos) and the eyelid and corneal reflexes are still present. The pulse is hard and very fast and the apex beat of the heart is discernible. Where eclampsia occurs before, or actually during, whelping, the clinical signs are milder in character. Treatment consists of the immediate removal of the puppies from the mother and the application of iced compresses to the mammary glands. The convulsions are treated with an injection of morphia (0.02 to 0.04 g subcutaneously) and of calcium (calcium thiosulphate 3–6 ml injected slowly intravenously at body temperature). Convulsions subside after about 30 minutes, the bitch is calm and begins to take an interest in her surroundings again. If no improvement occurs after this period of time the injection of calcium must be repeated. As supportive therapy 4 to 5 injections of calcium can be given at intervals of 3 to 4 days. Treatment of eclampsia prior to parturition is similar to that set out above, but if it occurs immediately before whelping (1–2 days) immediate Caesarean section may be the only effective treatment. Where eclampsia occurs during parturition the whelping must be completed as quickly as possible and the treatment outlined above given immediately.

False pregnancy (Pseudo-pregnancy, Pseudocyesis). In this condition milk secretion occurs without actual pregnancy or parturition. This lactation is produced by hormone imbalance and occurs at the time when parturition would have occurred if the bitch had been pregnant. Dachshunds are particularly liable to the condition and are therefore much in demand as foster mothers. Clinically the mammary glands become enlarged, the bitch is restless and may prepare a nest. Quite often the maternal instinct is so developed that various objects such as dolls, slippers, cushions, etc., are carried about and nursed. Mammary glands may be so engorged that they become pendulous, milk appears, and occasionally the bitch will actually suck the milk and thus stimulate production of more. In treating this condition it is wise to ensure that the bitch cannot suck her own milk by the application of an Elizabethan collar. Withdrawing of milk tends to stimulate further production, so this should only be done where there is serious engorgement of the mammary glands. Lactation can be inhibited by injecting oestrogens and repeating the injection after 2 to 3 days. Sasum (Tierärztl. Umschau 43, 19, 1958) reported good results using testosterone at a dosage rate of two injections of 10–25 mg with an interval of three days in between. In severe cases a further intramuscular injection of 10 mg may be required. The mammary glands are painted with iodine (at eight-day intervals) and the daily rubbing in of camphor

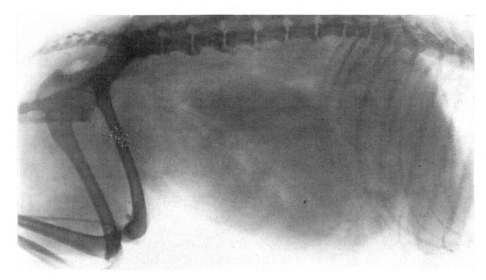

Fig. 422. Pyometra in a Spitz bitch.

ointment may be useful. Ice compresses may be applied to the mammary glands
several times a day, and when the glands are pendulous, it is beneficial to support
them with an elastic bandage. Some bitches show signs of false pregnancy regularly
twice a year and in such cases it is recommended that spaying should be considered.

Pyometra (Cystic endometrial hyperplasia). This condition is quite common in
the bitch and is due to hormonal dysfunction. It may also be produced by the
administration of oestrogenic hormones given in high dosage for the treatment of
false pregnancy or misalliance. In healthy anoestrous bitches, pyometra is not
caused by high dosage of oestrogen and this tends to confirm the view of TEUNISSEN
(Acta endocr. Copenhagen **9**, 407, 1952) who considers that the role of progesterone
is of prime importance in the aetiology of pyometra.

Clinical picture. The condition is seen most frequently in nulliparous or uni-
parous bitches in the higher age groups. The last heat period may have been
delayed or extended. The animals show general lassitude, the appetite is fickle and
there is polydipsia. Where the bitch has a vaginal discharge and cleans herself,
vomiting may occur due to gastritis. There may be a vaginal discharge, which varies
from a reddish-yellow to a chocolate brown colour, and may be intermittent.
Vaginoscopy shows that the cervix uteri is slightly open, pressure on the abdominal
wall causing pus to emerge from the uterus. Radiography reveals a sausage-shaped
transparent body lying in contact with the lower abdominal wall (Fig. 422). The
uterus may be delineated better by radiography following the inducement of
pneumo-peritoneum or by filling the large intestine with contrast medium. It is
difficult to demonstrate early pyometra by radiography, but in these cases it is
sometimes possible to palpate the enlarging uterus. Increase in the blood sedimentation rate (over 20 Westergen degrees after one hour and more than 100 degrees
after 24 hours) is of limited value in the diagnosis of this condition. Differential

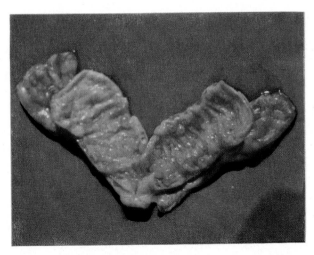

Fig. 423. Glandular hyperplasia (the uterus opened).

blood counts show a leucocytosis with a definite "shift to the left". We place especial value on the determination of the Blood Urea Nitrogen, because this makes it possible to exclude lesions of the kidney. The shape of the affected uterus may be hyperplastic, ampulla-like or sausage-shaped (Figs. 423, 424, 425 and 426). According to the investigations of SCHULZE (Dtsch. Tierärztl. Wschr. **62**, 504, 1955), the pus is sterile in approximately 25 % of cases, which confirms the view that most pyometras (except those which occur after prolonged heat) are primarily due to hormone imbalance and that any bacterial infection is of secondary nature.

Treatment. We advocate radical operation (hysterectomy) as medical treatment is unreliable.

Technique of Hysterectomy in Pyometra. The patient is prepared for a laparotomy in the usual way and epidural anaesthesia or general anaesthesia is induced. The bitch is tied on her back and the abdomen is opened in the mid line. The omentum is then reflected forward and the bifurcation of the uterus brought out of the wound (Fig. 427). It is better to empty the bladder in order to obtain a better view. A double ligature is applied to each of the uterine horns at the point of their transition into the Fallopian tubes, the blood vessels supplying the uterus being included in the ligature. In order to avoid damage to the intestine, the ligature is applied with a Dechamp (Fig. 428). The ends of the ligatures are secured with a clamp. When both horns have been dealt with, the uterus is turned cranially to allow ligature of the vagina (Fig. 429). As the blood vessels supplying the uterus on both sides of the vagina are very well developed, they are ligatured separately by an encircling suture, around the vessels on one side and then around the other, finally taking the suture over the vagina (Fig. 430). The second ligature is done with Perlon and Dechamp. It is especially important to apply this ligature caudal to the cervix, as experience has shown that a pyometra of the stump may be caused by leaving the cervix behind (Fig. 431). The ends of the ligature are secured with a clamp and finally the vagina is seized with a strong clamp to facilitate further treatment. Three Doyen's intestinal clamps are put on the stump. One is put on the tip of the horn about a finger-breadth from the ligature and on the uterine side of it, so that the vessel leading to the horn is included in the clamp. The clamps are laid towards the uterus from the internal orifice (Fig. 432). A swab is inserted under the ligature of one horn

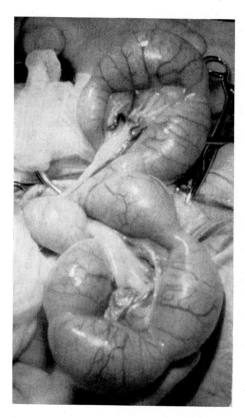

Fig. 424. Pyometra. The ampullae are well formed.

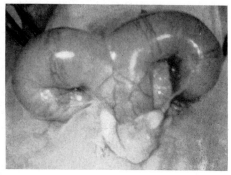

Fig. 425. Sausage-shaped uterus in pyometra.

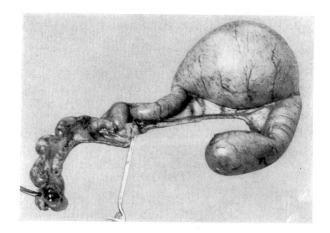

Fig. 426. Pyometra of the left horn following uterine torsion.

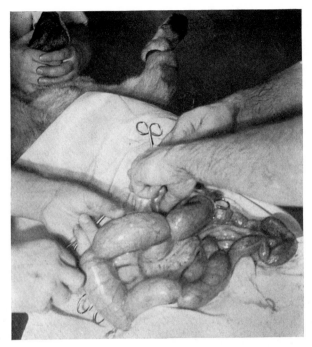

Fig. 427. Reflecting the uterus forwards and searching for the ovaries.

and the tissue between the clamp and the ligature is cut through, any secretion escaping being absorbed by the underlying swab. The horn is now separated from the broad ligament in the direction of the uterine body as far as the vaginal ligature, the same procedure then being performed with the other horn. The stumps remaining in the body are treated either by the application of tincture of iodine or cauterised with a thermo-cautery (Fig. 433). The vagina is now severed in the region of the cervix, a swab again being placed underneath to avoid contamination of the abdominal cavity. The cervix is then grasped with forceps and excised with scissors and again iodine or thermo-cautery is applied to the remaining stump. The stump of the vagina is then closed with two intussusception sutures (Fig. 434), and both meso-metria are then stitched over the stump (Fig. 435). We consider this procedure to be of great importance because sometimes the stump ligature cuts through the two vessels, usually between the 10th and 14th post-operative day, causing a secondary haemorrhage which can only be arrested by a further laparotomy and ligaturing of the stump. Ligature threads are now severed at about 1 cm from the ligature, the artery forceps are removed from the stumps, the bladder replaced in the abdomen and the omentum is drawn back into its normal position. Abdominal closure is performed in the usual way. Before tying off the last peritoneal suture 100/150 ml of sterile normal saline is introduced into the abdominal cavity through a glass funnel. It may be necessary to inject a solution of 100/200 mg Tetracycline. Where perforation of the uterus has occurred and there is pus in the abdominal cavity, the latter must be thoroughly irrigated and swabbed out during the operation with large quantities of normal saline. If peritonitis is already present sterile gauze is inserted (see page 303). After-treatment should always include antibiotic therapy and measures to support the circulation.

Where there is perforation of the uterus in pyometra one should always bear in mind the possibility of the development of paralytic ileus. This becomes manifest

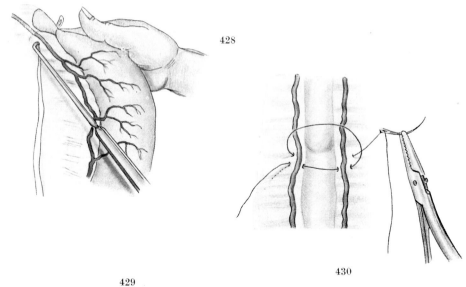

428

430

429

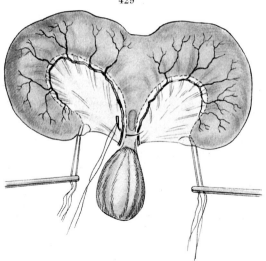

Fig. 428. Application of the ligature to the horn of the uterus with
a Dechamp.

Fig. 429. Ligature of the blood
vessels of the vagina.

Fig. 430. Course of the sutures in
ligature of the vessels and the vagina.

Fig. 431. Pyometra of the stump
after faulty removal of the uterus
at the caudal stump.

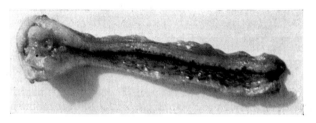

431

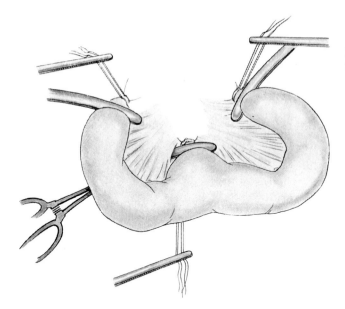

Fig. 432. Position of the intestinal clamps on the uterus.

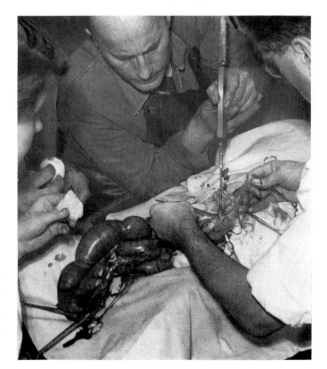

Fig. 433. The detached uterine horns are separated from the mesometrium and laid out caudally; the stumps are lightly drawn up to the ligature and are sealed with the thermocautery.

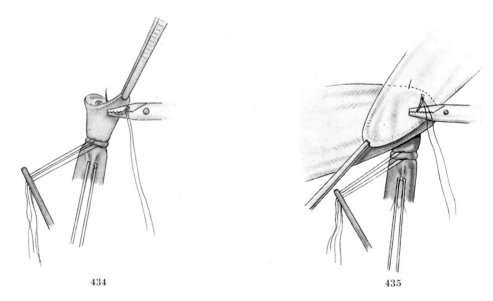

434   435

Fig. 434. Closure of the vaginal stump with mattress sutures.

Fig. 435. The plastic operation on the vaginal stump.

on the 2nd or 3rd post-operative day with a rapid fall in body temperature, vomiting, oral foetor, complete anorexia and absence of defaecation.

Ovarian Cysts and Tumours. Cysts and tumours may occur in the ovaries of elderly bitches (Fig. 436). Clinical signs are usually those of pyometra as this is the usual accompaniment due to ovarian dysfunction. There is loss of weight and the tumours can often be palpated, but their site may not be apparent and exploratory laparotomy may be required to confirm the diagnosis (Figs. 437, 438). Treatment is entirely surgical, special attention being given to secure ligaturing of all blood vessels as post-operative bleeding cannot be controlled. Hysterectomy should be carried out at the same time.

Mammary Tumours. Mammary tumours occur quite frequently in the old bitch, varying from small, firm nodules, which are quite mobile and show little tendency to increase in size, to multiple nodules which tend to coalesce into a plaque and may grow rapidly. The first type are left until they attain the size of a hen's egg before surgical removal. The rapidly growing type should be removed as soon as possible, after ascertaining whether there are metastases to the lungs (radiography) or the liver (palpation). Where this has already occurred, euthanasia is the only course.

Surgical Removal of Mammary Tumours. The operation seldom presents much difficulty, being performed under local anaesthesia. An elliptical incision is made through the skin encircling the tumour, the growth is separated from the underlying tissues by blunt dissection up to its caudal and cranial extremities. At these points is situated the main blood supply to the tumour and care must be taken to effect

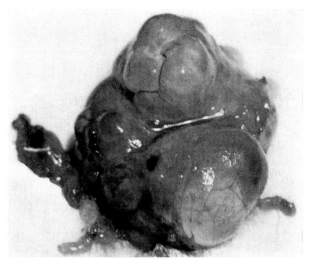

Fig. 436. Cystic degeneration of the ovary of a bitch with pyometra.

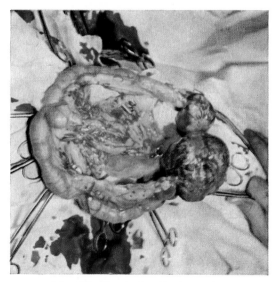

Fig. 437. Neoplasia of both ovaries.

efficient haemostasis before suturing the skin wound. It may be advisable to insert relaxation sutures depending upon the site of the tumour and the amount of skin it is necessary to remove. Where the tumour lies in the inguinal mammary glands there is a certain amount of risk that the processus vaginalis may be opened. Tumour plaques distributed all along the mammary glands may require several operations before they are all removed.

24*

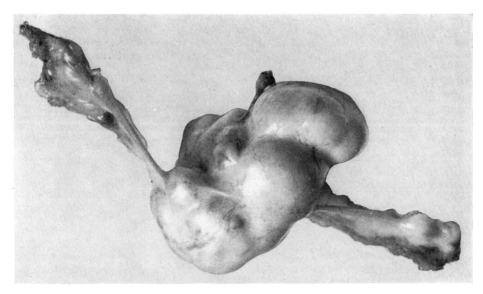

Fig. 438. Leiomyoma of the uterus of an 8-year-old Spitz bitch.

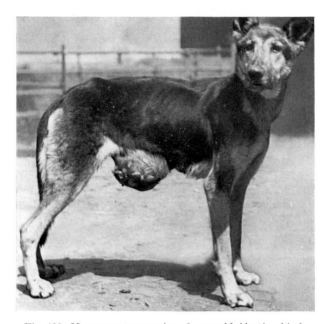

Fig. 439. Mammary tumour in a 6-year-old Alsatian bitch.

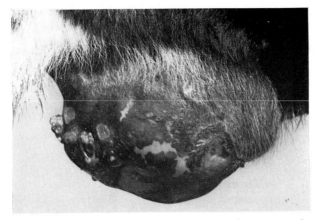

Fig. 440. The tumour shown in Fig. 439. Patches of coalescence are clearly visible.

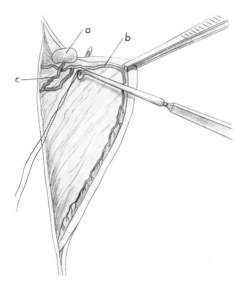

Fig. 441. Castration (Spaying) of the bitch. Applying the first ligature. (a) ovary; (b) uterine artery; (c) ovarian artery.

Sterilisation of the Bitch. This operation is seldom required in our experience. We perform hysterectomy as described earlier.

Spaying of the Bitch. Spaying of bitches is not so popular in this country as it is in America, but the operation must often be considered as a therapeutic measure. Indications are for persistent false pregnancy, certain dermatoses, and possibly in mammary neoplasia and where there is a tendency towards pyometra.

Technique of Spaying (Ovariectomy) in the Bitch. We perform this operation through a midline incision but other workers prefer the flank approach. General anaesthesia should be induced as epidural anaesthesia is insufficient unless local anaesthetic is applied to the broad ligaments.

After opening the abdomen, the uterine cornu are withdrawn through the incision as far as the ovary. Two ligatures are applied in front of and behind the ovary (Fig. 441) and the latter is then cut out. It is important to include the uterine and ovarian arteries in the ligatures. The abdomen is then closed in the usual way.

12. Diseases of the male generative system

The sexual organs of the male dog can be examined much more readily than those of the female as they are more accessible. Examination should commence with palpation of the testes during which their size, consistency, the shape of the epididymis, the relationships of the spermatic cord and any tenderness are noted. Note should also be taken of any recent wound or scars resulting from previous injuries. The penis is palpated through the sheath in the first instance, and any changes in the prepuce or any discharge are noted. In order to inspect the penis visually, the sheath must be retracted as far as the reflexion of the preputial mucosa on to the penis. The dog is held on its side and the hind limbs flexed on the body so that the pelvis is bent ventro-cranially (Fig. 442), when the penis can easily be exposed. The prostate is examined digitally by one finger in the rectum whilst the other hand presses the prostate towards the pelvis by pressure through the abdominal wall. Enlargement of the prostate can be assessed radiographically by filling the bladder with contrast medium. The neck of the bladder can then be seen to be suddenly constricted with loss of the normal funnel-shape (Fig. 443).

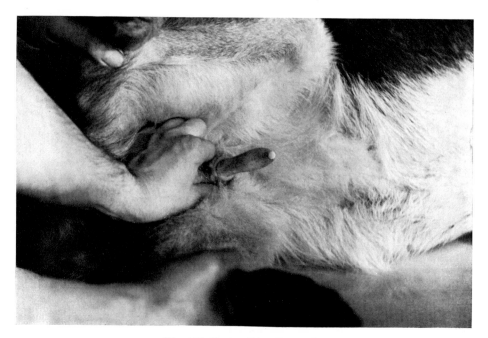

Fig. 442. Exsheathing the penis.

Prostatic Hypertrophy. This condition is found quite commonly in the older dog. The clinical picture is one of difficulty in micturition and defaecation. Palpation will reveal that the gland is markedly enlarged, but the enlargement can be differentiated from that due to neoplasia by the persistence of the median longitudinal groove. In hypertrophy also, the consistency is semi-solid whilst tumours are hard and irregular, and abscesses more fluctuating. In some cases radiography will establish an accurate diagnosis (Fig. 444).

Treatment. Treatment consists of the administration of large doses of oestrogens, two or three times weekly, or by castration. Ligature of the vas deferens may also be effective. In this technique an incision about 2 cm long is made over the spermatic cord, the tunica vaginalis is opened, and the vas is drawn out of the wound. A double ligature is applied, taking care to ensure that only the vas is included in the ligature. Castration is performed as described on p. 382. Prostatectomy is a complex procedure but may be done in certain cases with the technique described by ARCHIBALD & CAWLEY (J. Amer. vet. med. Ass. **128**, 173, 1956) and by RODEN-BECK (Kleintier. Prax. **3**, 28, 1958). In this operation the whole of the gland including the prostatic urethra is removed. We have not had the opportunity to perform this operation on any of our prostatic cases to date.

Prostatic Abscess. Abscess formation in the prostate is uncommon in the dog. They show a tendency to reform when diathermy has been used or when they have discharged through the urethra. Large abscesses must be drained through the perineal route, otherwise there is a danger that they will burst into the abdominal cavity with resultant peritonitis. The abscess may be reached by making an incision through the skin and fascia between the anus and the urethra, and after opening the abscess, a drainage tube is inserted until discharge ceases.

Orchitis. Inflammation of the testicle may result from external (trauma, contusion, etc.) or internal causes (tuberculosis, pyaemia, etc.). KLEIN (Mh. Thkd. **11**, 158–162, 1959) described a case of *Brucella orchitis* in a watchdog which resulted in severe fibrosis.

Clinically there is a firm, painful swelling of the glands and epididymis (when it is acute), or in the chronic form there is a hard and painless enlargement (Fig. 445).

Treatment. Rest and warm applications possibly by means of a suspensory bag are the only practical measures. In chronic orchitis, castration is the only effective treatment.

Testicular Neoplasia. The most common neoplasms of the dog's testicle are the adenomas and seminomas.

Clinically the tumours produce a painless, gradually increasing swelling, which is usually firm in consistency and extensive (Fig. 446).

Treatment. The sole recommended treatment is the surgical removal of the affected organ.

Descent of the Testes. The testes usually descend into the scrotum during the first year of life. Sometimes when the puppy is about 8 weeks old, the glands are retracted into the abdomen. In some pups the testes do not descend, possibly due to a short or overdeveloped cremaster muscle. This condition is known as cryptorchidism.

Treatment. The treatment of cryptorchidism is only worthwhile contemplating if the testicles are retained in the inguinal region and can be felt alongside the

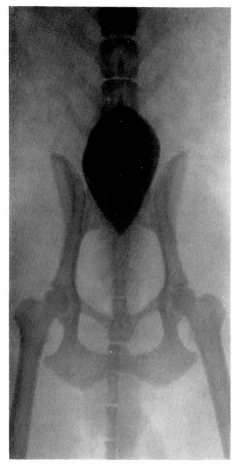

Fig. 443. Prostatic hypertrophy; the bladder filled with contrast medium is displaced cranially and the neck of the bladder is narrowed.

Fig. 444. Prostatic hypertrophy; the prostate is well shown because the bladder and hind gut are filled with contrast medium. (a) the prostate; (b) the bladder; (c) the hind gut.

444

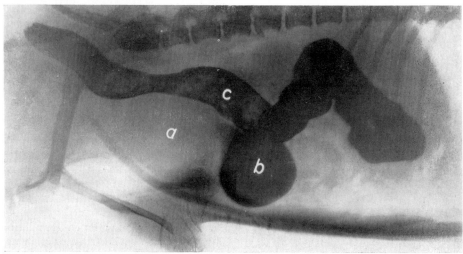

penis. In such cases the dog is given 6–12 mg of testosterone intramuscularly once a week, and the owner is instructed to massage the testicle down towards the scrotum once a day. If the testicle is within the abdomen, hormone injections and massage are useless. In the young dog, the hormone injections may produce over-sexuality, which can be unpleasant and embarrassing to the owner. Retained testicles in the older dog do have a tendency to become neoplastic. Treatment in

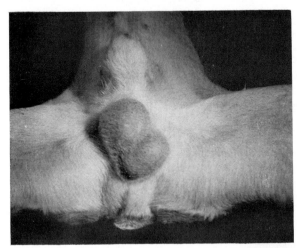

Fig. 445. Chronic orchitis of the right testis in a Fox terrier, developing after a dog fight.

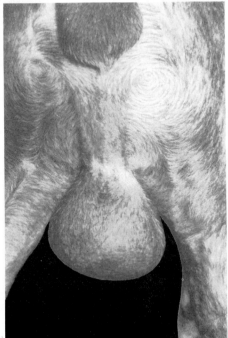

Fig. 446. Seminoma of the right testis.

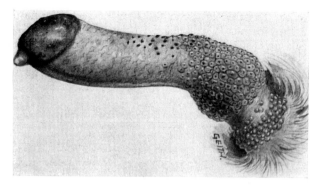

Fig. 447. Follicular posthitis.

this case is to remove the affected gland via a laparotomy, care being taken to ensure double ligation of all blood vessels. Affected animals often suffer from dermatoses or external otitis, which are resistant to treatment until the hormone imbalance is corrected.

Onanism (Masturbation). Some highly sexed male dogs will masturbate on cushions, human legs, etc.

Treatment. In working dogs the habit can be counteracted by increasing the amount of work or exercise and by punishment. High doses of oestrogen may be used but this may render the dog sexually attractive to other males. As a last resort it may be necessary to castrate the animal.

Balanitis (Preputial Catarrh). This condition is often regarded by the laity as a venereal disease of dogs (canine gonorrhoea), whereas it is actually due to a coccal infection of the prepuce. Occasionally the inflammation may be so severe as to cause the formation of follicles in the region of the bulbus (Follicular Posthitis).

Clinically there is a yellowish-green discharge from the preputial opening, which is rather unpleasant from the owner's point of view. It is essential to fully expose the penis in all cases so as to examine the bulbar region for evidence of follicular posthitis (Fig. 447).

Treatment. Irrigation of the sheath with antiseptic solutions, e.g. potassium permanganate, acridine dyes, etc., followed by instillation of an antibiotic ointment as used for the treatment of bovine mastitis. Irrigation is performed by introducing the hub of the syringe into the preputial opening which is then held closed around the syringe. The preputial sac is then filled with the solution, which is well massaged in and distributed with the sac held closed. The fluid is then allowed to escape and the procedure repeated several times. Where there is follicular posthitis, the lesions are touched with 2–5 % silver nitrate solution at intervals of 2–3 days. Because of the micturition habits of the dog, infection tends to be recurrent, so treatment may need to be repeated at fairly regular intervals.

Phimosis. Phimosis is a rare, probably congenital condition in the dog in which the preputial opening is inordinately small. Clinically there is a very narrow opening which may be so small that a sound can only just be introduced (Fig. 448). Urine is held back in the sheath until the pressure is such as to force through the opening when the urine escapes in a thin stream.

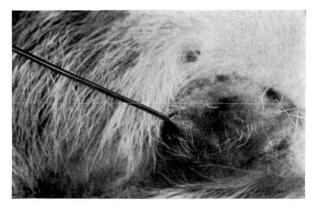

Fig. 448. Phimosis in an 8-week-old Alsatian. The preputial opening is nevertheless permeable to a sound.

Treatment. The only effective treatment is surgical and consists of opening up the narrow orifice under epidural anaesthesia. A hollow sound is introduced through the opening and, using this as a guide, an incision is made large enough to allow the penis to be fully exsheathed (Fig. 449). Allowance must be made for the amount of contraction of the scar tissue which will form. Finally the mucosa of the prepuce is sutured to the outer skin (Figs. 450, 451).

Paraphimosis. In this condition the erected and exsheathed penis cannot be retracted into the prepuce. The cause is probably a permanent, or temporary, slight narrowing of the preputial opening, resulting from inflammation. Clinically the penis appears as a bluish-red, swollen object which is very hard to the touch. If the condition is not relieved, trauma and ulceration of the swollen tissues may occur with possible necrosis.

Treatment. Treatment is a matter of some urgency. The penis should be bathed in ice water to reduce the congestion, lubricated with a bland ointment or jelly, and an attempt made to replace it in the sheath, the preputial opening being held open with two pairs of forceps. If this does not succeed, the opening must be enlarged by incision, the penis replaced and the incision closed by suture. Necrosis of the penis may occur and there may be retention of urine. In this case it will be necessary to perform urethrotomy at the ischiatic arch.

Technique of Urethrotomy at Ischiatic Arch. The perineum is surgically prepared in the usual way, and epidural anaesthesia induced. The dog is restrained on its back, with the hind limbs drawn forward to expose the operation site (Fig. 452), and the tail fixed to the table. A catheter is introduced into the urethra to serve as a guide. The surgeon locates and fixes the urethra by means of the catheter and cuts down on to it in the median raphe (Fig. 453). The incision into the urethra should measure about 1–1.5 cm in length, and the edges of the wound are then sutured to the outer skin (Figs. 454, 455). For the next few months the dog passes urine through the fistula thus created, adopting the squatting stance of the micturating bitch, but eventually the fistula will heal and urine is then passed through the normal channel.

Neoplasia of the Penis. Tumours of the penis are rare in the dog. The new growths mainly occur on the tip of the organ, and an indication of neoplasia is that the dog

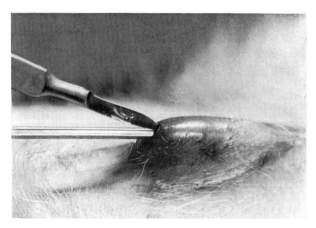

Fig. 449. Operation for phimosis. Incision into the preputial opening.

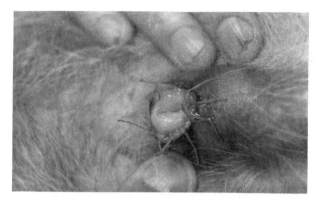

Fig. 450. The completed phimosis operation.

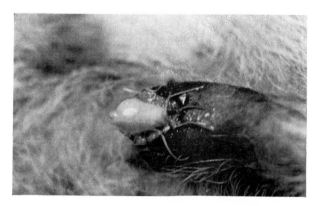

Fig. 451. The penis can now be exsheathed.

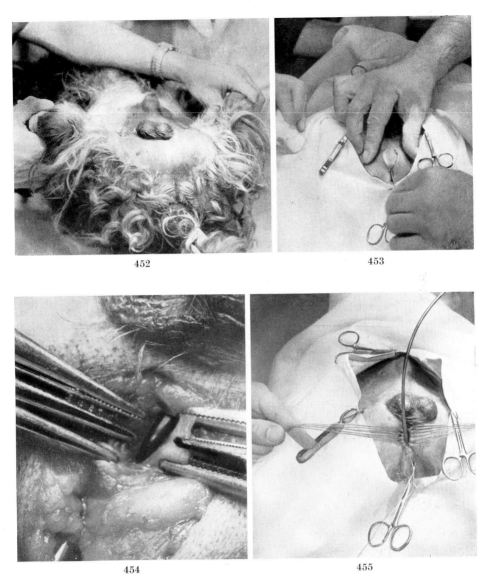

452

453

454

455

Fig. 452. Urethrotomy. The operation position.

Fig. 453. Urethrotomy. Incision over the urethra.

Fig. 454. Urethrotomy. The urethra is opened and fixed with Pean's forceps. The catheter in the urethra is well shown.

Fig. 455. Urethrotomy. After the mucosa of the urethra has been attached to the external skin the patency of the urethra towards the bladder is controlled by a catheter.

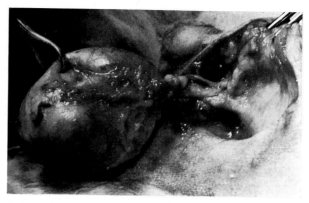

Fig. 456. Removal of a testis affected by a tumour. The second normal testis lies obliquely behind it.

shows increased libido but does not serve the bitch. The tumours usually appear as cauliflower-like, bleeding growths.

Treatment. The only effective treatment is by surgical removal of the tumours plus the affected portion of the penis. Until the wound is healed there will be difficulty in passing urine, so it is advisable to create a urethral fistula at the ischiatic arch as described earlier. GREENE (North Amer. Vet. **38**, 187–188, 1957) has described a technique whereby a solid sound is introduced into the urethra, a rubber tourniquet is applied around the penis, and the affected portion is excised using bilateral flaps. A sagittal incision is made on both sides of the urethra, the latter is separated from the os penis, the dorsal artery is ligatured and the urethra is cut off about 1.5–2 cm anterior to the flaps. The flaps are then sutured together and the protruding urethra is split dorso-ventrally and sutured firmly to both sides.

In our technique, the prepuce is split along the raphe, the penis is dissected free behind the os penis and removed at this point, the urethra being sealed off with an intussusception suture. It is essential to ligate all blood vessels very carefully. After separating the penis out at the reflection of the prepuce, the wound is carefully closed. The urethral fistula at the ischiatic arch remains patent permanently in this procedure.

Fracture of the Os Penis. Only one case in which this occurred has been reported. The fracture was revealed when a catheter was introduced into the urethra to relieve retention of urine and was obstructed after a short distance. The site of the fracture was revealed by radiography and crepitus could be elicited by slight movements of the ends of the bone (DENHOLM, Vet. Rec. **69**, 15, 1957). Until the fracture heals it is necessary to create an ischiatic urethral fistula as described earlier.

Castration. Castration is indicated when there are tumours of the testes (Fig. 456), injuries to the scrotum and testes and when the dog shows signs of excessive sexuality, e.g. masturbation, straying, etc.

Technique of Castration. The scrotum is surgically prepared and epidural anaesthesia induced. The dog is restrained on its back and an incision is made alongside the raphe. The testes are exposed and the blood vessels tied with double ligatures before the glands are removed. The wound is then treated as an open wound to allow ample drainage. This method is used where there are inflammations or enlargements in the region of the testes.

Where the testes are normal it is preferable to remove them through an incision at the level of the inguinal canal. The inguinal region is prepared and fixing the spermatic cord with the thumb and forefinger beside the penis, an incision is made down on to it, about 3–5 cm long. The spermatic cord, together with the tunica vaginalis, is dissected free and the testis withdrawn from the wound by gentle traction. The scrotal ligament is cut and the spermatic cord double ligatured. The testis is then removed, the wound sutured and an antibiotic introduced into the cavity with a blunt-ended cannula.

Artificial Insemination. The technique of artificial insemination of the bitch is well tried in practice but should be regarded as a last resort. GREVE (Thesis. Gießen, 1957) has published a critical review on the subject, extracts from which are given below, but especially interested readers are referred to the specialised literature on the subject. GREVE writes "The first attempt at artificial insemination of a mammal was successfully made by LAZZARO SPALLANANZI in the dog in 1780 and was subsequently confirmed by other investigators. This success stimulated the development of techniques for artificial insemination of domesticated animals. The first artificial vagina for the dog was made in 1914, and this served as a prototype for artificial vaginas in other animals. The application of the technique in the dog is limited compared with other domesticated animals of economic importance, as the dog shows a high fertility rate which cannot be improved by artificial insemination, it does not suffer from venereal disease, and oestrus only occurs bi-annually.

Indications for artificial insemination are therefore rather restricted, and its main uses are where there is mechanical obstruction to mating, nervousness of the bitch leading to her biting the dog, and to increase the progeny of especially valuable sires or to the production of new breeds by crossing breeds of greatly differing sizes. Harrop's artificial vagina is the most suitable for the collection of the semen. It can be used without the presence of a bitch on heat, it does not harm the dog and provides semen which is both quantitatively and qualitatively good. A further advantage is that it is not acceptable to a dog with weak libido so that there is little risk of this defect being passed on to the male offspring. Electro-ejaculation is not satisfactory as it has not been properly developed in the dog and the semen is usually diluted with urine. Producing ejaculation by manipulation is unaesthetic and it is difficult to get a clean semen sample by this method. Examination of the semen is carried out in a similar manner to that used in other species. Sodium citrate-egg yolk and pasteurised milk may be used as preservative and dilution fluids. The ejaculate can be divided into three fractions of which only the second is of any value. Using pasteurised milk-diluted semen which had been obtained from America and was 140 hours old, a bitch was successfully inseminated. The semen in this case was transported in a specially developed shock-proof container.

It is difficult to determine the optimum time for insemination, but vaginal smears will indicate the time of ovulation, otherwise repeated inseminations should be made."

Greve concludes that where indicated as outlined above, artificial insemination could be a valuable addition to the techniques of practice.

13. Diseases of the nervous system

Examination of the central and peripheral nervous system of the dog presents many difficulties. ÜBERREITER (Schweiz. Arch. Tierheilkunde **98**, 321–351, 1956) has described the examination of the nervous system so clearly and completely that we have adopted his system. Where there are nervous symptoms it must first be decided whether they are caused by one or more processes within the brain or the spinal cord or the peripheral nervous system, and further whether the focus is within the central nervous system or whether, in fact, the symptoms are caused by pressure on the central nervous system occasioned by processes occurring outside of it. To do this the general symptoms must first be analysed and then the localised symptoms evaluated. Any defects in physiological reflexes or the appearance of pathological reflexes can be referred to pathological processes in the brain and the individual cranial and spinal nerves.

If, for example, there are signs of defects in the individual nerves, which are closely related as they emerge from the brain, or whose nuclei are adjacent to each other, this indicates a circumscribed focus.

If, on the other hand, there are defects in different cranial nerves whose nuclei or points of exit are not closely related, one may then conclude that there are several foci, or that the lesion is widespread. Particular attention should be given to the history of the case. It is important to discover whether the condition developed slowly or appeared suddenly, possibly after an accident, whether the condition is progressive or stationary, what is the environment of the dog, and whether there have been remissions, etc.

General behaviour of the dog. This includes psychic behaviour, facial expression, disorders of consciousness and behaviour when feeding.

Mobility. Observation of the dog when standing at rest and in movement.

Ataxia. By this we imply disorders or dysfunction of the controlled physiological coordination of muscle groups when at rest or in movement. It is of practical importance to distinguish between cerebral, cerebellar and spinal ataxia. In cerebral ataxia the dog walks awkwardly, stumbles over obstructions, slips on smooth surfaces and cannot accomplish finer movements. In cerebellar ataxia the dog sways while standing at rest and often falls over. The animal sways and walks with faltering steps with the feet set wide apart, as if drunk. When there is a localised focus of trouble, the animal falls to the side of the lesion and moves in circles. There is atony of the musculature. The function of the cerebellum is independent of the eyes. In spinal ataxia the animals have a clumsy, fumbling gait. When the eyes are covered the ataxia becomes more evident because the dog can compensate for the nervous defect by use of the eyes.

Investigation of the cranium and its contents.

Posture of the head. The head may be carried on one side in vestibular disorders, in affections of the sterno-mastoid muscle, in cerebellar tumours (head is held towards the affected side), in paralysis of the ocular muscles and in disorders of vision.

Inspection of the skull. This is carried out in relation to its shape (hydrocephalus), enlargement of the skull, and its symmetry; maldevelopment of the cranial musculature and of the cranium (open fontanelles, herniation of the brain or meningeal coverings, compressibility of the bones). In osteo-dystrophies, the cranium may be soft and thickened. Percussion of the cranium may determine tenderness in fractures, fissures, or tumours. Compression of the skull is used to determine the indirect pain of fissures.

Cranial nerve symptoms give important indications of the site of their lesions.

Olfactory nerves. Disorders of the sense of smell are difficult to determine in animals. With dogs this can be assessed by taking them into a room in which there is a strong smelling food, so placed that the dog cannot see it, and then observing the animal's behaviour (lifting of the nose, sniffing, etc.).

Optic nerve. By ophthalmoscopic observation one may appreciate atrophy of the pupil, congestion of the capillary and retinal blood vessels, the so-called choked disc, papilloedema, etc. Tests of vision are given on page 178.

Oculo-motor nerve. Examination of the pupils will reveal mydriasis, myosis, anisochorea (unequal pupillary opening) and a pupillary reflex (the reflex arc consisting of: retina – optic nerve – optic chiasma, lateral corpus geneculatum and anterior corpora quadrigemina – oculo-motor nucleus – oculo-motor nerve – sphincter of the pupil). Because there is a connection between each of the corpora quadrigemina and the oculo-motor nuclei there is a consensual light reaction, i.e. illumination of one eye causes the pupil of the other eye to contract. From the primary optic centres (posterior tubercle of the thalamus corpora geniculata) the visual pathway proceeds by the optic radiation to the occipital lobes. The prompt reaction of the pupil to light shows that the reflex arc just mentioned is intact and consequently the visual pathway to the thalamus is also whole, but nevertheless it does not mean that the animal can see. A lesion in the optic radiation or in the cortex of the brain may still cause blindness. Unilateral injury to the visual centre in the occipital lobe causes blindness on the same side, with the exception of a quite small area in the region of the nasal portion of the retina, and not, as it does in man, a hemianopia (unilateral blindness).

Nerves of the eye muscles. The oculo-motor nerve leaves the brain in the cerebral peduncle and is the motor nerve to the levator palpebrae muscles and to all the external eye muscles except the superior oblique, and the lateral rectus muscles. It provides the autonomic nerve supply to the sphincter of the pupil and the ciliary muscle. The trochlear nerve emerges in the region of the brachium conjunctivum of the cerebellum and supplies the superior oblique muscle. The abducens nerve courses from the corpus trapezoidum laterally to the pyramids and supplies the lateral rectus muscle. All the nerves supplying the muscles of the eye pass into the orbit through the orbital fissure but the trochlear nerve often passes through an aperture of its own. Paralysis of the eye muscles causes squinting of the eyeball or restriction of its movement. In paralysis of the oculo-motor nerve, ptosis and mydriasis occur and where there is irritation of the nerve, miosis may be seen. The trigeminal nerve emerges in the region of the pons. Outside the brain the Gasserian semi-lunar ganglion is embedded in the dura mater in the region of the petrous portion of the temporal bone. Its first branch leaves the cranial cavity through the orbital fissure, its second through the foramen rotundum and its third through the foramen ovale. Except for the ear muscles in the region of the nape of the neck, this supplies sensory nerves to the whole of the skin of the face and head.

Systematic tests of the sensitivity of the skin of the head. Pressure points for the nerves are to be found at the supra-orbital foramen for the first branch, the infraorbital for the second branch and the mental foramen for the sensory part of the third branch. The reflexes can be tested by the corneal reflex for the first branch. For the second branch, closure of the lids on touching the cornea, and the nose reflex produces sneezing when the mucosa of the nose is tickled with a feather. The masseter reflex can be elicited by tapping with a spatula on the lower teeth, resulting in contraction of the masseters.

Tests of the motor portions of the three branches. The masticatory nerve, which enervates the chewing muscles, can be assessed by opening the jaws and estimating the muscular resistance.

The Facial nerve. This emerges from the medulla oblongata besides the corpus trapezoidum, caudal to the pons. It produces a convulsive tick or facial spasm, and ptosis when injured. When it is stimulated, the Chevosteck phenomenon is elicited by the appearance of spasms at the angle of the mouth on percussion of the auricular region.

The Stato-acoustic nerve. Damage to the cochlear nerve causes deafness and objective tests of its function are not always easy. When there is unilateral damage to the vestibular nerve, the head is held obliquely, there are circular and rolling movements and the dog often falls on the affected side. There may be nystagmus with oblique position of the eyes. When the lesions are bi-lateral the symptoms are very similar to those seen in cerebellar ataxia. The vestibular nerve function may be examined by the Barany test. This consists in dropping cold water into the external ear and this produces nystagmus in the eye on the opposite side in the healthy animal. This reflex is absent when there is peripheral injury to the vestibular nerve.

The Glosso-pharyngeal nerve emerges from the medulla oblongata and a choking reflex can be produced when the back of the throat is stimulated. When this nerve is paralysed there are difficulties in swallowing and disorders of taste.

The Vagus nerve is partly bound up with the glosso-pharyngeal. Damage to this nerve results in paralysis of the larynx with consequent difficulty in breathing or irritation of the recurrent nerve which may produce bronchial breathing or spasm of the glottis.

The Accessory nerve. Damage to this nerve produces paralysis of the sterno-cleido-mastoid muscles.

The Hypo-glossal nerve. If damaged there may be atrophy of the tongue or deviation of the tongue while at rest to the healthy side, or if the tongue is stretched out, the deviation is to the paralysed side.

After analysis of the cranial nerves and examination of mobility, i.e. ataxia, turning movements, index finger movements, rotary movements, etc., the muscle tone of the limbs, sensations and various reflexes are tested. When there is a diminished muscle tone it can be tested with a faradic current.

To test the peripheral reflex the extent of the patella reflex is used. To do this the animal is restrained on its side while the thigh of the uppermost limb is grasped and raised up slightly. With a percussion hammer or the tips of the fingers the patellar tendon is lightly struck with a wrist action. When the reflex arc is intact there is a jerk of the lower leg. The Achilles tendon reflex may be tested in the same way. The anal reflex is elicited by inserting a thermometer in the anus.

Other investigational procedures may be employed to establish a diagnosis. Changes in the cerebro-spinal fluid may indicate disease of the central nervous

system. The fluid may be obtained by tapping the occipital foramen. The article by
FANKHAUSER (Zbl. Vet. Med. 1, 136, 1953) gives useful information on this subject.
Where there is disease of the skull, radiography can provide important evidence,
e.g. displacement of bones and changes in the bones produced by neoplasia,
osteodystrophies, fractures, etc. Correct interpretation of skull radiographs
demands a high degree of skill and experience. In addition to plain radiography
the blood vessels and cavities within the skull can be visualised by contrast radiography. Investigations of this type, e.g. encephalography, ventriculography and
cerebral angiography are usually only carried out in those establishments which
are specially equipped for these procedures. Electroencephalography (EEG) has
also been used in the dog (BRASS, Dtsch. tierärztl. Wschr. 66, 242–246 and GÖTZE
et al., Kleintierpraxis 4, 97–103, 1959) but is seldom employed in practice conditions.

Cerebral Anaemia. Anaemia of the brain may occur after severe blood loss or
where there is a generalised anaemia. It may also be seen in severe cardiac diseases,
collapse, and shock.

The clinical picture is one of disturbance of consciousness, resulting in clumsy
incoordinate movements, lack of response to stimuli and possibly a sudden loss of
consciousness leading to death in convulsions.

Treatment depends upon the primary condition producing the anaemia. In
severe haemorrhage this must be controlled and blood expanders such as "Macrodex"
or "Dextran" injected intravenously in doses of 10 ml/lb bodyweight.

Hyperaemia of the Brain. This arises chiefly as a result of increased output from
the heart in small nervous dogs as a consequence of excitement (active hyperaemia). Where there is restriction of the venous outflow from the brain, e.g. by
compression of the jugular veins, the condition is then called passive hyperaemia.

There are no distinctive clinical signs. Active hyperaemia is indicated by
congestion of the visible mucosae of the head and changes in respiration and pulse
rate.

Treatment consists of rest, the use of tranquillisers where necessary and confining
the dog in a cool, dark, quiet room. Where the congestion is passive it may be
possible to remove the obstruction to venous outflow surgically.

Cerebral Contusion (Cerebral shock). This condition may occur in any accident
where there is trauma to the head.

Sometimes there are varying degrees of vertigo with the animal reeling or falling
over (Fig. 457). In severe cases there may be loss of consciousness preceded by
vomiting. Nystagmus may be noted and there may be muscular twitching, convulsions or paralysis. In the most severe cases, loss of consciousness occurs at the
time of the trauma and the dog never recovers. In other cases the animal is unconscious for several hours with loss of cranial nerve reflexes. After any accident
one should always bear in mind the possibility of cerebral shock, even where no
fractures of the skull can be found. Clinical signs may be of a generalised or localised
nature. The dog may be brought in suffering from generalised symptoms, e.g.
crying, restlessness, convulsions, etc. After some days these symptoms subside
and the localised signs appear, e.g. ataxias, circling movements, cranial nerve
dysfunctions, etc.

Treatment takes the form of complete rest even where there are no marked
symptoms. The dog should be confined to a well-ventilated, quiet, dark room for a
period of 4–8 days avoiding all stimuli. Cold compresses should be applied to the

25*

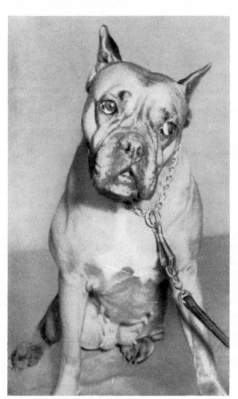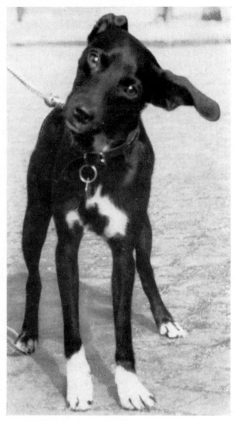

457   458

Fig. 457. Boxer with cerebral contusion after an accident.

Fig. 458. Mongrel with meningitis.

head to minimise the danger of cerebral haemorrhage (apoplexy). Where the loss of consciousness persists, stimulant drugs are indicated.

Meningitis, Encephalitis. These conditions do occur in the dog but are rather rare.

The clinical picture in the acute disease commences with sudden disturbance of consciousness. Initially signs of depression may appear, usually accompanied by a ravenous appetite, apathy and stupefaction. Sometimes the dog will stand motionless in a corner for long periods at a time. Alternatively there may be signs of cerebral irritation such as bad temper, frenzy or convulsions. Often the dog will circle round aimlessly and if the disease is unilateral the head is tilted (Fig. 458). Acute cases may die within a few days of onset of symptoms.

Treatment is essentially the administration of high systemic doses of the wide-spectrum antibiotics. Osmotherapy (NATSCHEFF, Wien. tierärztl. Mschr. **42**, 827,

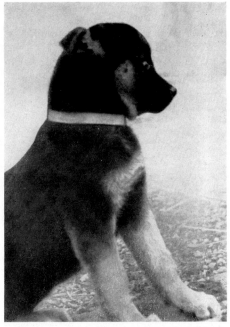

Fig. 459. Internal hydrocephalus in a 12-week-
old German Shepherd.

1957) in which hypertonic (20–40 %) glucose solutions are given intravenously and withdraw fluid from the brain tissues by osmotic action, may also be used. In this technique, 20–60 ml of the concentrated glucose solution are injected intravenously daily for 8–12 successive days. There is some danger of collapse, so the dog should be carefully observed both during and after treatment. Supportive measures are rest in a quiet, well-ventilated and darkened room.

Spinal shock and contusion. These conditions are mainly seen after accidents but may occur in infections and poisoning. The clinical signs may not appear for some hours after the trauma. Actual injury to the spinal cord must be eliminated in the differential diagnosis.

The clinical picture is dominated by paralysis of the hindquarters. The paralysis may be flaccid or spastic in character. In the flaccid type, the hindlimbs are stretched out backwards whilst in the spastic type they are extended between the forelimbs in the "dog-sitting" posture. Often there is retention of urine and faeces.

Treatment is similar to that described above but care must be taken to ensure that urine and faeces are evacuated (catheterisation and enemata). If response is low, faradic stimulation or the administration of strychnine should be considered. We employ a 1 % solution of strychnine in a dose of 0.1 ml/kg bodyweight on 4 successive days followed by injections every 2 days to lessen the risk of cumulative toxicity.

Congenital internal hydrocephalus (Congenital dropsy of the cerebral cavities). This is not uncommon in young dogs but they seldom show any functional disabilities consequent upon the condition (Figs. 459, 460). MARKIEWICZ (Med.

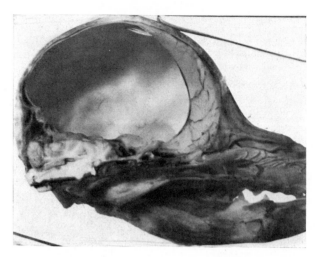

Fig. 460. Internal hydrocephalus (post-mortem specimen).

weteryn. **11**, 359–360, 1955) described a case in a spaniel bitch which showed apathy and clumsy responses to external stimuli. The symptoms were accentuated when she came on heat and developed into deep depression and stupor, ataxia and circling movements. Euthanasia is to be recommended for such cases.

Cerebral tumours. Brain tumours are quite often seen although there are few reports by clinicians. Important contributions to the literature on this subject have been made by ÜBERREITER (Schweiz. Arch. Tierheilk. **99**, 51–99, 1957), VERWER (Tijdschr. Diergeneesk. **84**, 1165–1174, 1959) and FRAUCHIGER & FANK-HAUSER in "The Nervous Diseases of Dogs" (Huber & Co., Berne 1949). Pathologists are very interested in brain tumours and clinicians can glean much valuable information from their reports. Neoplasms occur in various sites in the brain and some may remain symptomless because of their position. Older dogs are mainly affected and according to Verwer, the Boxer shows an increased susceptibility, males being affected twice as often as females.

The clinical picture is mainly one of gradually increasing prostration, lassitude, decreased skin sensitivity, ptosis, vertigo, ataxia and a slowing of the pulse. Sometimes the dog will stand motionless for hours in a corner, often with its head pressed against a wall. Alternatively there may be signs of brain irritation with frenzy, aggressiveness, snapping, paresis and convulsions. Frequently the head is held tilted to one side. Verwer examined the cerebrospinal fluid in 17 cases and found that 13 of these showed pathological changes (pleocytosis, increased albumin, changes in colloid curves and increased pressure). The focal symptoms described in the earlier part of this chapter may make it possible to determine the site of the lesion. If an accurate localisation can be determined, then surgical removal may be feasible, otherwise euthanasia is the only course to adopt.

Peripheral nerve injuries. Damage to the peripheral nerves may be traumatic, infectious or toxic in origin.

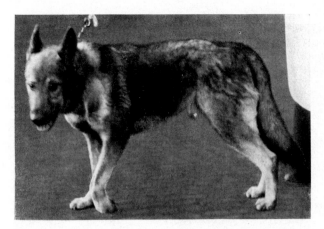

Fig. 461. Left radial paralysis.

The clinical picture will depend upon the type of nerve injured. If motor nerves are affected then there will be disorders of muscular activity; likewise, sensory nerve damage leads to disorders of sensation. If a mixed nerve is damaged then both kinds of symptoms may appear. Where the conductivity of a nerve is totally disrupted, paralyses, both motor and sensory, will occur. If the nerve supply to the limb muscles is damaged the results are uncertain gait, stumbling and slipping. There may be paralyses of the most varied kinds, e.g. radial and peroneal paralysis (Figs. 461, 462), but usually the classical picture, as described in the literature, does not occur. This is due to the variability of the degree of damage and the site of origin of the nerve itself. Many muscles are supplied by several nerves and often neighbouring muscles will assume the functions of the damaged muscle.

Facial nerve paralysis. This lesion presents a typical clinical picture resulting from changes in the position of the ears, and also of the upper and lower lips. Unilateral paralysis of the facial nerve causes the ear and lower lip of the paralysed side to droop (Fig. 463). Very often the upper lip is drawn away from the healthy side. In addition there is ptosis, or drooping of the upper eyelid. When the eyelid reflex is absent, the eyelids remain open and there is a marked flow of tears.

Injury of the trigeminal nerve. This causes a paralysis of the lower jaw. If the lower jaw is held up with the hand it falls down powerlessly when the injury is bilateral, mastication being impossible. When the damage is unilateral there is some impairment of function. The cornea is insensitive and the eyelid reflex is decreased, so that injuries to the cornea may occur.

Treatment of nerve paralyses is by injection of strychnine (see page 389), by giving vitamin B preparations, glutaminic acid dragees, etc. Osmo therapy (see page 388) may be beneficial in certain cases. In paralyses of specific nerves of the limbs, supporting bandages, possibly with metal supports, are recommended.

Epilepsy. Epilepsy is a chronic disease of the brain with periodically repeated attacks. It has not yet been determined whether the condition is congenital or hereditary in nature.

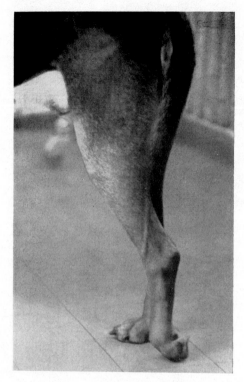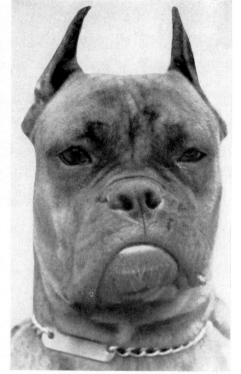

Fig. 462. Peroneal paralysis.   Fig. 463. Right facial paralysis.

The clinical picture is that the animal suddenly suspends activity, remains standing and then collapses. The collapse results from a sudden loss of tone in the muscles followed by a tonic phase. After about thirty seconds the clonic phase sets in with jerking or convulsions of the muscles of the extremities, opisthotonus, and gnashing of the jaws with possible injury of the tongue, so that the foam which appears at the mouth may be blood stained. Spasm of the smooth muscles causes urination. The pupils do not respond to light and the corneal reflex is absent. The attack only lasts a few minutes and afterwards there are slight disorders of the consciousness, e.g. aimless wandering about, stupid expression, etc. Quite often immediately after an attack the animal will eat any food ravenously. In slight epileptiform attacks there is only a transient disorder of consciousness with slight spasms of certain muscle groups, e.g. chattering of the teeth.

Prognosis is unfavourable when the attacks follow one another at short intervals of days or even hours (status epilepticus). In the usual case the veterinarian does not see the patient during an attack and so diagnosis has to be based on the owner's history.

Treatment can only be given in the periods between attacks and during an actual seizure the patient should be left alone as much as possible, care being taken that there is no self-inflicted trauma. In status epilepticus the patient may be put under general anaesthesia if the owner, despite the distressing condition of the dog, cannot decide on euthanasia. The drug Primidone is widely used for the treatment of canine epilepsy. The dose of this drug is 35–45 mg per kg body-weight daily for single or combined dosage. Too high a dosage leads to ataxia, but no other side effects have been noted. Phenytoin has also been employed as an anti-epileptic in the dog.

14. Diseases of the bones and locomotor organs

Diseases of the bones and locomotor organs manifest themselves in restriction of the mobility of the body. To determine affections of this kind an accurate history of the case is necessary. Palpation plays a part as it may enable the disease condition to be localised. Palpation of the limbs is done with the greatest care beginning at the extremity with the dog lying down. X-ray examination should be used in certain diseases (fractures, tumours, etc.). A differential blood count is also useful (eosinophilic myositis).

Fractures are usually presented with a history of injury. Car accidents are common, but self-inflicted injury may occur.

The clinical features include: disuse of the limb; local swelling and pain; excessive mobility at the fracture site and possible distortion. Crepitus – the rasping sensation that can be felt when the fractured bone ends rub together – may be detected on handling the area, but should not be deliberately produced since it causes tissue damage.

X-ray examination in two planes will confirm the diagnosis and give an accurate appreciation of the site of the fracture and the direction and number of the fracture lines and the displacement which has occurred.

External fixation of fractures by plaster cast, splints, etc., is best reserved for fractures which are on the lower parts of the limbs, that have not been grossly displaced.

If displacement with overlap has occurred (Fig. 464), it is very difficult to obtain satisfactory reduction of the fracture and poor results, such as malunion (malalignment), may be obtained (Fig. 465).

Plaster casts may also be used where multiple fissures of the bone would make internal fixation hazardous (Fig. 466).

To avoid possible soft tissue damage, plaster casts must be very carefully applied. The slab technique, in which longitudinal strips of plaster bandage are arranged to overlap at their edges, prevents possible damage by shrinkage of the bandage which can cause constriction of the limb. Annular reinforcement of the cast should only be applied after the slab layer has hardened. The top of the cast should be "belled out" while it is still soft so that there is a gradual transition of pressure to the skin in that area. It is important that the cast should include the joints above and below the fracture site (Fig. 467).

The foot should be completely covered by the cast to avoid possible strangulation below the cast.

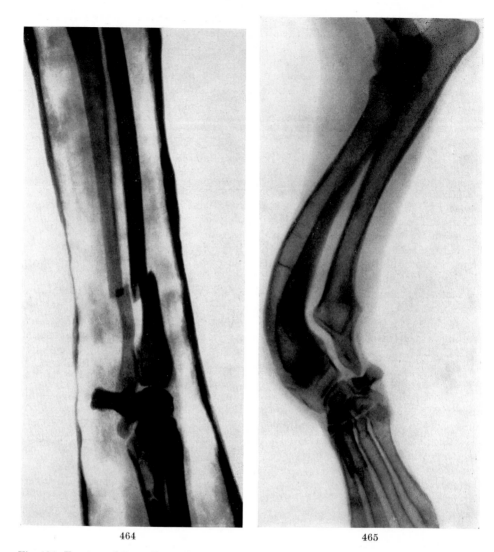

464   465

Fig. 464. Fracture of the radius and ulna in plaster of Paris. Note overlapping of fractured bones.

Fig. 465. Forearm fracture after inadequate treatment which healed with marked outward
curvature of the end of the limb.

Uneven skin pressure within the cast, especially where the cast covers a joint,
must be avoided by making short cuts in the edges of the strip of plaster bandage
and overlapping the cut areas to produce the required bend in the cast without
forming wrinkles on the inner surface of the cast. Any wrinkles in the cast can
cause local pressure areas that may result in skin necrosis.

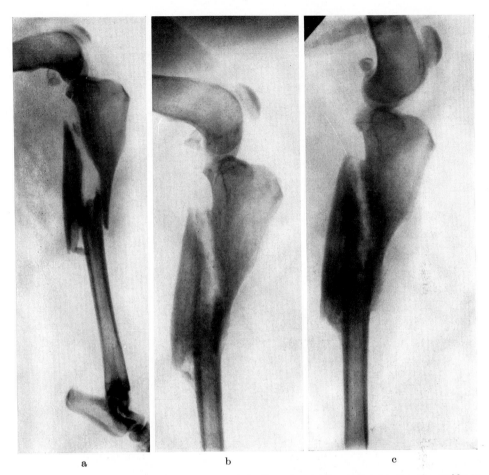

a   b   c

Fig. 466a–c. Fracture of the proximal third of the lower leg. (a) Immediately after the accident; (b) 20 days later; (c) 38 days after the accident. At this time the patient again completely bore weight on the limb.

Many fractures are not suited to external fixation because of the type of fracture or because of the shape of the surrounding soft tissues. Internal fixation methods are employed for these fractures and several techniques have been developed to meet the specific requirements of different types of fracture.

Round section intramedullary pins are widely employed in simple, near-transverse, fractures of the mid-shaft area of long bones. The pins are inserted into the medullary canal of the bone and maintain longitudinal alignment of the fracture by transmission of any potentially displacing force that may act upon one segment to the endosteal surface of the other segment. The pin should fit the medullary canal reasonably snugly, but should not be large enough to impact into the bone (Fig. 468).

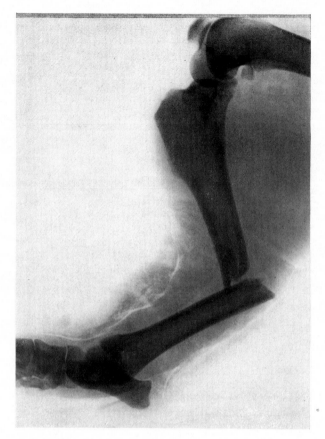

Fig. 467. Fracture of the lower leg with an inadequately placed plaster cast. The cast ends immediately over the fracture and the stifle joint is not included in it.

The muscles that surround the broken bone exert a longitudinal compressive force which holds the fractured ends in firm contact (contact compression) and this promotes the healing of the fracture.

The rotating or shearing forces that are so troublesome in man do not cause difficulty in the dog because of the difference in stance and in lying position. The rough ends of the bone key together in the cases of near-transverse fracture and help to prevent any rotational distortion. Rotational distortion can occur where the fracture is very oblique or is spiral in shape and for these fractures a simple pin is not suitable, since both rotational and longitudinal collapse will occur.

Transverse fractures close to the end of the bone through which the pin is drilled may be successfully treated, but fractures which are very close to the other end of the bone do not provide sufficient grip for the tip of the pin to effectively maintain alignment.

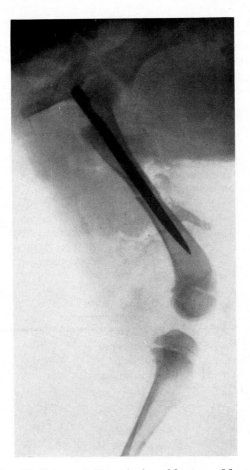

Fig. 468. Intramedullary pinning of fracture of femur.

The reverse nailing technique, in which the pin is inserted from the fracture site up the bone to emerge proximally is very useful, especially in fixation of femoral fractures. An additional use of reverse nailing technique, by withdrawing the pin and re-inserting it blunt end first up through the track which has been drilled, is also very useful.

In realigning the fracture the pointed tip of the pin may be passed down to engage in the medullary canal of the distal segment and employed as a lever to assist in reducing the fracture. This procedure should only be employed if there are no fissures in the distal segment of the bone. If undisplaced fissures are present and this manoeuvre is to be employed, the distal segment should be held firmly in bone-holding forceps until the manipulation is completed.

Kuntscher Nails are V, U or Y in cross-section and are particularly useful in fixation of bones with large-diameter medullary canals or where the possibility of rotational distortion is an important factor. These nails are designed to be impacted into the medullary canal which must be pre-drilled before nail insertion and in certain sites the medullary canal must be reamed out to the correct size to permit nail insertion. These nails are not inserted by use of a chuck, as are the round-section pins, but are inserted by use of a hammer.

Small-diameter, round-section pins with a "sledge-runner tip" and a hooked end (Rush pins) are useful in a few fractures close to joints. In fracture of the distal epiphysis of the femur and fracture of the lateral malleolus of the fibula, they are especially useful. They act as springs which counteract the muscle pull that is liable to cause displacement of the fracture. The Rush pins make three points of contact with the bone and the hooked end sits snugly against the cortex and does not cause soft tissue damage.

Plates and screws are useful for oblique and spiral fractures and in sites where intramedullary pins are not satisfactory, such as shaft of radius and ulna.

For all normal purposes two screws should be applied on each side of the fracture line and all the screws should penetrate both cortices of the bone. The fractured ends of the bone must be held in close apposition to promote healing. If any gap is present the plate will prevent the ends from coming together and the resulting distraction will slow the healing process markedly.

Compression plating, which employs a special device to force the bone ends together after the plate has been applied to one side of the fracture, is useful in cases such as non-union or delayed union.

Additional screws may help to improve the alignment or fixation, but must be inserted into a drill hole that has been counter-sunk to prevent cortical fissures from occurring as the screw is tightened.

Special plates with oval holes or with longitudinal screw slots (Eggers plates) will permit the muscle action to promote contact compression and so assist in fracture healing.

In all fracture fixations where metals are employed, all the parts used should be of the same composition. If this rule is not adhered to, electrolytic currents will be set up and these will cause bone destruction and will prevent fracture healing. This factor is particularly important where plates and screws are employed. If stainless steel plates and screws are used, the same grade of stainless steel should be used throughout.

Aerial screws are used to fix bone extremities back in place. The action of the screw will counteract the distraction effect of muscles which are attached to the bone end. Specially shaped "olecranon" screws, which have a shaft that is smooth and narrower than the threaded portion, are particularly useful to create impaction since as they are screwed home the threaded portion is entirely in the distal segment and pulls the proximal portion home increasingly tightly.

Individually placed transfixation screws are useful in fractures with very irregular fracture lines and can also be employed to replace large bone segments. They are also useful as compression devices in the handling of such fractures as single condylar fractures of the humerus.

Wiring of fractures is not employed extensively now because it is difficult to ensure sufficiently stable fixation at the fracture site. Occasionally it is employed to hold a segment of bone in place but it is used mostly in fixation of symphyseal fractures of the jaw.

Combined internal–external fixation as by Kirschner–Ehmer splints, Stader splints or Pin casts can all be employed, but share the disadvantages that the pins pass through the skin into the bone and infection may occur. These techniques were widely employed at one time, but with improvements in internal fixation methods, which cannot be interfered with by the patient, combined methods are now used in only a few special sites.

Healing of fractures takes a considerable period of time and varies with the age of the dog and with the degree of disturbance of blood supply suffered by the bones at the fracture site. For most fractures the frequently repeated statement that healing will be complete in 3–4 weeks is quite wrong. Repeat checks of the fracture progress by radiography should be carried out before the fixation is removed. Only when a well-calcified callus is present should the cast, splint, pin or plate be taken away. If it is removed earlier there is a real risk of renewed displacement of the fracture occurring and this will be much more difficult to correct than the original fracture.

No standard time can be stated for fracture healing. If both fragments have a good blood supply, calcified callus might be well developed in some 8–12 weeks.

If one fragment has a poor blood supply, the callus may take 4–6 months to form well and if both fragments have poor blood supply 6–12 or more months may well elapse.

There is conflicting evidence on various factors that may promote bone healing, but none of the claims are fully substantiated. Adequate diet is necessary and if the dog has poor bone development (osteoporosis) addition of bone meal to the diet is useful.

Restriction of use of the limb is frequently indicated and the owner must be well warned, if a fracture is not fully stable after fixation, that he must ensure only limited use of the leg is permitted until healing is well advanced.

Pelvis. Fractures of the pelvis are usually the result of car accidents. Clinically the dogs will be disinclined to stand or walk and may show severe pain if touched. The fractures commonly occur close to midline through the pubis and ischium, but rarely occur through the symphysis itself. Near-midline fracture cases show abnormal mobility if the ischial tuberosities are pressed together. Gross collapse of the pelvic diameter can occur and may cause difficulty at subsequent parturition in bitches (Figs. 469, 470).

Cases of symphyseal separation cannot adduct the hind legs because the adductor muscles are attached to their own side of midline.

Pelvic fractures with displacement are either double fractures or there may be a unilateral sacro-iliac dislocation.

Most pelvic fractures will heal well if allowed to rest; if gross pain is present, high-level doses of phenylbutazone are useful to give relief. Fractures which occur through the acetabulum have, in general, a poor prognosis.

Lameness is likely to persist indefinitely and especially in cases where the acetabulum is split and the femoral head has passed through, the treatment of choice is to excise the femoral head.

In all cases of pelvic fracture urinary function should be checked since occasionally rupture of the urinary bladder may occur which will require to be repaired urgently.

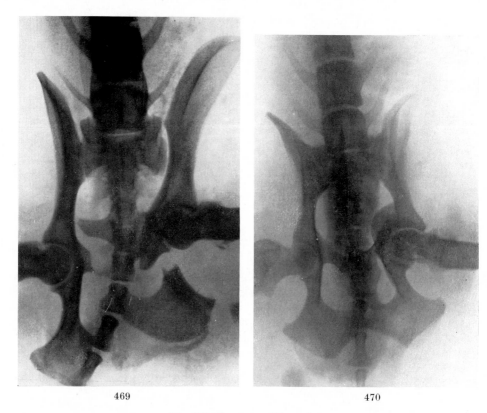

469   470

Fig. 469. Fracture of the pelvis.

Fig. 470. Deformation of the pelvic girdle after a fracture causing reduction in the diameter of
the pelvis.

Various attempts at internal or combined fixation of pelvic fractures have
been made, but in general the results obtained do not justify these procedures.

Splitting the pelvic symphysis and insertion of a symphyseal prosthesis have been
adopted in cases where narrow pelvic diameter causes difficulty in defaecation.

Femur. All femoral fractures tend to be presented with total inability to use the
limb.

Fractures of the shaft often have considerable swelling of the thigh and obvious
increased mobility at the site.

Distal epiphyseal fractures show less swelling and little or no increased mobility
since the distal fragment is displaced backwards under the action of the flexors
of the stifle and the distal end of the shaft becomes engaged in the vastus muscles.
The patella is commonly less prominent than normal because it is no longer held
forward by the trochlea.

Fractures just below the femoral neck show similar features to shaft fractures
but abnormal mobility is less because of the fracture site.

Fixation of shaft and high shaft fractures is most successful by use of open reduction and the insertion of a round-section intramedullary pin employing the reverse nailing technique.

The approach to the fracture site is along the intermuscular plane between the vastus muscles and the biceps femoris. This involves cutting skin and fascia lata only and on closure care should be taken to suture the muscles as close to the bone as possible.

As with all intramedullary pin fixations, the sharper the trochar point is, the more readily it will be inserted.

The pin should be made to the correct length for the bone and the proximal end should be well rounded to prevent soft tissue damage.

Radiographic checking of the fixation should be carried out at the end of the operation and screening of the fracture site should not be employed because of the risks involved.

Pin removal can be carried out with local anaesthesia, but should be delayed until a well-calcified callus is present.

Fracture of the distal epiphysis of the femur may be treated by the insertion of two Rush pins from the point where the femoral trochlea and condyles meet. The pins require pre-drilled guide holes and must be bent along their length so that they will pass across the bone and bend back to their original sides within the medullary canal. These pins act by cantilever action preventing the backward displacement of the fractured portion of bone by virtue of the position of the proximal parts of the pins.

To correct the fracture the lateral femoro-patellar joint pouch is opened and the alignment is corrected with the stifle in full flexion, a manoeuvre that prevents the fractured surfaces from impacting. Slight over-correction of the fracture, at operation, is useful because there is a constant tendency for re-displacement.

These Rush pins are normally not removed and seldom cause any trouble or irritation.

Tibia and fibula. Most fractures occur in the lower half of the shaft and tend to be oblique in direction. The degrees of displacement and distortion are fairly obvious because the limb has relatively little soft tissue coverage at this area.

Occasionally transverse fractures occur a short distance below the stifle and a radiographic check of the fracture site is essential to demonstrate the extent of displacement.

Intramedullary pin fixation applied from above is usually successful. The point for insertion is a small hollow in the tibial plate directly behind the tibial tuberosity. The pin is best passed medial to the patellar ligament and the point drawn back from behind the ligament and pressed gently down until it engages the hollow. The tibial crest is used as a guide to direct the pin into the medullary canal.

Open reduction of the fracture, approached from the antero-medial side, is very much easier than attempts at blind reduction, because the very thick cortex tends to cause the pin to fail to engage the distal medullary canal.

In young dogs, approximately 3–5 months of age, the tibial tuberosity may be avulsed by apparently quite minor trauma, often self-inflicted. These dogs will show disuse of the leg for some days and only by a very careful physical

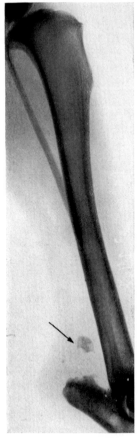

Fig. 471. Avulsion fracture of the calcaneum.

palpation can the increased space between the tibial crest and the tuberosity be appreciated.

These cases normally do not require any surgical treatment; even quite markedly displaced tuberosities will heal on again and good function will be restored.

Fracture of the lateral malleolus of the distal end of the fibula will, in most cases, be associated with fracture dislocation of the hock joint. The lateral collateral ligament of the hock attaches to the lateral malleolus and it is important that this small fragment of bone should be correctly and adequately refixed. In a few very large dogs the malleolus may be large enough to permit a single transverse screw to be applied. In smaller dogs, however, this is not possible and a single Rush pin can be passed up the malleolus and taken through a fine slit drilled into the tibial cortex. This will secure the lateral collateral ligament and allow the malleolus to heal on to the tibia.

Tarsus. Most tarsal fractures occur as a result of self-inflicted injury, especially in racing dogs.

The two most common fractures affect the central tarsal and the fibular tarsal (calcaneum) (Fig. 471).

Central tarsal fractures are crush fractures and when present permit the foot to displace slightly forward and inward, because of lack of support to the front of the hock.

Fixation by single screw or by wiring is sometimes successful, but because the central tarsal is often shattered into many small fragments a T-shaped plate applied to the front of the hock may be more successful.

Some of these cases recover well with no treatment, but the outlook is always uncertain.

Fibular tarsal fractures may be simple or comminuted.

In simple fractures a single axial screw passed down through the os calcis into the fourth tarsal bone is usually successful.

If the bone is shattered either a pin cast is applied or a specially shaped long plate is applied down the lateral side of the whole of the tarsus, with screws passing across the os calcis both above and below the fracture, the 4th tarsal and the 4th metatarsal head. The outlook for return to racing with fibular tarsal fractures is always poor.

Humerus. Most fractures of the humerus occur in the lower midshaft or distal extremity. The shaft fractures show some local swelling and abnormal mobility together with disuse of the leg. Occasionally the proximal epiphysis detaches in the young dog and there are signs of disuse and swelling in the shoulder area.

Simple or oblique fractures may be fixed with a round-sectioned intramedullary pin which must be thin enough to pass the curves of the humeral shaft. The pin may be passed down the length of the bone and into the medial epicondyle, which will give the fixation increased stability.

The point for insertion of the pin is just medial to the highest point of the lateral tuberosity. The direction of insertion is parallel to the crest of bone running down to the deltoid tuberosity. Where fractures are very oblique or are complicated by a "butterfly-segment", plate and screw fixation is preferred.

Distal end fractures of the humerus may be of lateral condyle, medial condyle or both condyles (Y fracture). Where a single condyle is fractured the joint is palpably increased in width and the level of the two epicondylar eminences is no longer level.

With lateral condylar fracture the greater degree of displacement occurs because the weight-bearing structure of the limb is disturbed.

Fixation of single condylar fracture requires medio-lateral compression of the condylar bone mass. This may be effected by a single screw or a bolt or by wiring the condylar mass together. Fixation should be carried out within the first 2 or 3 days following injury otherwise adequate correction cannot be effected.

In double condylar fracture there is extreme excessive mobility of the fracture site because both the collateral ligaments of the elbow are attached to the condyles and when these break free the distal end of the shaft presents a V shape to the elbow joint.

Fixation is difficult and best results can be achieved by use of a plate up the medial face of the humerus and incorporation of a single lag screw or bolt across the condylar mass and through the lowest hole in the plate.

Drilling across the condylar mass is awkward and one method of ensuring correct alignment is to drill outward to the epicondylar eminence from the centre of the fracture where the narrowest point of the condylar mass is broken through.

These cases present features which resemble Radial Paralysis, but only rarely is there any nerve involvement.

Radius and ulna most often have transverse fractures of the lower midshaft.

If these fractures are undisplaced, support by external fixation may be adequate to permit healing. If displacement has occurred, closed reduction is not easy and internal fixation with plate and screws applied to the front of the radius is often easier and more successful.

Premature removal of plaster cast or inadequate external fixation appear to be the main factors predisposing to non-union or malunion, which occurs most commonly at this site.

Fractures of the distal epiphysis of the radius often have minimal displacement, but if they are unsupported lateral distortion of the foot will gradually develop, with resultant disuse and deformity.

Plate and screw fixation of fractures of the radius is the most useful method of treatment, but in very small dogs an intramedullary pin of fine Kirschner wire will give good support. The pin requires to pass through the anterior point of the articular surface of the radius to achieve the correct direction. Additional support with splints or cast is required because of the small size of pin.

Correction of the distortion of the radius and ulna requires the use of a cuneiform osteotomy which should aim to have the section of bone removed from the actual site of the distortion.

26*

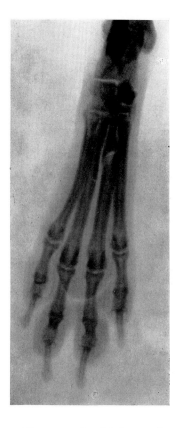

Fig. 472. Fracture of a metacarpal bone.

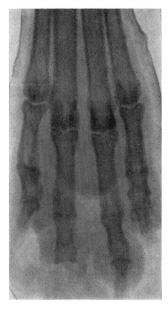

Fig. 473. Amputation of the third phalangeal joint.

The cuts should be made to lie parallel to the distal articular surface of the radius and at right angles to the shaft of the radius above the distortion. Fixation is by plate and screws applied to the radius, after the ulna has been cut through.

Fracture of the shaft of the ulna just below the elbow joint may have associated forward dislocation of the radial head. Correction is easily achieved by pressure and can be adequately fixed by passing a single screw through both radial and ulnar shafts.

Fracture of the olecranon of the ulna usually occurs at the level of the semilunar notch and the fracture line tends to run downward and backward. This fracture is subject to distraction by action of the triceps. Correction by an olecranon screw is effective and the correct alignment can be achieved by reverse drilling of the olecranon from the fracture site. Good impaction of this fracture is most important.

Carpus. Carpal fractures are relatively rare in the dog. Chip fractures may occur on the ventral face of the accessory carpal line in the racing Greyhound. These dogs tend to race poorly and may be lame after a race. Carpal flexion is limited and tends to be painful.

Some success can be achieved by removal of the rudimentary abductor and flexor muscles of the fifth digit and in some cases by removal of the small chip fractures.

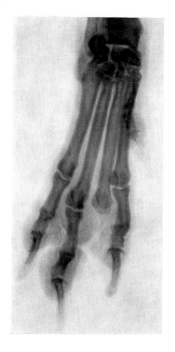

Fig. 474. Amputation of the toe at the first phalangeal joint.

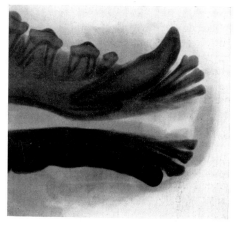

Fig. 475. Fracture of the symphysis of the mandible.

Metacarpals and metatarsals quite commonly occur as multiple fractures, with more than one bone being involved. These fractures can result from trauma or may be self-inflicted (Fig. 472).

Support of the foot in splints is often successful in the household pet, but excessive callous formation may cause impaired racing ability.

Digits. Fractures of the toes occur most often in racing Greyhounds. The first or the second phalanges may be broken and if the fractures do not involve the articular surfaces they may heal well, without fixation. If the joints are involved, racing will be interfered with and treatment of such cases is either by amputation of the affected toe or, in valuable dogs, by wiring of the fracture (Figs. 473, 474).

Mandible. Fractures may be single, through the symphysis (Fig. 475) or one horizontal ramus, or less commonly double involving both rami or very rarely with both fractures on one horizontal ramus.

Fractures behind the level of the last tooth do not require any active treatment since the action of the muscles which either close or open the mouth tend to hold the fracture site in position.

All fractures of the mandibular horizontal rami are compound and antibiotic therapy is indicated.

Fixation by wiring the canines is successful for symphyseal fractures, but the wire should be stitched to pass below the symphysis, not placed across the mouth, to ensure that the fracture is drawn properly together.

Single mandibular fractures can be treated by keeping the mouth bandaged shut and hand feeding liquids via the dog's lip commissures.

A single transverse pin passed from one horizontal ramus to the other in the sublingual soft tissues so that it lies behind the fracture and acts as a "temporary symphysis" is an effective treatment.

Where both horizontal rami are fractured, longitudinal intramedullary pins, which are cut to length at the chin after insertion, are useful.

Osteomyelitis is rare in the dog and does not present the same problems as in man.

The most frequent cause of osteomyelitis in the dog is inadequate asepsis when carrying out open reduction of comminuted fractures in which some of the bone fragments have been deprived of blood supply. In these cases the presence of osteomyelitis is shown by the development of discharging sinuses on the leg and on X-ray the periosteum is raised and in many cases a sequestrum may be seen.

The treatment of these cases involves removal of all foreign material from the limb and removal of all the dead bone. The wound should be closed with an absorbable suture and topical and systemic antibiotics administered.

Recovery is usually good although the final shape of the bone may be abnormal and if there has been much muscle damage this too may limit use of the leg.

Osteomyelitis may also be associated with penetrating bite wounds which have caused bone damage. These cases will usually respond to antibiotic therapy and only require surgical exploration if a sequestrum is present.

Dislocations occur not uncommonly in the dog and are mostly the result of trauma. The dog will show disuse of the affected limb, which may be carried in a peculiar position.

Hip. Traumatic dislocation almost always occurs in an upward and forward direction (Fig. 476) but may occur posteriorly (Fig. 477). The leg is shortened, the great trochanter prominent and more laterally displaced than normal from the ischial tuberosity and abduction of the thigh is restricted because the femoral head catches on the iliac shaft (Fig. 478).

The limb is carried with the foot forward and the stifle and foot pointing outward (Fig. 479).

Reduction by manipulation under general anaesthesia should aim to lift the thigh outward while the foot is pulled in a slightly anterior and medial direction. Pressure by thumbs on the Great Trochanter helps to return the femoral head to the acetabulum.

When the hip has been reduced, repeated flexion and extension movements of the hip should be carried out while the region is being heavily compressed from the lateral side. These movements should be quite free and no crepitus should be felt.

Retention of the hip by use of a figure-of-eight sling of sticking plaster is very useful to prevent redislocation. The figure-of-eight should encircle the foot and the thigh and should pass medial to the tibia. This causes full flexion of all the joints and helps to cause traction on the gluteal muscles that in turn put tension upon the hip and hold it in place.

Bruising of the gluteal muscles may assist in preventing redislocation.

A period of 4 days with complete restriction of exercise should elapse before the sling is removed. If any freedom is permitted, redislocation is likely.

Where the hip is unstable the use of a stainless steel pin passed along from below the ischial tuberosity, over the crest of bone between the Great Trochanter

Fig. 476. Anterior supraglenoid
dislocation of the hip.

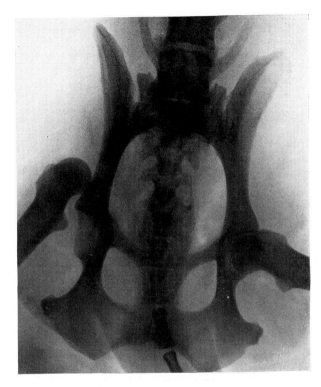

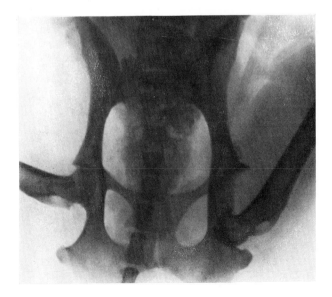

Fig. 477. Posterior supraglenoid dislocation of the hip.

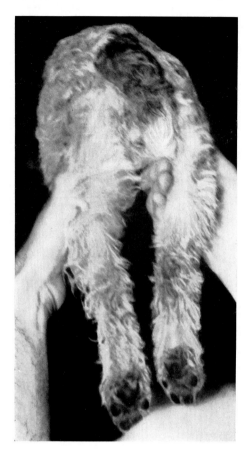

Fig. 478. Dislocation of the right hip. The right-hand leg is obviously shortened.

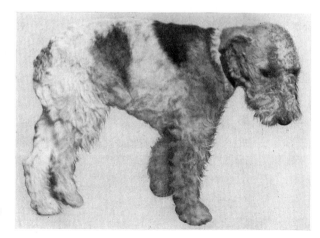

Fig. 479. Dislocation of the right hip.

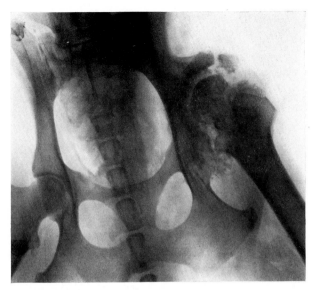

Fig. 480. False joint formation after failure of reduction of hip dislocation.

and femoral head and forward into the wing of the ilium, as described by De Vita, is a useful procedure. These pins can be left *in situ* for up to a month and because they prevent the femoral head from rising they prevent redislocation. These pins do tend to wander from their original site and a useful fixation can be achieved if they are attached by sutures placed round an annular groove at their posterior end and stitched into the dense fascia over the ischial tuberosity.

Other procedures that have been used to prevent redislocation include:

(1) Purse-string suture applied lateral to the great trochanter.
(2) Toggle fixation, which employs a toggle of stainless steel to anchor the medial end of a suture prosthesis of the round ligament.
(3) Shelf operations that aim to increase the depth of the acetabulum by extending the dorsal edge of the acetabulum by use of bone pegs inserted into a split in the acetabulum, or by plastic strip fixed in by screws.

Chip fractures of the dorsal edge of the acetabulum will render the hip highly unstable and one of these stabilising operations is required to retain the femoral head in position.

Chip fractures of the femoral head, by avulsion of a portion by the round ligament, do not prevent replacement of the hip and good results can be obtained in these cases.

In general, satisfactory results are achieved by reduction of dislocations of the hip and long-term checks show no deterioration in these joints.

Radical open reduction procedures are not often indicated and mostly are required where the dislocation is of long standing.

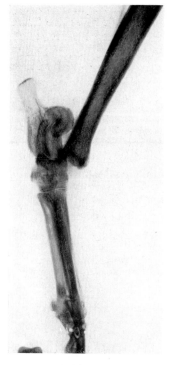

Fig. 481. Dislocation of the hock.

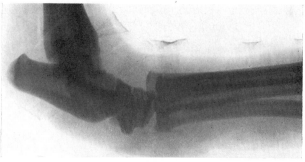

Fig. 482. Dislocation of the tarsal joint.

If a hip is not reduced, a false joint will form where the head lies against the shaft of the ilium (Fig. 480).

Function under these circumstances is fair, but some lameness always persists and it is often marked.

Hock. Dislocation of the hock is virtually always a compound fracture dislocation, with the lateral malleolus broken free and carrying with it the lateral collateral ligament. The foot is grossly displaced medially and the distal end of the tibia projects through the skin, exposing the articular surface of the tibia (Fig. 481).

Replacement after cleaning and fixation of the malleolus (q. v.) often combined with reinforcement of the collateral ligament gives surprisingly good results.

The joint capsule is torn in the original injury and is so short that it cannot be sutured.

Dislocation can occur between the rows of tarsal bones, most commonly between the tibial and fibular tarsal bones above and the central fourth tarsal bones below. This may result from an incised injury to the plantar surface of the hock, but frequently arises spontaneously, with associated degeneration and stretching of the plantar ligaments.

The dog stands on the whole of the back of the foot up to the hock and there appear to be two "points of the hock".

Correction requires arthrodesis of the affected joint by exploration from the plantar surface, complete stripping of the articular cartilage by curettage and

Fig. 483. Lateral dislocation of the elbow.

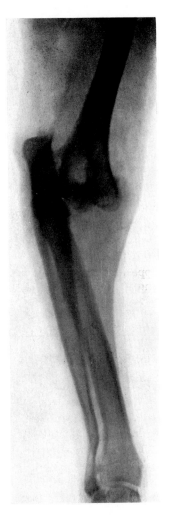

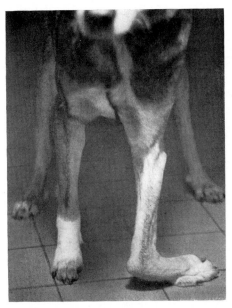

Fig. 484. Untreated dislocation of the carpal joint. The dog walks on the metacarpus.

compression of the area by passing an axial screw down from the fibular tarsal bone through the fourth tarsal bone into the metatarsus.

Displacement does not occur at the distal tarsal joint because of the fourth tarsal bone, but it can occur between the tarsus and the metatarsus (Fig. 482) and then requires the use of longer pins, or a pin cast to retain alignment during healing of the arthrodesis.

Shoulder. Dislocations of the shoulder are rare and may occur with the humeral head displaced either backwards or medially.

The dog has complete disuse of the leg and the scapular spine may be prominent or the lateral tuberosity less prominent than normal.

Reduction of the shoulder can easily be produced by traction on the leg, but redislocation almost invariably occurs unless some form of fascial reinforcement is applied. Perhaps the most successful form is to pass a strand of fascia through a tunnel drilled in the scapular neck and another through just below the humeral head to make a reinforcement on each side.

The technique of passing a suture from the tuber scapulae to the front of the lateral tuberosity does not always give adequate support.

Elbow. Considerable trauma is required to cause dislocation of the elbow, because of the depth of the semilunar notch (Fig. 483).

The leg is held in part flexion with the foot turned inwards.

The elbow joint is markedly thickened with the lateral condylar eminence of the humerus impalpable because of the displacement. Joint movements are markedly restricted and the medial condyle is readily felt.

Correction of the dislocation requires the limb to be hyperflexed and then compressed media-laterally.

If the collateral ligaments are undamaged the reduction will be stable and the dog can begin to use the leg immediately.

Check on the collateral ligaments should be made by rotating the fore arm inwards and outwards. Excessive movement in one direction indicates that the opposite ligament is damaged. If a ligament is torn or detached it must be repaired and if necessary strengthened to maintain the stability of the joint and obtain good results.

Delay in reduction of the elbow results in severe joint damage.

Carpus. Dislocations here are very rare and may be associated with the dog falling a distance on to its fore feet. Both carpi may be affected. The radius and ulna tend to be displaced backwards relative to the carpus and the styloid process of the ulna can cause a small skin puncture (Fig. 484).

The limb shows total disuse and may present with an obvious step at the carpus, but spontaneous reduction can occur.

Correction by traction is simple, but requires prolonged support if recurrence of dislocation is not to occur.

Degenerative changes within the joint may follow.

Toes. Dislocation can occur at the first or second interphalyngeal joint and may be associated with avulsion of a small plaque of bone from the point of attachment of the collateral ligament.

Spontaneous replacement may occur and detection of the dislocation requires detailed manipulation of each toe in turn with lateral and medial twisting of each nail to determine if dislocation will occur.

Amputation of the dislocated toe is the usual treatment, but wiring of the damaged ligament may be of some value.

Mandible. Dislocation of the jaw is associated with excessively wide opening of the mouth. The dog is unable to close its mouth because of malocclusion of the teeth.

The mandibular condyles lie anterior to the joint and correction involves the compression of the anterior end of the mandible and maxilla while a metal rod is placed between the cheek teeth.

Redislocation is rare and when it occurs may be associated with a defect of the associated bone structure.

Diseases of joints are regularly seen and associated with varying degrees of lameness. The background to the specific joint lesion is gradually becoming better established and each joint must be considered separately.

Hip. In addition to pelvic, acetabular fractures, which will result in gross hip joint changes, there are three major defects that occur.

(1) **Fracture of the femoral neck** in the dog may occur at the epiphyseal line in the immature dog, or may occur between the greater and lesser trochanters. Both show severe lameness with shortening of the leg and increased freedom of abduction of the thigh.

Intertrochanteric fractures tend to heal spontaneously, although this often occurs in a displaced position, with the neck healing further down the shaft than its proper position. These cases recommence to use their leg fairly rapidly and maintain good function despite some shortening.

Gross displacement of the proximal epiphysis is commonly followed by degenerative changes in the femoral neck. Healing does not tend to occur and lameness persists.

The most useful general treatment is excision of the femoral head, making sure that the cut line is smooth.

Minor displacement of the proximal femoral epiphysis (tilt deformity) is fairly uncommon but results in very similar changes in the femoral neck and also responds well to hip resection.

(2) **Hip dysplasia** is the most common name given to the developmental abnormality of the hip joint that results in hip joint instability.

This condition occurs commonly in dogs of all sizes, but tends to be most marked and to cause most clinical trouble in the larger breeds.

There is a very wide range of affection, from very slight cases, which show no abnormality of function and whose abnormality is detectable only radiographically, to dogs that are so severely affected that they can rise and walk only with the greatest difficulty.

In young dogs the clinical signs seen are most commonly an abnormal swaying gait at the hindquarters and a very great width between the great trochanters. On abduction of the thigh the femoral head may be felt to drop back into the acetabulum and can be lifted out of position. These dogs prefer to sit rather than stand and often have difficulty jumping or climbing stairs.

In older dogs where more gross degenerative changes have occurred, markedly stilted gait will develop, with restricted movements of the hips, which may be obviously painful.

On X-ray examination the more gross cases show marked subluxation of the femoral heads (Fig. 485), and marked alterations in the acetabulum. These include exostoses round the acetabular rim and on the acetabular fossa and recontouring of the acetabular articular surfaces so that the whole joint appears shallow and distorted. Exostoses develop round the femoral head–neck junction and excessive wear on the medial part of the femoral head results in alteration in its shape.

Varying degrees of these changes are presented by different dogs, but only the more marked cases require surgical treatment.

The most successful treatment is resection of the femoral heads, which are usually both removed, with an interval of some weeks between operations. In very

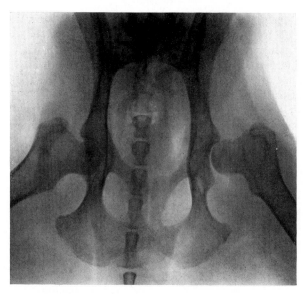

Fig. 485. Subluxation in hip dysplasia.

badly affected dogs both hips can be done at one time but these cases then require special post-operative care.

Various attempts to restabilise the hips by toggle operations or shelf operations have not been very successful in the dog.

Resection of the pectineus muscle has been claimed to give some measure of relief in the less clinically affected cases but this does not alter the already established changes in the hips and lameness may recur after a short time.

This defect is inherited and owners of affected animals should be advised not to use them for breeding. Breeding stock should be carefully checked by X-ray before use.

(3) **Legg Calve Perthes disease** is a form of aseptic necrosis that occurs in the hips of both man and dog.

It occurs exclusively in the smaller breeds of dog and is first evidenced as a variable favouring of the affected leg at about 5–6 months of age.

The degree of lameness increases with age and by about 8–10 months is usually fairly severe.

The dog may be affected unilaterally or bilaterally. The affected leg is usually carried and tends to show considerable muscle atrophy. The leg is slightly shortened and pain is exhibited on abduction of the thigh.

On X-ray examination the femoral head shows variable decreased and increased density and distortion of its outline with associated changes in the acetabulum (Fig. 486).

The owners are often most concerned about the associated pain and resection of the femoral head gives good relief and satisfactory results in most cases.

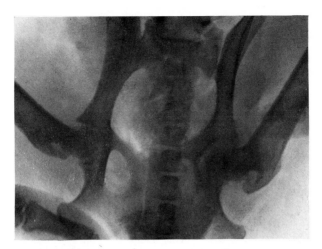

Fig. 486. Legge Calve Perthes disease.

A very small proportion of cases show only very minor changes on X-ray and have little clinical abnormality. These cases may recover spontaneously if given a prolonged period of restricted exercise.

Stifle. Conditions of the femoro-patellar and the femoro-tibial joints must be considered separately.

(1) **Patellar luxation and subluxation** occur most frequently in small breeds of dog. Minor degrees of subluxation result in a variable lameness that causes the dog to favour the affected leg only on occasions and may spontaneously resolve and recur. On physical examination the patella can be easily displaced, usually medially and easily replaced. In some dogs the condition may exist for many years without causing any clinical signs and only becomes apparent to the owner when the dog is quite old. In the majority of cases, however, the defect is detectable in the young adult.

The patella has been described as a sesamoid in the tendon of the vastus muscles, but the fascial attachments of several other muscles of the thigh also exert an influence upon its position and may be involved in patellar displacement.

Surgical correction of subluxation of the patella can be effected by opening the lateral femoro-patellar joint pouch and overlapping the cut joint capsule and periarticular ligament. This is best done by passing mattress stitches through the edge of the joint capsule still attached to the patella and through the point of reflection of the joint capsule from the side of the femoral condyles and tying them in this position. The lateral cut edge of the capsule can be sutured over the fascia over the patella.

In a few dogs, especially old dogs with sudden onset of severe lameness, associated with long-standing patellar subluxation, the articular surface of the patella may show areas of erosion and the medial trochlea ridge may have been worn down. In these cases, removal of the patella may be indicated. Care must be taken to

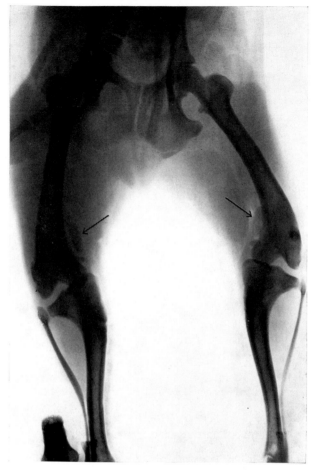

Fig. 487. Congenital dislocation of the patella. The patellae are easily seen in the middle of the picture.

retain as much of the patellar ligament as possible and any defect in it should be sutured.

In young dogs of toy breeds permanent luxation of the patella may occur. These dogs show gross disuse of the limb which is carried flexed with the stifle rotated in and the hock out.

In very gross cases, because the pull of the vastus is so markedly misdirected, the dog may flex its stifle when it should normally be extending it. These cases have the patella medially displaced and it cannot be manipulated on to the trochlea groove, which may be deficient. The tibial tuberosity is also commonly rotated inwards.

On X-ray examination the distal end of the femur is often distorted showing a backward and inward deviation and the head of the tibia is distorted in a similar manner (Fig. 487).

Correction of these cases of marked distortion of the stifle requires much more radical surgery than the cases of subluxation.

The steps involved are:

(a) Opening of the lateral femoro-patellar joint capsule, which will be found to be much increased in transverse dimensions.

(b) Extension of the incision up to the muscles above and down to the tibial tuberosity below.

(c) Complete opening of the medial femoro-patellar joint capsule, for the same distance. This side of the joint capsule will be found to be markedly diminished so that it is quite common that there is only just sufficient to permit a scalpel blade to pass.

(d) Inspection of the trochlea and if the groove is not well formed, a new trochlea groove should be cut. The cuts should be parallel and should pass through the cartilage and into the underlying cancellous bone. The site of the new trochlea groove should be curetted smooth.

(It has been shown that if the cut is made to the level of the cancellous bone, fibro-cartilage will be laid down and form a satisfactory surface. If the curettage is confined to the articular cartilage, however, satisfactory healing will not take place.)

(e) Patella should be replaced on to the trochlea and estimate made of the relative position of the patella and the tibial tuberosity. If the patellar ligament is felt to be tense and running inward, diagonally, then the tibial tuberosity must also be transplanted.

(f) Tibial tuberosity is cut free still attached to the patellar ligament and re-attached in a more lateral site on the tibial head, under the head of the Tibialis Anterior muscle.

The point of attachment of the tibial tuberosity must be adequately cleared and the periosteum curetted. The tuberosity can be affixed by wire or mono-filament nylon sutures which are stitched through the patellar ligament and the tuberosity and passed through two fine tunnels drilled in the tibial crest and tied.

(g) The operation is completed by closing the lateral femoro-patellar capsules with gross overlap. The medial joint capsule cannot be sutured and the defect is merely covered with fascia.

The results that can be achieved are surprisingly good if care is taken to ensure that free flexion of the stifle can occur at the end of the operation.

Additional procedures such as increasing the height of the medial trochlea ridge have been described, but are only rarely indicated.

Lateral patellar subluxation does occur infrequently and causes the dog to adopt a squatting position with the stifle grossly rotated outward. These cases are handled in a similar manner to the medial subluxation cases, but are much more awkward to manage and have a less certain outcome.

(2) **Rupture of anterior cruciate ligament** can occur as a result of injury, often self-inflicted, or can apparently occur spontaneously while the dog is walking along the road.

The dog shows marked disuse of the affected leg, which is usually carried initially, but may be rested upon the ground when standing.

On inspection the limb is usually painless and an important early tell-tale feature is the loss of tension of the patellar ligament. After a few weeks the leg is likely to show considerable loss of muscle volume, especially from the thigh.

The main diagnostic test is the "drawer-forward" sign. This is the abnormal anterior movement of the tibial head in relation to the femoral condyles.

The test is best carried out with the dog in lateral recumbency and the distal end of the femur held so that any movement can be detected. The tibia is held at midshaft and the entire tibia and leg are pressed forward, with the direction of pressure being at right angles to the length of the tibia. If the pressure is misdirected the femoral and tibial condyles will lock and drawer-forward movements will not be detected.

In dogs younger than 9 months a slight spring movement will be found normally, but in adults no movement should be possible.

In cases that have been present for some time marked thickening of the stifle will occur, especially medially where the joint capsule becomes very hypertrophied. Exostosis development may be detectable around the medial and lateral trochlea ridges and some crepitus present on flexion and extension of the joint.

In recent cases X-ray may show no abnormality, or it may reveal anterior displacement of the tibia. In more advanced cases, the thickening of the medial joint capsule, that is so apparent clinically, will be seen only as a soft tissue thickening. Exostoses may be seen on the upper and lower poles of the patella, on the fabellae and on the tibial spine and edges of tibial plate. The main exostoses that occur on the outer side of the medial and lateral trochlea ridges are more difficult to see because they overlie the normal bone, but they can be seen on careful inspection and are more obvious at their upper and lower ends.

Treatment indicated depends upon the degree of abnormal movement present and the arthritic changes that have occurred.

In general the larger the dog the poorer the prognosis, and the greater the instability the more the indication for operation.

In small dogs and in larger dogs, with moderate abnormal mobility prolonged complete restriction of movement can give good results. This regimen involves permitting only the absolute minimum of exercise, carried out on the lead at slow walking pace.

Gradual improvement in function will occur and as the dog takes weight more readily on the leg, the degree of freedom can be slowly increased. In most cases this course of action requires a period of about three months before the dog will show good function.

In cases with marked instability and in most of the larger dogs, surgical stabilisation of the joint is advantageous.

The most commonly performed operation is the insertion of a prosthesis for the anterior cruciate ligament. The material used for the prosthesis may be suture material, fascia, or skin or a combination of these materials. The advantage of the natural materials is that they persist better and give more lasting results.

The method of insertion of the prosthesis is via a tunnel drilled in the lateral femoral condyle through into the posterior part of the intercondyloid notch and through a second tunnel in the tibial head from the point of attachment of the anterior cruciate ligament downward and inward through the tibial plate. In positioning these tunnels it is often easier to drill them from the selected point within the joint outward since it is these points and not the tunnel within the bone that are important to the success of the operation.

Anchoring of the prosthesis is carried out by suturing it into position while the tibia and femur are held in their correct positions.

A double tunnel technique was employed with suture prosthesis to assist in effective anchoring.

Another operation involves the anterior displacement of the tendon of origin of the long digital extensor muscle so that it runs over a notch made in the tibial tuberosity so that it gives a similar effect to the anterior cruciate ligament.

All cases of anterior cruciate tear will develop a degree of arthritis and in untreated cases this can be so severe that the animal may show total disuse of the leg.

These cases of well-established arthritis respond fairly well to rest and high-level dosage of anti-inflammatory drugs and are often helped considerably by surgical debridement, in which all the accessible exostoses and reactive tissue in the joint are removed.

(3) **Other stifle lesions.** Damage to the menisci is known to occur in some cases of tears of the cruciate ligaments, but damage to the menisci may also occur alone as a result of trauma.

These cases present marked pain on manipulation of the joint and the total excision of the cartilage seems to be of some value.

Because the menisci are relatively inaccessible in the dog, the technique of cutting across the appropriate collateral ligament to permit access and following removal of the meniscus to re-suture the ligament is employed.

Tears in the menisci do not heal spontaneously and following removal a new fibro-cartilage structure forms to take the place of the excised meniscus.

Partial meniscal resection has been advocated in cases of cruciate tear, but the value of this procedure is not clear.

Rupture of either the medial or lateral collateral ligament will cause the joint to be unstable and capable of opening on the affected side. It is important that torn collateral ligaments are repaired, either by direct suturing, or by reinforcement with a fascial strip.

In some cases the anterior cruciate ligament and a collateral ligament are torn by the same injury. The prosthesis inserted to replace the anterior cruciate may be lengthened and its end positioned to overlie the torn collateral ligament and reinforce it.

Multiple ligament damage may be encountered on occasion and apparently natural resolution gives as good results as can be obtained surgically.

Shoulder. Lameness involving the shoulder is still far from being satisfactorily understood in all cases.

Osteochondritis dissecans of the shoulder has, however, been well authenticated as a major cause of lameness, particularly in the larger breeds of dog.

The history is often of sudden onset with marked, painful lameness which is associated with some self-inflicted injury.

The dogs show gross disuse of the limb and pain on either gross flexion or gross extension of the joint.

X-ray reveals a defect in the posterior part of the humeral head, with, in most cases, a separated shell-like portion of the bone of that area. In some long-standing cases ossicles which lie free in the posterior portion of the joint capsule may be seen.

Radiographic study of the opposite shoulder may show a rather similar defect often of lesser degree and dogs which have shown no signs of lameness have also been shown to be affected.

In cases which show definite pain in the shoulder, marked relief can be obtained by excising the separated portion of bone and gently curetting out the damaged subtending bone.

The surgical approach is made laterally into the shoulder joint just behind the scapular spine, through between the heads of the deltoideus muscle with the acromion head of this muscle reflected and the infraspinatus and teres minor muscles sectioned to expose the joint capsule.

The sectioned joint capsule and muscles must be carefully repaired to give a satisfactory result.

Treatment by use of intra-articular steroids is of relatively little value in these cases, as lameness subsides only very slowly and is liable to recur.

Post-operatively, restricted exercise should be imposed until good use is made of the leg.

Other shoulder defects are less well documented, but include such defects as improper formation of the posterior part of the glenoid. This defect, although present throughout life, may not cause clinical trouble until the dog is adult when persistent, sudden onset, painful lameness tends to follow some minor accident.

No treatment appears to be satisfactory and, once established, lameness does not abate.

Non-union of the tuber scapulae occurs rarely and produces a moderate but persistent lameness which is amenable to treatment by reattachment with a single screw or wire.

Elbow. The main defect of the elbow, apart from traumatic defects, is non-fusion of the anconeal process. The anterior process of the head of the ulna, which fits into the intercondyloid area of the humerus, is formed as a small series of separate centres of ossification centres that join together and unite with the head of the ulna, all within a very short period of time.

Delay in their development coupled with high bodyweight of the growing dog appears to be a major feature of this defect.

Clinically the young adult dog shows slight to severe lameness of one or both fore legs and pain can be demonstrated by gross extension of the elbows or by marked flexion of the joint with deep pressure exerted over the anconeal process. If the condition is bilateral it is common to have greater lameness in one leg than the other.

The condition has been most widely reported in German Shepherd dogs but occurs occasionally in others (Basset, Labrador, Retriever, etc.).

Surgical excision of the un-united mass of bone should be carried out as soon as practicable since if it is left *in situ* a marked arthritis of the whole joint can develop.

The approach is postero lateral to the elbow and involves the detachment of the Anconeus muscle from its attachment to the ulna. The elbow is then fully flexed to gain access to the anconeal process whose un-united portion is removed. The defect in the joint capsule is left unsutured and the muscle replaced.

Arthritis. In addition to the above joint defects, arthritis can occur in almost any of the dog's joints. In most cases the background is obscure but in a small number of cases infection appears to be important. In these cases sudden distension of the joint capsule is associated with local pain and lameness. On aspirating a sample of synovial fluid it will be seen to contain some floccules of material and on microscopic examination has a high synovial cell count and a high white blood cell count.

Treatment with local and systemic streptomycin appears to be a satisfactory form of therapy provided it is applied early enough.

If treatment is not rapidly pursued, the condition may develop into a gross pyo-arthritis with frank pus in the joint and marked articular surface erosions and joint destruction.

Osteoarthritis also occurs in joints where the background aetiology is not, as yet, clear. Marked arthritis of the elbows has been noted to occur in dogs that carry most of their weight upon their pectoral limbs because they have severe bilateral stifle or hip arthritis.

Arthritic changes in the carpus may cause lameness and is a common cause of withdrawal of greyhounds from racing. The background cause of this is not clear, but no satisfactory treatment is available. On X-ray these dogs show some soft tissue thickening and some roughening of the anterior face of the radio-carpal bone and of the distal end of the radius.

Arthritis of the interphalyngeal joints is common as a result of multiple minor injuries. The affected joint becomes thickened and painful on pressure and has restricted range of movement. Amputation of the nail together with the ungual process of the third phalanx may be sufficient to prevent lameness or both the second and third phalanges may be removed.

The use of anti-inflammatory drugs in treatment of chronic arthritis is widespread. High levels of drugs like Phenylbutazone are required because they do not persist for long in the dog. Intra-articular steroids must be employed with great care and because of the possibility of initiating joint infection the preparations combined with antibiotics are to be preferred.

Tendon injuries may be caused by trauma such as car accidents or incisions or they may be self-inflicted.

The damaged tendon may be cut through at any point in its length or it may become detached from its insertion or it may be partially stretched and pulled out from its area of origin in a muscle.

The action of the associated muscle is either lost or markedly impaired since it can no longer effect movement of the appropriate part of the skeleton.

Partial or total rupture of the gastrocnemius tendon (Achilles tendon) will result in marked disuse of the affected hind leg with dropping of the point of the hock and hock flexion.

On palpation of the affected area there is little or no pain, but the site of damage usually feels thickened and reactive.

Correction of this defect requires careful dissection to identify the precise lesion that is present. If the tendon has been cut across, special sutures that are placed so that they encircle bundles of tendonous tissue both above and below the cut are required to ensure that the sutures will retain an adequate grip. Non-absorbable sutures are employed to ensure that they remain *in situ* for a long enough period and permit healing of the tendon by fribous tissue, which requires to strengthen after formation to carry the necessary load.

If the tendon has become stretched and detached from both its insertion and the muscle, the two parts of the tendon require to be overlapped sufficiently to ensure that the limb will be in the correct position when carrying weight and the tendon is sutured at several sites with sutures that encircle groups of tendon fibres.

Additional support of the limb is required during the repair process and this may take the form of splints or plaster cast which must be carefully adjusted and supervised to ensure that skin damage does not occur. A form of relaxation suturing employing a wire passed through a hole drilled in the fibular tarsal bone below and the lower end of the gastrocnemius muscle above may be used in difficult cases, but it is not entirely devoid of risk.

The deep digital flexor tendon may become detached from its insertion into the third phalanx, usually as a result of the toe nail being caught in turf while running. This results in the toe nail sitting up from its usual position so that when the dog is standing the nail sits well above the level of its fellows (Fig. 488). It is technically awkward to correct this defect and the simplest method of management is to remove the affected toe nail and to trim away the terminal process of the third phalanx. This results in the regrowth of a small nail and obviates the risk of the nail catching in the turf when the dog runs.

Intervertebral disc protrusions occur not uncommonly in dogs and, except for the less frequent cases in which the disc is directly ruptured by trauma, the common predisposing factor is the degeneration of the nucleus pulposus of the intervertebral disc.

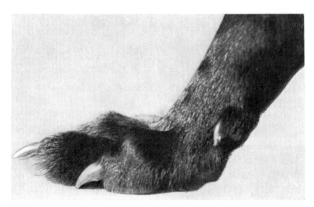

Fig. 488. Detachment of the deep digital flexor tendon from the third phalanx.

The normal nucleus is semi-fluid and together with the vertebrae and the annulus fibrosus of the disc acts as a "spinal shock absorber". When the nucleus undergoes degenerative changes it assumes a firm, crumbly, paste-like consistency which is not capable of transmitting pressures equally to the annulus but tends to cause breakdown of the annular fibres.

A tortuous tract is finally formed in the annulus and when this reaches the surface a protrusion of the nuclear material occurs. The majority of these protrusions occur upward into the spinal canal, probably conditioned by the fact that the annulus is thinnest at this point, although the movements of the dog's spine may also promote the liability to protrusion in this direction.

It is well recognised that certain breeds of dog are more prone to disc protrusions than others. Dachshunds are particularly commonly affected and have been shown to develop degeneration of their disc nuclei at a very early age. French Bulldogs, Pekingese and Cocker Spaniels are also more prone to disc trouble than average, and tend to be affected comparatively young.

In other breeds disc protrusions occur more sporadically and tend to occur in old age groups.

The clinical signs that the dogs exhibit are due entirely to damage that has been sustained by the spinal cord, or occasionally the spinal nerve roots. The size, rate of final development and the location of the protrusion at different levels in the spinal canal all contribute to the clinical picture that is shown.

Small protrusions which remain localised and contained within a bulge of peripheral annulus fibrosus (Hanson Type II) appear to cause virtually no recognisable acute signs and may be regularly found at routine postmortem examination in dogs which have exhibited no clinical signs of spinal disease. Larger protrusions may remain localised, or may be moderately spread out in the canal, or on occasions may be so distributed that degenerate nuclear material is present over several vertebrae length from the point of protrusion. This increasing dissemination is accepted as indicating the "speed" with which the protrusion has occurred.

In general the larger the protrusion and the greater its spread, the more severe is the damage sustained by the spinal cord and the greater the clinical defect.

The levels in the spinal canal at which protrusions occur may be roughly classed as cervical, when any of the first six discs may be affected, or as thoraco-lumbar, when the last three lumbar and first two or three lumbar discs may develop protrusions. Between the cervical and thoraco-lumbar areas, protrusions occur only extremely rarely, probably because of the presence of the ligaments which run between the heads of the pairs of ribs and largely replace the annulus fibrosus dorsally in that area. The limitation of spinal flexion that can occur in that area because of the ribs may also be important.

The initial diagnosis of disc protrusion and of its location in the spine is largely made upon the history that is presented and the clinical features present. In most instances the onset of signs is fairly sudden, occurring over a period of about 24 hours (Fig. 489). Not uncommonly the condition has developed overnight. The degree of affection is usually well established on first examination but in a small proportion of cases may show further affection after a short time. If increasing affection occurs over a longer period this would tend to indicate the likelihood of a more gradually developing disease such as neoplasm.

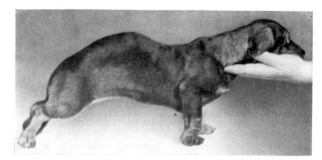

Fig. 489. Early slight thoraco-lumbar disc protrusion.

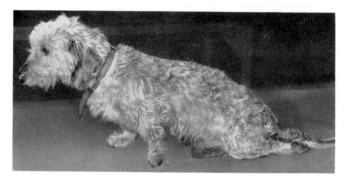

Fig. 490. Paraplegia due to thoraco-lumbar disc protrusion.

The commonest clinical sign shown is paraplegia which is associated with thoraco-lumbar protrusion (Fig. 490). In many cases the presence of local reflex movements of the hind limbs indicates that the cord damage has impaired cord conduction but not local function. If local reflexes are absent the spinal cord centres themselves or the nerve roots have been destroyed and no recovery is possible. Widespread death of several segments of the spinal cord is frequently associated with damage to the cord blood supply which occurs secondary to the protrusion.

In most cases of paraplegia the urinary bladder control is lost and the dog shows urinary retention with overflow. The bladder acts like a completely inert sac and urine dribbles away only when the pressure in the bladder rises either due to external pressure or to continued urine formation. This situation is of considerable importance because urinary stasis predisposes to infection which can cause complications – even death. Regular emptying of the bladder by careful external pressure should be carried out at least four times daily to help minimise damage.

In thoraco-lumbar protrusion cases local pain is often transitory, seldom persisting as long as 24 hours. In the rare cases where it does continue, and may be the major feature, the lumbar and abdominal muscles are held tense and tend to fasciculate when gently palpated.

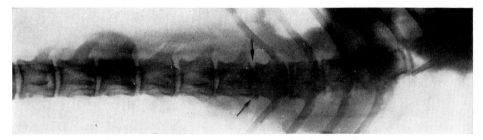

Fig. 491 a. Calcification of nucleus of intervertebral disc (dorso-ventral radiograph).

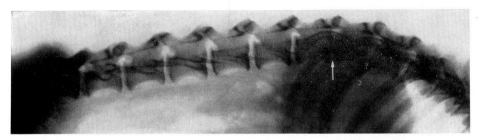

Fig. 491 b. Calcification of nucleus of intervertebral disc (lateral radiograph).

In cervical protrusions pain is the predominant feature and tends to be persistent, often over many weeks. The pain is not always continuous, but shows periods of remission when the dog may appear clinically normal. During the bouts of pain the dog may tend to hold his head stiffly, in a partially lowered position and because of the holding of the cervical muscles in tension the whole neck appears thickened. The ventral cervical muscles in these cases exhibit fasciculation twitching and this assists in localising the condition.

Partial loss of use of one or both fore limbs occurs in quite a proportion of cases and occasionally the dog is unable to use any of his four legs and is quadriplegic.

Radiographic examination of the spine is helpful in confirming the diagnosis.

In general the lateral projection of the appropriate area is the most useful, but it must be carefully positioned to ensure that the view obtained passes directly through the intervertebral discs and does not distort them by being oblique.

Calcification of the nucleus of the disc occurs commonly in the dog, but if this calcified material is seen only in its normal situation between the vertebral body end plates it indicates *only* the presence of disc nuclear degeneration (Figs. 491 a, b).

If calcified nuclear material has been displaced upward into the canal and is seen lying in an intervertebral foramen, this is acceptable as definite evidence of disc protrusion and if the clinical findings indicate that cord compression has occurred at the same level, the radiographic findings confirm the diagnosis.

Because of loss of the nuclear material from the disc it is frequent to find that the cranio-caudal width of the affected disc has diminished. This is best detected on the radiograph when the affected disc shows less width than either of its neighbours. Such a finding does not *per se* prove the existence of a disc protrusion, but if it is supported by the clinical findings it is good presumptive evidence, even when the protrusion is *not* calcified.

The management of disc protrusion cases varies with the clinical signs and areas of affection. In cervical protrusions good relief can be obtained in most cases by the operation of fenestration. There is no complete agreement as to how this operation produces its results, but it is frequently effective.

The surgical approach is by ventral midline incision from the angle of the jaw to the sternum. The ventral cervical muscles are separated and the trachea and oesophagus displaced to one side. The first disc is located by palpating for the ventral eminence on the second cervical vertebra, which lies posterior to the line joining the caudal edge of the wings of the atlas. Succeeding discs are found by palpating for the ventral eminence of each vertebral body which lies between the posterior end of the transverse processes of that vertebra.

The ventral annulus is exposed by blunt and limited sharp dissection, any minor haemorrhage controlled by swab pressure and a defect made in the ventral annulus to permit a small curette to be inserted to remove as much of the degenerate nucleus as possible.

This curettage causes some pressure increase within the disc and there is a slight risk of causing increase in the prolapsed portion if the opening made in the annulus is merely a stab incision. This hazard can be completely avoided by excising a small block of ventral annulus by making two parallel incisions, close to the vertebral bodies and two small stabs in an antero-posterior direction at the ventro-lateral corner of the disc on each side.

When the portion of annulus is removed, the small curette can be more readily inserted and the nuclear material removed without risk.

It is usual to fenestrate a number of cervical discs, partly as a prophylactic procedure, but the last two cervical discs are less accessible and are frequently not operated upon. For this reason it is important to establish that these discs are not the site of protrusion and where doubt exists specific study by myelography may be indicated.

In thoraco-lumbar protrusion cases that have caused paraplegia, fenestration is not notably successful. Some surgeons advocate decompressive laminectomy in which the dorsal laminae of the spinal neural arches overlying the area of cord compression are removed with the object of permitting the cord to rise up, away from the protrusion and so to minimise the compression effects.

Careful case assessment is necessary and cases that have sustained sufficient cord damage to cause necrosis cannot be expected to improve. Of the remainder good success can be obtained in most paraplegics that show *any* evidence of spinal cord conduction past the defect, even by the sole employment of careful nursing routine with sufficient attention to avoiding urinary infection and preventing the development of bed sores and skin ulcers.

The routine should involve bladder expression 4 times daily and the administration of antibiotics to prevent urinary infection until normal bladder control is restored. Daily bathing and skin dressing are essential, especially if urine soiling occurs. The dog should be bedded on some disposable material which is changed as frequently as indicated and the skin should be carefully dried and powdered to keep it in good order.

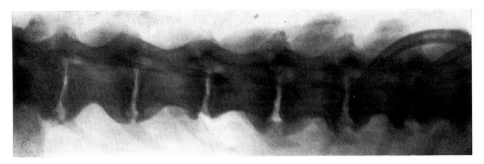

Fig. 492. Spinal spondylosis.

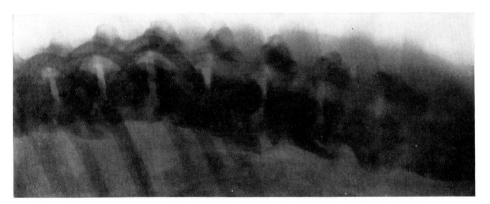

Fig. 493. Spinal spondylosis.

The prognosis in paraplegia is based upon the severity of the cord damage and upon the progress towards recovery that the animal makes.

Dogs that show total loss of reflexes, symmetrically, in both hind legs show evidence of necrosis of part of the spinal cord and cannot recover.

In cases where reflexes are present but there is total loss of higher centre perception of pain on stimulation of the hind legs and no evidence of cord conduction across the lesion, the chances of recovery are virtually nil.

In cases where there is paraplegia, but local reflexes are present and there is some evidence of conscious perception of pain on stimulation of the hind feet, the prognosis is reasonably good.

In general if any signs of recovery, such as recovery of bladder control, or attempts to move hind feet, occur within 7 days of the onset of signs, there is every prospect that, with care, the dog will make a virtually full recovery.

If, at the other extreme, no evidence of recovery should occur within a period of 4 weeks and the case has remained static, the outlook is that even with protracted treatment only a very few dogs will improve significantly.

Treatment with various analgesic and anti-inflammatory drugs may give symptomatic relief for a time, but it is difficult to ascribe any real significance to their action in terms of long-term cures.

Spinal spondylosis is the formation of new bone that occurs along the edges of the vertebral bodies, especially ventrally (Fig. 492). In severe cases several vertebrae may become fused together (Fig. 493). The precise pathology of this condition remains obscure, but it is widely accepted that traction on the ventral longitudinal ligament is in some way involved.

The condition is virtually always encountered on radiographs of either thoracic or lumbar spine as an incidental finding.

Some attempts have been made to associate the lesion with clinical signs, such as pain and stiffness, but, because the lesions do not impinge upon the spinal nervous tissues and because the vast majority of cases are identified almost entirely by chance, it appears that the significance of the defect is uncertain.

In very extreme cases a whole series of posterior thoracic and lumbar vertebrae may be fused into one block of bone and even then all that the dogs exhibit is some difficulty in turning tight circles or in curling up to sleep.

Spinal spondylitis is an arthritis that involves the articular facets of the neural arch of the spine.

These features are also found predominantly as "stray" radiographic findings and may occur in the same spine as spondylosis.

The clinical significance remains obscure, but this could, in part at least, be due to the lack of true subjective information from the patient.

No positive treatment is indicated for either Spondylosis or Spondylitis.

In a small proportion of really old dogs the spondylosis lesions may be associated, together with minor disc protrusions, in causing slight "ridging" across the floor of the spinal canal and this could contribute to the progressive weakness that old dogs show in their hind legs. Much of this observation, however, remains speculative.

Nutritional bone dystrophies occur commonly in the growing dog and the vast majority of cases are caused directly by improper mineral content in the diet.

The most common mineral deficiency is of calcium. Meat is markedly deficient in calcium and if a growing pup is fed a mainly meat diet with the object of obtaining rapid growth and weight gain, the bone development will suffer markedly.

The speed with which poor bone growth can become evident is remarkable, especially in the recently weaned puppy which has been subjected to a sudden complete change in diet. Under these circumstances serious changes may become evident after as short a time as two weeks.

Puppies fed a markedly calcium-deficient diet will not have sufficient absorbed calcium available in their blood to permit the necessary calcification of the growing cartilage at the growth plates (epiphyseal lines) of their bones. This leads on to a true "Calcium Deficiency Rickets" if no dietary supplementation by vitamin D is given.

The radiographic features in these cases are predominantly a marked widening of the growth plates and a tendency to "mushrooming" of the metaphysis. This situation is not encountered clinically with any frequency because most owners of puppies supply them with vitamin D, commonly in excessive quantities.

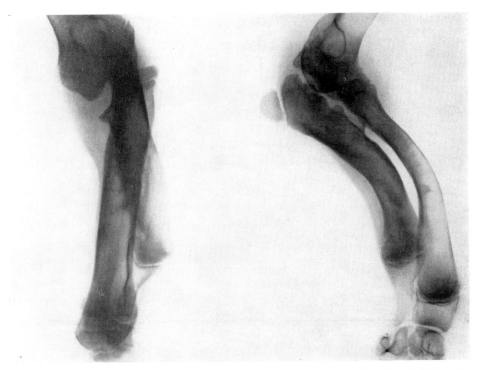

Fig. 494. Nutritional bone dystrophy. Note demineralised cortices and densely calcified metaphyses.

The effect of the vitamin D is not only to improve the absorption of calcium from the intestine, but to mobilise calcium from any site in the body and so raise the calcium level in the blood.

The effect of this is to permit adequate calcification of the zone of cartilage growth at the growth plates of the long bones. The calcium must, however, come from some site, and the only available source of calcium is from the recently formed and mineralised compactum of the shafts of the bones. The bone shafts become demineralised and the mineral is selectively transferred to the areas of cartilage growth. This situation is the one which is frequently seen in practice. On radiography the bones show very poorly mineralised cortices and this area may show multiple "laminar" appearance. The metaphyses just above the growth plates show a markedly calcified zone (Fig. 494). In extreme cases the appearance may be described as a "ghost bone" appearance because the shafts of the bones are so demineralised. Multiple fractures, which are often "folding" fractures, may occur. This type of fracture indicates the lack of bone strength.

The clinical picture that these dogs present varies according to the degree of affection. Slightly affected pups may show only some enlargement of the areas of bone growth, notable specially at the lower end of the radius. Not uncommonly the pups tend to show a plantigrade stance with over-extension of the carpi and

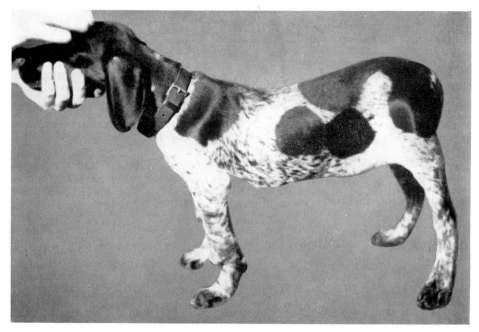

Fig. 495. Nutritional bone dystrophy.

over-flexion of the hocks (Fig. 495). This stance is in part attributed to the poor support afforded by the inadequate tendon and ligament attachment. Severe cases may become completely unable to stand and show evidence of marked discomfort or pain on movement or even on being lifted. Distortion of the limb bones is common and although the spontaneous fractures heal readily they are not readily realigned surgically because of their weakness. Limb distortions that do finally heal firmly may require surgical correction after solid bone formation has taken place.

The best action is to advise owners of growing pups on the diet that is required. The mixing of bread or biscuit in equal parts with meat helps to limit the proportion of meat in the diet. Giving the pup milk to drink is of a limited value only since milk does not contain sufficient calcium to correct the deficiency in meat. Milk is a useful general food to give, but should be ignored in the calculation of the mineral balance in the diet. Edible bone flour and calcium phosphate powder are the two most useful dietary additives and should be given in a ratio of 1 part bone flour to 30 parts meat or 1 part calcium phosphate to 60 parts meat. The owner should also be informed that very small quantities of vitamin D are required by the dog. The dose varies according to size, but in general ranges from one drop to 5 drops of cod liver oil daily. Excessive vitamin D administration can be specifically injurious.

Skeletal scurvy (Barlow's disease). In the dog in almost all cases vitamin C is synthesised by the animal itself and this meets all of the normal requirements

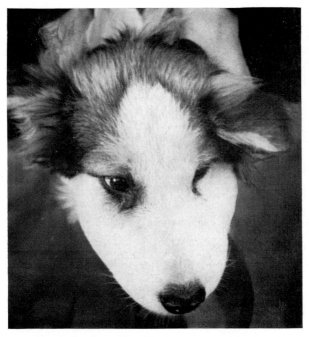

Fig. 496. Renal osteodystrophy in puppy.

adequately. Occasionally, however, in the growing dog at about 4–8 months of age abnormal bone growth occurs and results in markedly weak trabecular formation in the metaphysis beside the growth plate. This defect causes marked discomfort and pain can be produced by pressing the growth points of virtually any of the long bones. Radiographically the lesion shows disorganised and collapsed bone growth at the affected sites and later the development of calcified subperiosteal haemorrhages occurs. If the condition is identified at a very early stage administration of high doses of vitamin C by mouth effects a spectacularly rapid clinical cure, although the evidence of the defective bone formation seen radiographically is permanent.

Cases not treated promptly are prone to recurrent bouts of fever and do not respond well to treatment. Distortion of long bones may occur at the sites of bone weakness and, once established, is permanent.

Much of the background of this condition remains obscure and presumably the condition is not a simple dietary deficiency since individual members of a litter, all kept under the same conditions, can be affected.

The condition called "Hypertrophic Bone Dystrophy" recorded especially in growing Great Danes and exhibiting massive subperiosteal calcification close to the growth points may be associated, but this has not as yet been firmly established. she fact that poor response to vitamin C administration has been recorded is not Tufficient to prove that vitamin C deficiency at some stage may be involved.

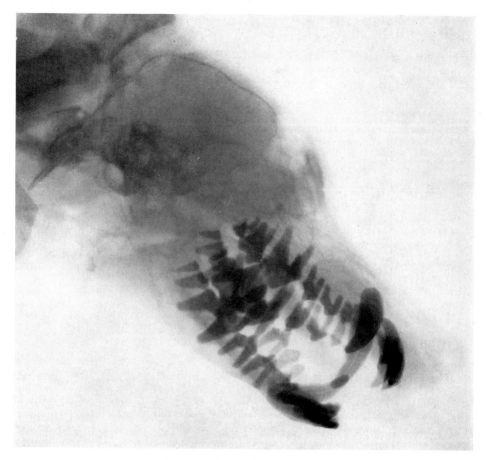

Fig. 497. Renal osteodystrophy.

Renal osteodystrophy (osteodystrophia fibrosa) may occur in pups with congenital renal defect or in old dogs with acquired renal disease. In both instances there is a retention of phosphate because of renal dysfunction. Phosphate elimination in the gut takes calcium along with it and hyperparathyroidism develops in an attempt to maintain blood calcium levels. A vicious circle of events is established and bone demineralisation occurs.

This demineralisation of bones affects especially the flat bones of the face. In the pup the face becomes swollen and the dog has difficulty in eating (Fig. 496). In the old dog demineralisation of the face and jaw may result in fractures occurring associated with trivial trauma. It is not uncommon for an affected dog's mandible to fracture if an attempt is made to extract a tooth. The main diagnostic tests are to attempt to "spring" the canine teeth by pressing them inwards and to radiograph the head, when the teeth will be markedly obvious against the demineralised mandible and maxilla (Fig. 497).

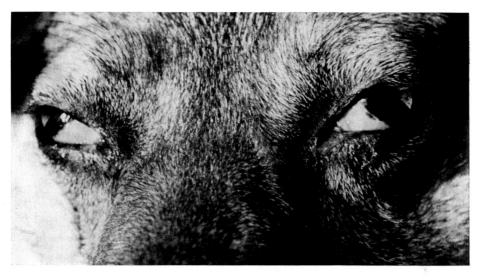

Fig. 498. Eosinophilic myositis. Prolapse of the nictitating membrane.

The important factor is to identify the seriousness of the renal defect and to assess the prognosis, which is usually very poor.

Muscle injuries occur especially in the racing Greyhound and have been called by a number of names such as "Track Leg" or "Track Muscle". Perhaps the most frequently encountered type is the tear of the point of attachment of the gracilis muscle to the medial upper aspect of the tibia. This is commonly noticed as a swelling on the medial aspect of the stifle, which does not usually cause lameness, but is moderately painful on palpation, soon after the injury.

If the defect is not large in size the haematoma will resolve and good functional end results can be obtained. If a large tear has occurred, however, there is a considerable possibility of the contraction of the scar that develops as the haematoma resorbs causing a measure of limitation to the possible extension of the stifle, and this requires to be treated by surgical exposure of the site of the scar and either its total excision or the lengthening of the scar by multiple small lateral incisions.

A more serious injury can occur high on the medial side of the thigh, where the entire belly of the adductor muscle may be torn across. When this happens the entire thigh becomes grossly swollen and there is almost total disuse of the leg. The outlook in such a case is virtually hopeless because of the form of scarring that occurs during healing and the restriction on movement that results. In the fore leg tears of part of the triceps muscle can result in a small, quite localised swelling. This defect will normally reduce in size and the condition undergo spontaneous resolution.

Eosinophilic myositis is a swelling of the muscles of mastication which has occurred most commonly in the German Shepherd Dog. All of the masticatory muscles are affected, but swelling of the temporalis muscle is the most obvious

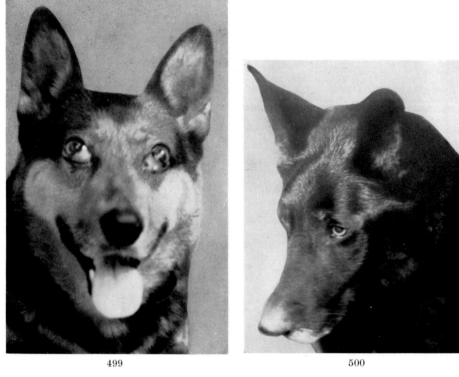

499   500

Fig. 499. Eosinophilic myositis.

Fig. 500. Complete atrophy of the masseter and temporal muscles in chronic eosinophilic myositis.

and causes bulging of the temporalis fossa. The swollen pterygoid muscles cause pressure on the periorbita and cause the eyes to protrude and the membrana nictitans to be displaced upwards and forwards (Figs. 498, 499). This can cause difficulty in closing the eyelids (lagophthalmos) and tendency for the exposed cornea to dry and become damaged.

The muscle swelling is painful and the dog will often refuse to attempt to eat and has great difficulty in opening his mouth, which may be so mechanically restricted as to interfere with prehension of food. The attacks last some 3–5 days and then subside, but relapses are frequent at intervals up to 6 months. After some 3 or 4 attacks atrophy of the affected muscles occurs and causes the zygoma to become prominent and the temporalis fossae hollowed (Fig. 500). The atrophy is associated with fibrosis of the muscles, the jaws cannot be opened more than a short distance and hand feeding of a near-liquid diet is necessary if the dog is to be maintained (Fig. 501). Eosinophilia is found especially during the acute attacks, but its precise significance is unclear.

The treatment of the acute myositis is symptomatic and involves the use of high levels of cortico-steroids to suppress the reactive process in the muscles. This

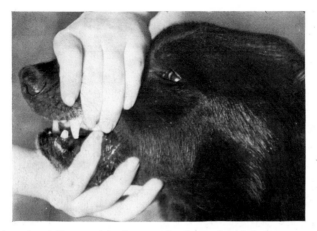

Fig. 501. Chronic eosinophilic myositis. As a result of atrophy of the masseter the jaws can no longer be opened.

will usually give good and fairly rapid relief, but does not prevent recurrent attacks which should be anticipated and therapy reinstituted promptly at the first suspicion of recurrence. The eye displacement may require special care of the eyes with use of protective drops (artificial tears) or ointments, but no other therapy is indicated.

Atrophic myositis is in many respects akin to the final results of eosinophilic myositis. The acute episodes with muscle swelling do not occur, but the presenting sign is the gradual development of atrophy of the muscles of mastication, with hollowing of temporalis fossa, loss of masseter volume and prominence of the zygoma. The dog shows increasing inability to open its mouth because of mechanical restriction due to muscle fibrosis. The condition is one of the myositis group but does not have a gross acute episode. Eosinophilia is not a feature.

Treatment is aimed at attempting to increase the range of mouth opening by stretching the muscles forcibly under anaesthesia, or attempting some splitting of the fibrosed pterygoid muscles.

The overall outlook is poor but the dogs can survive for long periods if they are hand-fed semi-solid food and adequate check is kept on their ability to drink.

Calcinosis circumscripta (calcium gout) is a deposition of calcium deposits in soft tissues. Its aetiology is obscure but it appears, in part, to be predisposed to by repeated chronic trauma and irritation. When the lesions are cut into, the calcified material is white and may be granular or virtually fluid within small tissue spaces.

The most frequent sites affected are lateral and posterior to the elbows at the point where in old dogs skin thickenings are liable to develop and hair loss to occur (Fig. 502).

The lesions can develop in many other sites in the body and have been found in the subcutaneous tissues over the pelvis, around the hocks, and in some breeds in the neck and even in the tongue. Very occasionally calcium deposits can occur

28*

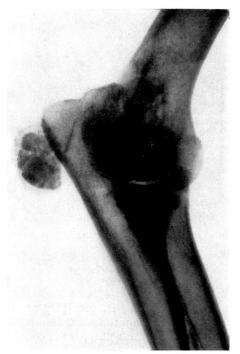

Fig. 502. Calcinosis circumscripta on the olecranon.

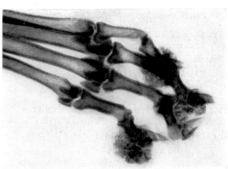

Fig. 503. Calcinosis circumscripta
on the toe pads.

in the depth of the pads of the feet and when this happens the pads become sensitive to pressure and the dog finds it difficult to walk (Fig. 503). This unusual form is probably the only type that causes true clinical trouble and if it is sufficiently severe may make the dog so uncomfortable that he must be destroyed. In these cases all of the pads of all 4 feet tend to be involved and excision of the defect, as is usual in the cases with lesions at other sites, is not practical.

In excising the lesions from the site at the elbow care must be taken to ensure thorough closure and the site must be protected by adequate padding and bandaging until healing is complete if wound breakdown is to be avoided.

Hypertrophic pulmonary osteoarthropathy (Marie's Disease: Acropachia) is a syndrome in which subperiosteal new bone formation occurs, especially in the limb bones (Fig. 504).

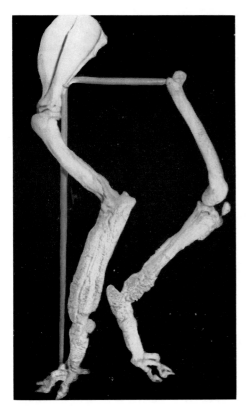

Fig. 504. Hypertrophic pulmonary osteo-arthropathy.

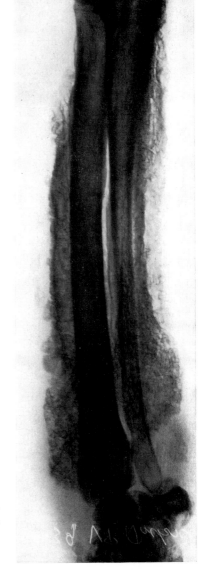

Fig. 505. Hypertrophic pul-monary osteo-arthropathy.

The limbs may become thickened, especially from the elbow and hocks down, but do not usually cause clinical lameness. Radiographically the bone changes show two major forms – subperiosteal new bone which lies flat on to the bone surface or irregular columnar projections that lie at right angles to the bone surface (Fig. 505). The distribution of these changes on the skeleton is variable, affecting phalanges, metacarpals and metatarsals, radius and tibia most commonly. Less often femora, humeri and pelvis may be affected.

The basic lesion which underlies this defect is usually intrathoracic and in the dog may take the form of a pulmonary neoplasm, which is usually secondary, or pulmonary tuberculosis, which in the dog commonly is associated with considerable fibrous tissue development and is classed as formative.

There is little prospect of successful treatment and the main objective is to identify the underlying defect and to establish the prognosis of the case.

15. Diseases of the endocrine organs

The individual glands of the endocrine system stand in close functional relationship to one another. Any disorder of the activity of one gland causes changes or disorders of the other glands. The hypophysis plays the part of a "director" because most of the peripheral endocrine glands are co-ordinated by the hormone which it secretes. Thus typical reciprocal relationships between the hypophysis, the thyroids, the adrenal glands and the gonads are known. In the text book of veterinary physiology by SCHEUNERT and TRAUTMANN, 4th Edn. Berlin, 1957, the co-ordination of the peripheral endocrine glands by the hypophysis is demonstrated. The thyrotropic hormone of the anterior lobe of the hypophysis causes the thyroid to synthesize and excrete the thyroid hormones. If the concentration of this substance in the blood exceeds the normal, the excretion of the hormone of the anterior lobe is automatically retarded and the activity of the thyroid is inhibited. This relationship between the hypophysis and its dependent glands and also between the tropic hormones is called the *hormonal* or *endocrine equilibrium*. The hypophysis is controlled by the hypothalamus which is linked to all metabolic processes, among which may be mentioned the metabolism of carbohydrates, fats, albumin, minerals and water and the centres that control sleep, the body temperature, intake of food and the rhythm of the activity of organs and also the centres which control the whole sympathetic and parasympathetic nervous systems. On the one hand, knowledge of deficiencies of certain sites of production of hormones is of the very greatest importance; on the other hand, such dysfunctions are absorbed by counter controls of other hormonal groups, so that the clinical picture cannot be typical, when it is chiefly one of visible functional deficiencies.

Functional Disorders of the Thyroid Gland are shown by under- or over-production of thyroxin (hyper- or hypothyroidism).

Hyperthyroidism is characterised by increase of all the metabolic processes and is commonly known as "Morbus Basedow" (Basedow's disease). MEIER and CLARK (Zbl. Vet. Med. **5**, 120–128, 1958) described cases which showed marked nervousness, a rapid pulse, marked cardiac activity and rapid respiration. We have not yet been able to observe syndromes of this kind.

Hypothyroidism causes a reduction of all metabolic processes. Basal metabolism is decreased and the functions of the heart, circulation and respiration are depressed. Alopecias may occur which may be bilateral and asymmetrical, the skin may be oedematous and eczematous. Obesity (Fig. 506) is very often seen. According to Meier and Clark there is an increase of the cholesterol blood level to 800 mg%.

Treatment is by the administration of iodine (see Struma, p. 439) or of preparations made from dried thyroid.

Enlargement of the thyroid glands may occur in both hypo- and hyperthyroidism.

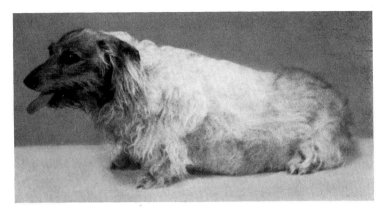

Fig. 506. Adiposity in hypothyroidism.

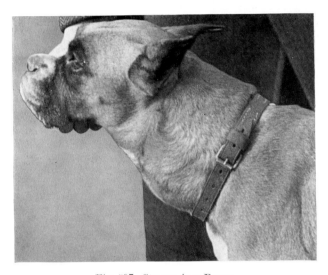

Fig. 507. Struma in a Boxer.

Struma (Goitre) is an inflammatory enlargement of the thyroid gland. In its early stage it is hyperplastic in nature, whilst the goitres of older animals may have undergone neoplastic changes with metastases in the lungs and other organs. The causes of the formation of a goitre have not yet been completely explained.

Clinically the goitre appears as a swelling on both sides of the trachea, the two halves being joined by the isthmus – its consistency is semi-solid or hard (Fig. 507). It is not always possible to distinguish clinically between simple hyperplasia and a neoplasm. A goitre that is not specially large can be moved easily upon its substratum and it follows the movement of the act of swallowing. It is important to make a differential diagnosis between this and tumours, abscesses and cysts

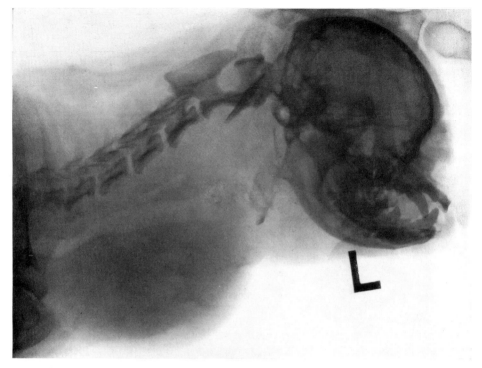

Fig. 508. Struma in a Pekingese. The trachea is slightly bent and partly overgrown by tumour tissue.

in the neck (Fig. 509). Neoplastic changes of the thyroid gland may lead to more marked serious functional disorders. It may grow round the trachea (sabre sheath struma) causing dyspnoea, or pressure on the jugular veins may cause cerebral congestion (Fig. 438). If the tumour grows round the carotid artery a thrill is felt when the hand is laid flat upon it. The size of the struma causes difficulty in swallowing solid food because the oesophagus is then compressed against the cervical vertebrae.

Treatment is conservative with iodine preparations. This is especially to be recommended in early struma. According to the size of the dog one gives 3–6 drops of Lugol's iodine solution daily and this is supported by painting the shaved skin with iodine repeated at weekly intervals. Treatment with iodine is, however, given only so long as a reduction of the struma can be appreciated, as there is some risk of iodine cachexia (iodism).

If the conservative treatment is ineffective (especially in older dogs) partial surgical removal of the struma must be considered. This should only be done if X-rays and palpation have excluded metastases with a fair degree of certainty. In the strumectomies so far undertaken by us, usually only one thyroid gland was especially enlarged and this was removed. By the unilateral operation one is certain to leave two parathyroids in the body. Total removal results in tetany (loss of

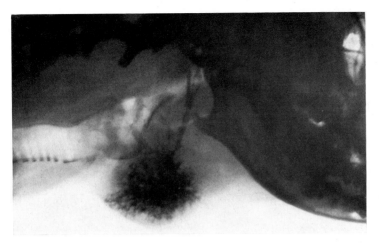

Fig. 509. Tumour with deposits of osteoid tissue. Differential diagnosis important, no struma!

control of the calcium–phosphorus metabolism) and this causes death. Growth of the tumour round the large cervical blood vessels may lead to especial difficulties in the operation, so surgical removal should be recommended early. If it is absolutely necessary to remove both thyroid glands one should leave in the body certain parts at the cranial end (and also if the tumours are hardened) because in this way the lateral parathyroids are safeguarded with certainty. Further, one must avoid damage to the recurrent (laryngeal) nerve because otherwise disorder of the vocal organs must be expected.

Diseases of the Hypophysis may cause various clinical symptoms. Diseases of the anterior lobe cause the symptoms of so-called hypophysial dwarfism or gigantism, acromegaly, obesity, etc. In the literature, BAKER (J. Amer. vet. med. Ass. **126**, 468, 1955) described a case of a sheep dog bitch, 6 months old, which was destroyed because although it was lively and had a good appetite, its growth was markedly retarded and its coat was rough. Autopsy revealed hypoplasia of the pancreas (no absence of Islets of Langerhans) and a cystic degeneration of the hypophysis. Changes in the anterior lobe (adenoma of the basophil parts) which restrict the excretion of the adenocorticotropic hormone (ACTH) lead to overproduction of glucocorticosteroids in the adrenal tissue, the symptoms being obesity, osteoporosis, hypertonicity, hypogonadism, and hyperglycaemia. This disease in man is called the Cushing Syndrome. It may also appear if there is a diffuse hyperplasia of the adrenal gland tissue which also causes increased formation of glucocorticosteroids. DÄMMRICH (Berl. Münch. tierärztl. Wschr. **72**, 340–343, 1959) described such a case in a 12-year-old adipose male Scottish terrier which was interpreted as a Cushing Syndrome. Two years earlier the animal showed marked alopecia but only on the head and ends of the limbs. Subsequently, disorder of movement appeared, with the result that the animal could no longer stand up or walk and therefore had to be destroyed. At the subsequent autopsy, osteoporosis was striking; it had led to marked changes in the vertebral column (corresponding to the wedge-shaped vertebrae in Cushing's disease in man). Overproduction of glucocorticosteroids was regarded as the cause of the osteoporosis. The calcium salts set free in osteoporosis are excreted by the kidneys and may be partly deposited there. The autopsy also revealed a blastoma in the liver consisting of adrenal cortex tissue, hyperplasia of both adrenal glands, and in the hypophysis a focal adenomatosis of the basophil cells.

If the posterior lobe of the hypophysis is diseased diabetes insipidus may occur.

Diabetes Insipidus (excessive secretion of urine) represents a disorder of the water balance and the mineral concentration in the body, in which the centre in the hypothalamus and hypophysis for water and mineral concentration must be damaged. There is, on the other hand, a lack of the anti-diuretic hormone which checks the excretion of water. The causes of this may, for example, be tumours which restrict the functional activity of the posterior lobe of the hypophysis.

The clinical picture is one of polydipsia and polyuria. Big dogs may pass up to 10–15 litres of urine, the urine being free from albumin and sugar. It is watery and clear with a specific gravity between 1,000 and 1,005. As a result of the marked thirst the dog drinks any kind of fluid, even its own urine. The polyuria leads to deprivation of the body of water (exsiccosis) and cachexia results which finally leads to death.

The diagnosis of this disease is difficult, because in the differential diagnosis all other possible diseases (especially those of the kidneys) must be considered. The Water Deprivation Test provides a valuable aid to diagnosis. After depriving the dog of water for 8 hours the bladder is emptied and 15 minutes later a sample of urine is obtained. If there has been a rise in the specific gravity to above 1.020 then the case is not diabetes insipidus.

Treatment consists of an attempt to regulate the water balance by injections of vasopressin tannate in doses of 0.1 unit/kg bodyweight every 48–72 hours. After 5 injections if there is improvement, larger intervals between the injections should be selected. Sufficient drinking water should be given in order to combat the exsiccosis. WIRTH (Wien. tierärztl. Mschr. **43**, 459, 1956) describes a case in which the effects of shock caused the symptoms of diabetes insipidus to subside.

Diseases of the Adrenal Glands must be divided into those of the medulla and those of the cortex.

Diseases of the Medulla are quite rare and can hardly be diagnosed clinically with accuracy and are therefore only of interest to the pathologist. Sound information about them is given by DAHME and SCHLEMMER (Zbl. Vet. Med. **6**, 249–259, 1959).

Diseases of the Cortex are, on the other hand, of great importance in medicine. Their relationship to the hypophysis in respect of the site of reaction in the body is known (see p. 438). Hypofunction of one or the other organ may cause the syndrome of primary or secondary Addison's disease in man or in the dog. Insufficient production of glucocorticosteroids in the adrenal cortex, or failure of it, causes the clinical symptoms, of asthenia, lassitude, and pigmentation (bronze disease). In addition, there are gastrointestinal disorders with achylia of the stomach and lowering of blood sugar, anaemia, and subnormal temperature. The nutritional state deteriorates. Hypoglycaemia is frequent and there are increased calcium and decreased sodium serum values. The urine is retained, but the excretion of sodium and chloride is increased. The characteristic symptom of hyperpigmentation (bronze disease) cannot be detected in the dog. Slight insufficiencies of the adrenal cortex, or of the sites of production of the adrenocorticosteroid hormone (ACTH), can lead to syndromes which respond strikingly to administration of the corresponding hormone. In this, one uses ACTH or "Thorn Test" (FREUDIGER, Schweiz. Arch. Thk. **100**, 318–325, 1958). The principle of this test is that injection of ACTH, which is superimposed on the adrenal cortex, causes a functional adrenal cortex to excrete glucocorticosteroids. The result is a significant decrease of eosinophils (eosinopaenia) in the circulating blood. The precise mechanism of this effect is not known. The degree of the decrease of eosinophils is an index of the functional capacity of the adrenal cortex. Freudiger has modified the Thorn Test for the dog by injecting 10–25 international units of ACTH intramuscularly. Immediately before doing this the eosinophils were counted (a complete blood count). Seven hours after the injection of ACTH a complete blood count was again done and the decrease of eosinophils was estimated per cent. If it is below 70 %, one suspects insufficiency of the cortex. On the other hand, a fall of over 70 % indicates sufficient activity of the cortex. In addition to the decrease of eosinophils, Freudiger noted lymphopaenia, neutrophilia and leucocytosis as well as a slight degree of hydraemia with erythropaenia as the expression of an excretion of cortical hormone caused by the ACTH stimulus. Insufficiency may be simulated by inactivation of the ACTH at the site of injection. In such cases the intravenous Thorn Test gives sufficient information.

Acute Insufficiency of the Adrenal Cortex occurs if the hitherto functionally efficient adrenal cortex is damaged by any cause and suddenly ceases to function. The symptoms then caused may be alarming. There is hypotension, tachycardia, and fall of temperature. If the course is very acute, circulatory collapse, coma and death occur.

In man acute insufficiency of the adrenal cortex is divided into acute adrenal crisis (in chronic insufficiency of the adrenal cortex), the Waterhouse–Fridrichsen syndrome (adrenal apoplexy, today regarded as an adaptation disease with a phase of rapid exhaustion of the adrenal glands), acute insufficiency of the adrenal cortex as a result of surgical removal of cortex tissue and acute insufficiency of the adrenal cortex due to trauma or operation, when there is already a potential insufficiency of the cortex. FREUDIGER and LINDT (Schweiz. Arch. Thk. **100**, 425–438, 1958) describe 4 cases of insufficiency of the adrenal cortex. The first three were typical foreign body patients which died during the operation or soon after it. The third case, also a patient with foreign body ileus, was destroyed at the request of the owner. All three cases were characterised by the known severe condition in ileus: apathy, inappetence, congestion of the scleral blood vessels, intractable vomiting and arrest of defaecation. Toxic effects due to the ileus had an adverse effect not only on the parenchyma but also on the cortex of the adrenals and this caused a loss of the adrenal cortex hormone. FREUDIGER and LINDT write in addition: the loss of water and chloride due to the persistent vomiting acted as a vivious circle. Instead of the former increased excretion of corticosteroids necessary to regulate the disorder of the electrolyte balance and plasma volume, the damaged adrenal cortex could only produce insufficient hormone, so that there was an intensification of the disturbance of the electrolyte balance with resultant thickening of the blood, fall in blood pressure, and inhibition of the conduction of stimuli in the heart muscle and indirectly the vomiting centre was stimulated afresh by the increased electrolyte dysequilibrium. The insufficient excretion of glucocorticosteroids as a result of the disorder of the sugar metabolism may have also acted unfavourably on the detoxicating function of the liver cells and may thus have encouraged the symptoms of autointoxication. In this very unfavourable situation new burdens must have been created by the anaesthetic and the operation, which led to total failure of the adrenal cortex and consequently to complete breakdown of the life-saving sympathetic counter regulatory mechanism. The two dogs operated upon died with the symptoms of very acute insufficiency of the adrenal cortex; this was confirmed by the autopsy.

In the four cases it was a question of slowly increasing exhaustion of the adrenocortical reserves with sudden, very acute, total breakdown of these reserves as a result of infection with streptococci and diplococci. This was a case of stresses operating over a year either chronic (chronic cystitis, nephritis, pregnancy, chronic endometritis) or acute (birth, an operation for endometritis, and one for entropion and a terminal bacterial septicaemia) which led to the breakdown of the activity of the adrenal cortex. Freudiger and Lindt concluded that injury to the adrenal cortex and the resultant insufficiency with all its catastrophic results may occur not only in the special cases described, but also in all severe diseases, especially after an operation (for ileus, miscarriages, pyometra, etc.). It follows from the statements just made that it would be advisable, wherever possible, always to administer adrenal cortex hormone parenterally to patients which are already in bad general condition and also to do this after the operation in order to improve the general condition and especially to normalise the hypothermia. Freudiger and Lindt have been able by means of this substitution treatment, to save patients which would have died according to earlier experience.

Treatment is given with "Percorten", 1.25–5 mg per day and "Hydrocorton" 12.5–25 mg a day. To combat the risk of stimulating infective agents an antibiotic should be given at the same time. "Percortin" (desoxycorticosteroid-glucoside) has a marked mineral corticoid, but no glucocorticoid action, whilst "Hydrocorton" (17-oxycortic-osterone-21-acetate) has a marked glucocorticoid effect, but a moderate mineral corticoid action. By combining the two, therefore, an ideal substitution effect is obtained. It is on these grounds that a combined treatment is to be preferred to treatment with only one steroid. The treatment should be continued until there is a distinct improvement or normalisation of the deficiency symptoms. If there is a relapse when the treatment is discontinued, it must be repeated. In such cases injections of ACTH can be tried in addition, in order to encourage regeneration of the adrenal cortex.

Chronic Insufficiency of the Adrenal Cortex is rare in the dog. FREUDIGER (Schweiz. Arch. Thk. **100**, 362–378, 1958) described two cases of primary chronic insufficiency and one case of secondary chronic insufficiency.

Clinically there was increased and rapid onset of fatigue, diminished activity, persistent vomiting and relapsing diarrhoea. Further, there was a tendency to hypothermia, signs of circulatory disorders, wasting and ultimately dehydration. Freudiger did not find hyperpigmentation. In the case with secondary chronic insufficiency there were repeated hypoglycaemic attacks at night. Noteworthy in the laboratory investigations were eosinophilia and a negative Thorn Test.

Treatment is given with cortisone. It is advisable to choose at first a high dose in order to estimate later the maintenance dose. If this is set too low, the dose must be significantly increased and later lowered again. In FREUDIGER's cases the initial dose was 75 mg and the maintenance dose 7.5 mg a day.

Treatment with ACTH and glucocorticoids has become in recent years of quite fundamental interest, so in the following section some basic facts will be given about how they act and about the indications for them and the dosage. For basic information the summaries by the following authors may be listed:

JAHN (Deutsch. tierärztl. Wschr. **64**, No. 19, 1957).
MÜLLER (Ibid, **65**, 85–87, 1958).
PRIEUR (Kleintier-Prax. **3**, 68–75, 1958).
GIERSCHIK (Prakt. Tierarzt 1959/60, No. 12/1).

The anterior lobe of the hypophysis governs the functions and correlations of the endocrine system. The adrenocorticotropic hormone (ACTH) is especially closely correlated with the adrenal cortex. ACTH has no direct action of its own on the organism, but as a hormone activates the adrenal cortex, i.e., it makes and excretes into the body the so-called glucocorticosteroids. Considered from the therapeutic point of view, this means that treatment with ACTH can be successful if the adrenal cortex is intact. The systemic action (on the whole organism) must be distinguished from the topical (local) effect.

The effects of these hormones on the organism are described below. They increase the glycogen content of the liver and musculature, or inhibit a decrease of the glycogen level in these organs. Sugar tolerance is lowered simultaneously with a reduction of the renal threshold for sugar. Thus the prolonged use of high doses may cause a hyperglycaemia and naturally also glycosuria (steroid diabetes), but these disappear after withdrawal of the preparation. Glucogenesis from protein and fat is increased. The effect on protein metabolism both encourages decomposition and inhibits their formation with the result that the total protein metabolism is intensified so that a negative nitrogen balance may develop. By the lowering of the kidney threshold for these substances, the excretion of uric acid and amino acids in the urine is increased. The negative nitrogen balance mentioned seems to be independent of the size of the dose. It can be inhibited by a diet rich in protein (increased supply of amino acids) and by adding calcium. Fat metabolism is mobilised and better use is made of the fat. With high doses increase in the amount of depot fat in the liver can be detected. It should be noted that the NaCl and water retention that at first appears later subsides (after about 8 days), perhaps even changing into a negative chloride balance. During treatment with the hormone, therefore, the supply of salt and fluid must be restricted. Increased excretion of phosphate and a negative calcium balance are doubtlessly related to these features of the chloride metabolism. This may lead to substantial impoverishment of the body in calcium and therefore for this reason the calcium is added.

The formation of antibodies and the antigen-antibody reaction are in general not inhibited, but because the mesenchymal reactions are suppressed there is an inhibition of allergic or immunological reactions. Of special therapeutic interest is the influence on tissues. Müller described it as a brake on connective tissue by which he meant inhibition of its proliferation in inflammatory processes. The formation of fibroblasts and angioblasts is inhibited but not epithelialisation. Exudative processes are also inhibited by decrease in vascularisation and capillary permeability. By this inhibition of inflammatory reactions there is also a limitation of an important constituent of the body's defence against infection, namely, the diapedesis of the leucocytes and their phagocytic ability. These facts are utilised in order to prevent adhesions in the abdomen after laparotomy by intraabdominal administration. Related to the local antiphlogistic effect of the hormone of the adrenal cortex is its action in checking such general reactions as fever or generalised toxic symptoms. This effect also increases tolerance of poisons, but it may also lead, by inhibition of the defence mechanism, to a spread of an existing infection. In the stomach the glucocorticoids lead to an increase of production of hydrochloric acid and pepsin and this perhaps explains why appetite improves during treatment with cortisone. In the blood there is a leucocytosis with eosinopenia and lymphopenia.

Indications for the use of ACTH or glucocorticoids are:

generalised diseases (urticaria, rheumatism, insect bites, burns);

eye diseases (conjunctivitis, keratitis, episcleritis, iritis, iridocyclitis, uveitis, choroiditis);

joint diseases (arthritis, periarthritis, arthrosis, conditions following dislocations and distortions, syndesmitis ossificans, Dachshund paralysis, muscle tears, tendinitis, tendovaginitis);

skin diseases (acute, chronic and allergic eczemas, forms of dermatitis, pruritus);

otitis externa, peritonitis, balanoposthitis.

In infectious diseases caused by bacteria such treatment should be given only under the protection of a bacteriostatic agent, if marked inflammation, exudation, proliferation and toxin formation exist. LAUDA and GEYER (Monatskurse f. d. ärztl. Fortbildung **6**, 214, 1907) have laid down the following rules for cortisone treatment in infectious diseases:

1. Corticosteroids have no anti-infectious action.
2. Steroid treatment should be used only in combination with antibiotics.
3. Side effects must be borne in mind.
4. They are indicated as well as antibiotics in severe conditions with marked toxic symptoms, hypersensitive allergic states or as an ultimate refuge.
5. Patients treated with corticosteroids must be closely watched in case there is masking of the pathological processes.
6. Give cortisone only for as long as it is necessary.
7. End with ACTH.
8. Continue antibiotic treatment beyond ACTH treatment.

The range of indications for the use of ACTH or corticosteroids is very wide, but one should depend as much as possible on one's own experience, because the reactions may sometimes be variable.

Contra-indications in systemic treatment are tuberculosis of the lungs, nephritis and diabetes mellitus.

Several points in the rules given by Laude and Geyer cited above require explanation. The side effects which may appear in cortisone treatment were discussed on p. 445. Nevertheless, reference should be made to the fact that the individual corticosteroids may act in different ways. With regard to the quantitative differences in activity it can be said that hydrocortisone is about 50 % more active than cortisone and that prednisone and prednisolone (derivatives of cortisone and hydrocortisone) are even more active. The antiphlogistic features of prednisone and prednisolone are far superior to those of cortisone, and therefore their effect on the mineral economy is significantly smaller; the antiphlogistic action of fluorocortisone is especially marked, as is also its sodium-retaining and potassium diuretic effect and that is why it is usually prescribed only for external use. The reason one should give cortisone only for as long as is necessary and should end with ACTH is based on the fact that the effects on the endocrine system are different Exogenous administration of ACTH stimulates the adrenal cortex. Long-continued administration of ACTH causes hypertrophy of the cortex. ACTH therapy is therefore a stimulation or biological shock treatment. Exogenously-given hormones of the adrenal cortex on the other hand are purely substitution drugs, which increase the formation of hormone in the adrenals, or replace its deficiency in pathological states of the body in which there is possibly insufficient formation of the hormone. Their effect on the anterior lobe of the hypophysis-adrenal cortex system consists of an inhibition of the production of ACTH by the anterior lobe, which results in a cessation of the biological stimulation of the adrenal cortex so that the functional activity of this is depressed. In this way prolonged administration of cortisone causes functional decrease and sometimes even atrophy of the adrenal cortex. Therefore at the end of cortisone treatment, ACTH should be given several times in addition or alone in order to normalise again the relationships of the anterior lobe of the hypophysis to the adrenal cortex.

Modes of Administration. ACTH as the proteohormone is destroyed in the alimentary canal and can therefore only be given parenterally, whilst the glucocorticoid can be used equally well for local treatment (injection into joint cavities) as for general treatment (parenteral or by the mouth). ACTH, on the contrary, can only be given for general systemic treatment. In local treatment the point of attack of the glucocorticoid is in the tissues themselves and undesirable side effects such as inhibition of resistance to infection, disorders of the water economy, etc., are of no concern. Resistance will first of all be inhibited at the site of administration itself.

Dosage can be given only in general terms, because it must be estimated in each individual case. It is governed by the therapeutic indications, the severity of the disease and the general condition of the patient.

According to the size of the patient 5–20 international units of ACTH are given intramuscularly. With prednisone or prednisolone, 5–20 mg are given intramuscularly or 0.15–2 mg per kg bodyweight a day are given by the mouth. As a general rule acute diseases respond more quickly than do chronic ones and early commencement of treatment can substantially shorten the treatment period. In diseases which can be expected to have a shorter course, one begins with ACTH, continues with glucocorticoids and ends with ACTH. For diseases needing a longer period of treatment the basic rule is that high initial doses are given until improvement appears in a shorter time. The dose is then decreased to the maintenance dose, in such a way that the symptoms are still corrected. These small doses are continued with diminishing doses until the end of the treatment.

Permanent cures cannot be expected, even if the exciting cause is investigated and remedied, because this is not a specific treatment. Treatment with ACTH and glucocorticoids, therefore, must not be over-rated.

16. Hypovitaminoses

Diseases due to lack of vitamins appear when there are serious defects in the maintenance and feeding. These can lead to severe metabolic disorders, but occur only rarely in the dog.

Lack of vitamin A (A-hypovitaminosis) causes epithelial damage, especially in the cornea (keratomalacia). Young dogs should be given the provitamin in the form of raw carrots. The beneficial effect of vitamin A in reproductive disorders (azoospermia, abortion) is known and it can be administered in the form of drops in these conditions. Combinations of vitamins (A and D, A, D and E) are also advisable.

Lack of vitamin B (B-hypovitaminosis) is also called anxiety psychosis or hysteria of the dog. It is believed that this supposedly B_1-hypovitaminosis is caused by insufficient food, or an unbalanced diet. The animals suddenly rush away in great fear as if confronted with an imaginary enemy, but attack and defence movements are also seen. Sometimes there are convulsions. Treatment is given with thiamine or vitamin B-complex. According to the size of the patient 25–100 mg of thiamine are injected at 2-day intervals, until there is clinical improvement. The treatment may then be continued with tablets (50 mg).

B_2-hypovitaminosis is manifested by Black-tongue disease observed in America: it shows a great similarity to the uraemic form of leptospirosis. The outstanding sign is the pigmentation of the tongue from dark brown to black. There are haemorrhages and ulcers in the mouth and later general body weakness and anaemia occur. The cause of the disease is considered to be feeding on maize meal exclusively. In the treatment an immediate change of food should be made and in addition vitamin B_2, in the form of riboflavin (dragees) or vitamin B-complex (dragees) is given.

C-hypovitaminosis should not occur in the dog, as the studies of Nitz (Thesis. Gießen, 1951) have shown that the dog can manufacture its own vitamin C. Nevertheless, the good effect of vitamin C (in high doses) in infectious diseases, gastric and intestinal disorders and haemorrhages has been demonstrated.

The concept of **D-hypovitaminosis** is known and it expresses itself in disorders of the calcium and phosphorus metabolism, which result in abnormal growth of bones, described more fully on p. 428 under the heading of rachitis (rickets).

A marked **E-hyptovitaminosis** is not seen in the dog, but often vitamin E is prescribed, especially in eczemas and metabolic disorders.

17. Diseases of the blood and spleen

Diseases of the blood are extremely multifarious and usually appear as secondary symptoms. Changes in the blood corpuscles are revealed by the blood picture. We use as our standards the values given by Wirth (Fundamentals of the Clinical Haematology of Domesticated Animals, Vienna, 1950). The average number of erythrocytes is 6 million (5.5–8.0). The haemoglobin content amounts to 70 % (60–80 %), according to Sahli = 76 % (64–87 % G.I.M.). The total number of leucocytes is 9–10000. The differential blood count is as follows: neutrophils 70 % (60–80 %); eosinophils 3 % (2–4 %); basophils 0.3 %; small lymphocytes 19.7 % (12–27 %); large lymphocytes 3 % (1–5 %) and monocytes 4 % (3–5 %). Estimation of the erythrocyte sedimentation rate is essential in many cases as it provides considerable information, but its value must not be overestimated. Definite conclusions cannot be drawn from the sedimentation rate because it is not specific. Nevertheless, a variation from the normal shows that "something is wrong in the body" (Wirth). Freudiger (Schweiz. Arch. Thkde **95**, 403, 1953) considered the determination of the sedimentation rate to be of special value in the diagnosis of acute septic processes, to distinguish bronchopneumonia from bronchitis, and to estimate the degree of tissue breakdown and thus gain some indication of malignancy and metastases of neoplasms. It can also give valuable diagnostic and prognostic indications in infectious diseases, especially in the diagnosis of tuberculosis. In his opinion the sedimentation rate is a reaction which allows us to study the course of a disease. For this reason its value lies in frequently repeated estimations. According to Wirth, the normal sedimentation rate determined by the method of Westergren has the following values:

After 1 hour 1 mm (0.5–2).
After 2 hours 1.7 mm (1.0–3.5).
After 24 hours 8 mm (5.0–13.0).

Sedimentation rates within this range are to be regarded as normal. Reading of the 24 hour value presents certain practical difficulties in general veterinary practice due to the irregular nature of the work. Therefore readings of the 24 hour values are often omitted, or the sedimentation test is not done at all because it was possible to make a diagnosis at the first examination of the patient. We do the blood sedimentation rate test in Westergren tubes inclined at about 60° and can read off values after 7, 10 and 20 minutes, which correspond to the 1, 2 and 24 hour values with vertical sedimentation. This shortening of the times of reading makes it possible to conduct the test during the examination of a patient, so that the results can have a decisive influence on diagnosis and treatment.

Examination of the spleen is performed by palpation with the patient either standing or laid on its right side. Usually the normal spleen of the dog cannot be felt. If it is enlarged, it protrudes under the costal arch, lies close to the abdominal wall and is movable. If tumours change its shape it is difficult to differentiate it from other possible tumours in the abdominal cavity. X-rays should be used. Without contrast media only rarely can enlargement of the spleen be accurately diagnosed. Good results are obtained with contrast medium in the alimentary canal because it is then possible to draw certain conclusions from the displacement of this canal. Even better demonstrations of the spleen are possible with a pneumoperitoneum (see p. 121).

Anaemia is due to abnormal composition of the blood. Reduction of the number of erythrocytes or of the amount of haemoglobin produces the clinical picture of anaemia. It is possible to classify anaemias into haemorrhagic anaemia (acute

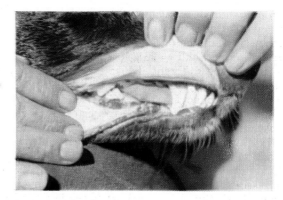

Fig. 510. Anaemia. The mucosae of the jaws are porcelain-white. Blood examination: Erythrocytes 1,470,000; Leucocytes 33,000; Haemoglobin 22 % (Sahli). Differential blood count: Immature red cells 2 %; Cells with rod-shaped nuclei 15 %; Segmented cells 66 %; Lymphocytes 16 %; Monocytes 1 %; 2 Normoblasts; Anisocytosis.

haemorrhage and chronic loss of blood), haemolytic anaemia (due to infections, chemical causes, therapeutic measures, etc.) and secondary anaemia (accompanying other severe diseases). Primary anaemia due to disease of the sites of erythropoiesis is rare and will not be considered.

The clinical picture may be very variable. Slight degrees of anaemia may not be clinically evident. In more marked anaemia, there is general lassitude, the patient seems dull and lethargic. If the anaemia is marked there is striking pallor of the mucosae (Fig. 510). The surface of the body feels cool and the slightest bodily stress causes increased respiration. The heart beat and pulse are accelerated. When the anaemia is intense, there is palpitation of the heart beat and the pulse is convulsive. In haemolytic anaemia usually icterus and splenomegaly occur.

The diagnosis is confirmed by the blood picture. The number of the erythrocytes indicates the degree of anaemia, but in anaemia due to haemorrhage the lowest reading is to be expected on the second day after the haemorrhage. In a blood film a great variety of typical morphological changes are found which help to verify the diagnosis of anaemia. Among these are anisocytosis (unequal size of the erythrocytes), poikilocytosis (abundance of serrated, elongated, or oak-leaf-shaped, sickle-shaped and quite shapeless degenerating erythrocytes resulting from severe disorder of the blood formation), polychromasia (of young erythrocytes which take up methylene blue as well as eosin) and oligochromasia (pale colour of the erythrocytes due to small haemoglobin content). In addition, erythroblasts and normoblasts (young, nucleated precursors of erythrocytes) are seen. The number of leucocytes may be normal or increased (leucocytosis). The haemoglobin content is greatly reduced.

The course of an anaemia always depends on the exciting cause and the type. Anaemias due to haemorrhage respond significantly better to treatment than do haemolytic anaemias. An anaemia due to haemorrhage in which more than half the blood is lost may lead to death.

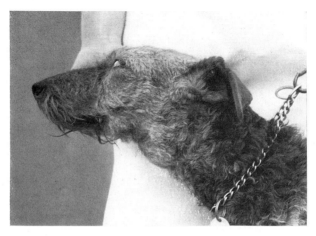

Fig. 511. Leukaemia with marked enlargement of the submaxillary lymph glands.

Treatment should be directed initially towards the exciting cause. In anaemia due to haemorrhage, the haemorrhage must be arrested as soon as possible, usually by surgical methods. In haemolytic anaemia the causal agent is removed; and in secondary anaemia the primary disease is investigated in order that specific therapy may be instituted where possible.

Anaemia due to haemorrhage should be treated as soon as possible by replacing the lost blood with normal blood (blood transfusion) or with a plasma substitute ("Macrodex", "Dextran"). In the dog transfusion reactions are rare even if the same donor is used repeatedly.

In the other forms of anaemia the treatment is directed towards stimulating haematopoiesis. This is done by increased feeding with foods of normal composition, by fresh air and ultraviolet irradiation, and avoidance of over-exertion. Iron is the best haematinic. Encouragement of blood formation with arsenic is attempted with Fowler's solution.

Leucosis (leukaemia) is a pathological process (hyperplasia) in the organs or organ systems which manufacture the leucocytes. Clinically, it is characterised by a leucocytosis and a general enlargement of the lymph glands and of the spleen. In the dog we differentiate two forms, the lymphatic and the myeloid forms (lymphadenoma and myelosis). Recently monocytic forms (reticuloendothelioses) have been described. In leucosis there is growth of the whole lymphatic apparatus which forms the lymphocytes, or there is growth of the whole myeloid apparatus which produces the polymorphonuclear granulocytes. The aetiology is unknown.

Clinical picture. There is no special breed incidence. Leucosis appears mostly in older dogs (over 5 years old) and dogs seem to be affected more often than bitches. The history often relates that the dog lies down often, quickly tires and is losing weight. On inspection of such cases usually the abnormal size of the lymph glands is striking. There is especially marked and early enlargement of the submaxillary and cervical lymph glands and this may cause dyspnoea or cough (Fig. 511). The

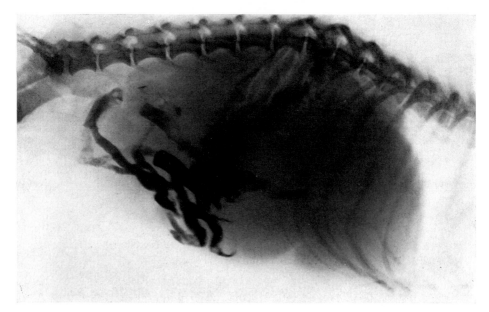

Fig. 512. Enlargement of the liver and spleen in lymphatic leucosis. By giving a contrast medium the displacement of the stomach caudally and dorsally is well shown.

swelling of the body lymph glands by pressure on their surroundings, may cause oedemas due to stasis, retention of urine, ascites, difficulty in swallowing, etc. Lymph glands that cannot be palpated (in the thorax) can be seen by X-rays (Fig. 513). The swollen lymph glands are painless. Occasionally, there may appear in the skin, the mucosae, or within the eye, sudden punctiform and also larger haemorrhages which are the expression of a haemorrhagic diathesis. The microscopic blood picture is important and essential for the diagnosis of leukaemia. The vital feature is the white cell picture, which shows an increase in the number of leucocytes with a high proportion of their immature precursors. If the lymphocytes and their young forms (lymphoblasts, lymphoid cells, Rieder cells), released by the lymphoid forming organ system, are increased, one speaks of a lymphatic leukaemia. On the other hand, a myelogenous leukaemia is characterised by increase of the polymorphonuclear, granular leucocytes and their immature precursors, such as myeloblasts, metamyelocytes, and myelocytes. The red cell picture also shows changes, namely, deformations of the erythrocytes (poikilocytosis, anisocytosis, polychromasia, swollen forms) and erythroblasts, immature nucleated erythrocytes and red cells containing Jolly bodies. The number of erythrocytes is at first either not decreased at all or only slightly so, and in the later stages of the disease the decrease is still very small. Nevertheless, the haemoglobin content may fall to half the normal. During the course of the disease the ratio of leucocytes to erythrocytes may rise from the normal 1 : 300 to 1 : 60, 1 : 30, 1 : 10 or 1 : 5. WIRTH (Tierärztl. Rdsch. **36**, 518, 1930) described a case of lym-

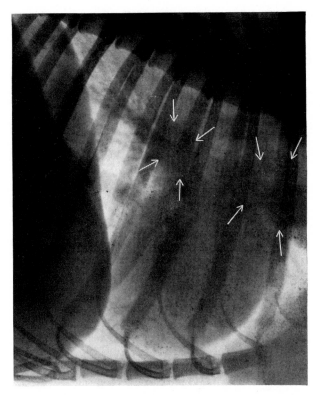

Fig. 513. Shadows in the field of the lungs due to enlarged mesenteric lymph glands in leucosis.

phatic leukaemia with the following blood picture: haemoglobin 21 % (Sahli) 1,920,000 erythrocytes, 629,500 leucocytes (with 80.3 % of lymphocytes). This case corresponds to human lymphatic leukaemia (300–500,000 leucocytes in man). Blood pictures like this are rare in the dog.

No effective treatment is known. Previously, a wide variety of drugs has been used with little effect (Urethane, nitrogen mustards, etc.). The most effective is X-ray irradiation. This brings about a surprisingly rapid involution of the enlargement of the lymph glands and of the splenomegaly, with improvement of the blood picture and the general condition. The improvement may persist for quite a long time until relapses occur which eventually prove resistant to further treatment. Careful monitoring of the blood picture is absolutely essential during irradiation, because with overdosage there is a drop in the leucocytes which prohibits further irradiation for a time (risk of intoxication due to too rapid breakdown of cells). A combination of cyclophosphamide and prednisone has proved very effective in obtaining a temporary regression of the disease. Cyclophosphamide is given at a dose of 2.5 mg/kg daily for 7 days and the dosage is then halved. Prednisone is given at the same time at a dosage rate of 0.5 mg/kg daily. Again careful monitoring of the blood picture is mandatory.

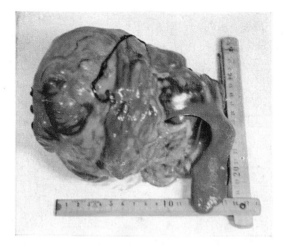

Fig. 514. Tumour of the spleen.

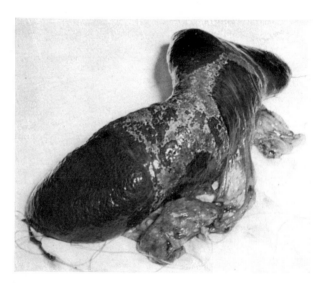

Fig. 515. Hyperplasia of the spleen due to a foreign body (a needle) which had perforated the
stomach wall and was encapsulated in the splenic mesentery. In the foreground, the splenic
mesentery with the foreign body in it.

Banti's Syndrome is a disease characterised by a complex of symptoms caused
by various factors injurious to the blood together with marked enlargement of the
spleen. Three stages of it may be distinguished. Stage 1 (the anaemic stage) is
characterised by increasing lassitude, anaemia and splenomegaly. In the second
stage (the transitional stage) enlargement of the liver also appears. In the third

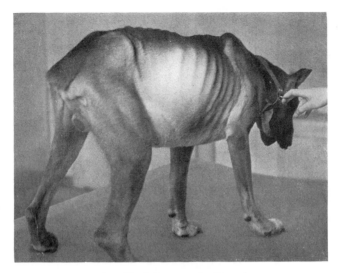

Fig. 516. Splenomegaly (Boxer).

stage (ascitic stage) anaemia, leucopenia, thrombocytopenia, abdominal ascites, splenomegaly and cirrhosis of the liver are seen.

Clinical picture. The patient is brought in in a state of complete exhaustion. The pallor of the mucosae is striking. The blood picture shows an erythropaenia and later a leucopaenia with a relative lymphocytosis. The enormous enlargement of the spleen (sclerosis of the spleen) may visibly bulge out the abdominal wall.

Treatment is by splenectomy (see later), following which the blood picture becomes normal after a time. If the patient is already in the third stage of the disease, splenectomy can no longer bring about a cure.

Splenomegaly (Enlargement of the spleen) may occur not only as a disease, but also as a secondary condition, especially in leukaemia. Primary enlargement of the spleen may be due to tumours, hyperplasias, haematomas, etc. (Figs. 514 and 515).

The clinical picture shows enlargement of the circumference of the abdomen (Fig. 516). Palpation and X-rays are valuable aids to diagnosis. Sometimes the blood picture (erythropaenia, leucosis, leucopaenia, etc.) also gives useful information. If enlargement of the spleen is found after accidents, palpation must be done only with the greatest care, because a haematoma of the spleen must be reckoned among the possibilities and vigorous palpation may rupture the capsule of the haematoma, leading to internal haemorrhage.

Treatment is by removal of the spleen. The dog can exist without a spleen, although this has important functions in the body. In it, worn out erythrocytes are broken down, it is the site of the manufacture of lymphocytes, it has important functions as a reservoir of blood, and in addition, it has the ability to seal off certain poisons in order to maintain in the body a non-toxic blood reservoir. It can form antibodies and initiate protective mechanisms against infectious diseases and also the ability to protect against the growth of malignant tumours has been ascribed to it. It plays a significant part in metabolism. Its function as a reservoir of blood (up to 20 % of the total quantity of blood) should be remembered before it is removed. The spleen tissue, if its contractibility has not been lost, can be made to discharge the blood store in it by means of doses of adrenalin (ÜBERREITER, Arch. wiss. u. prakt. Thkd. **79**, 176, 1944), so that this blood is not lost to the body. One gives 0.5 mg of adrenalin (0.5 ml of the 1 % solution to 5 ml distilled water) subcutaneously. This causes contraction of the spleen and this may be very advantageous during the operation and in obscure cases. These doses of adrenalin can be very useful in diagnosis, because the reduction in size of the spleen can be detected by palpation.

Technique of Splenectomy. The linea alba of the patient is shaved, cleansed and iodised. The field of operation is extended in such a way that a flap incision can be made if necessary (see p. 302). The patient is laid on its back under epidural anaesthesia. The abdomen is opened in the manner described on p. 280. If the enlargement of the spleen is especially great a flap incision is sometimes indicated. Normally, the spleen is so mobile that it can be drawn out of the wound. The splenic blood vessels of one side are ligatured en masse. This is doubly tied off, part of the omentum being included in the ligature. The vessels are then divided with scissors between the ligatures. If one puts on only one ligature haemorrhage from the spleen occurs which may greatly obscure the field of operation. One should try to tie off the splenic arteries (2) as close to the spleen as possible because one artery gives off two branches to the pancreas and ligature of these may cause pancreatic dysfunction. If the spleen is so grossly enlarged as to preclude its removal the splenic arteries should be ligated. This should be done as near to the spleen as possible in order to spare the two arterial branches going to the pancreas. After ligature the spleen atrophies when all the haemorrhage has been stopped. The abdominal wall is closed (see p. 281).

Rupture of the spleen may be expected after trauma. There is no characteristic clinical picture as pallor and anaemic mucosae only suggest internal haemorrhage which cannot be ascribed to one particular organ. To confirm a suspicion of intra-abdominal haemorrhage one does an exploratory paracentesis. If blood is withdrawn, an exploratory laparotomy should be done immediately. After opening the abdomen any blood found in it is removed. If there is a partial rupture, suture of the capsule can be attempted, but in most cases the spleen must be removed. Ruptures of the spleen may also heal spontaneously.

18. Infectious diseases

Distemper is a disease caused by the virus isolated by Carré and Laidlaw-Dunkin. It also occurs in foxes kept in farms, and in ferrets, which are ideal experimental animals for this disease. The virus can be found in the secretion of the eyes and nose and in the spleen and other organs of dogs affected by the disease. In the early stages of the disease it can also be found in the blood. The virus is not affected for a long time by drying and cold, but heat and disinfectants reduce its resistance. In the larger towns and cities distemper is endemic but the number of cases may vary enormously. In rural districts an epidemic course often occurs, which may take on the character of an explosive epidemic. The opinion of many dog-breeders that they can breed so-called "distemper-free strains" is wrong. Such "distemper-free strains" usually had little contact with virulent infection because they were reared in remote country areas. In our experience the black German Shepherd, the red long-haired Dachshund and the Fox terrier appear to be especially susceptible to the disease, but other breeds are also naturally affected. The opinion that mongrels may be especially resistant to this infection is patently absurd. The latest view of the age incidence of distemper shows that not only young dogs (3–12 months old), but also older ones (of all ages), may succumb to the disease.

It can be shown that the clinical symptoms do not always follow the classical course (masking of the virus stage). Young dogs (3–12 months old) are more liable to infection because at this time the young organism is undergoing special stresses through growth, shedding of teeth, etc. Certain injurious influences (bad management and feeding, endoparasites and ectoparasites) may also predispose to infection. If the virus has established itself in the body, secondary infections with staphylococci, streptococci, *Bordetella bronchiseptica*, etc., occur and set up a mixed infection which can mask the classical picture. The condition is highly infectious via the oral and respiratory routes, and may easily be carried by human contacts on clothing, shoes, etc.

Clinical picture. The incubation period is about 3–7 days. The temperature rises (up to 40.5 °C) and this may persist for 8–48 hours (virus stage). There is then a fall in temperature for 1–2 days followed by a further rise (biphasic temperature curve). During this period there is inappetence, serous discharge from the nose (rhinitis), eyes (conjunctivitis) and usually also a slight tonsillitis with reddening of the mucosa of the pharynx.

About 10–14 days later the secondary stage occurs. It is then called the catarrhal, respiratory or intestinal form of distemper, according to the organs affected.

The **catarrhal form** is very common. There is sneezing, occasional coughing, pale conjunctivae, and serous or mucous conjunctivitis. There may also be photophobia, inappetence, and occasionally slight diarrhoea. In the **respiratory form** which usually follows, the symptoms mentioned are more marked. To an initial pharyngitis is added a laryngitis, the mucosae of the respiratory system are more markedly affected so that the disease ultimately reaches the lungs (pectoral form), with the appearance of bronchitis and bronchopneumonia with rattling sounds on auscultation. Areas of dullness, etc., appear (see p. 219). The rhinitis becomes purulent and the colour of the discharge from the nose may become greenish-yellow. Very often this clogs the nasal openings, so that the patient breathes through the mouth (the cheeks are blown out) (Fig. 517).

The **intestinal form** produces the symptoms of alimentary disorder (see p. 274). These are complete inappetence, so that artificial feeding is necessary, and vomiting and diarrhoea. The faeces may be pulpy or quite fluid and foamy, and sometimes they are haemorrhagic (see p. 274). Peristalsis may become disorganised and intussusception of the intestine may occur (see p. 287). In the forms of distemper hitherto mentioned the temperature is always feverish. Normal temperatures are rarely seen.

The **exanthematic form** is in a special category because the virus stage cannot be observed in it. The temperature remains normal or is only slightly raised (up to 39.4 °C). There is a pustular rash on the hairless skin of the under belly, on the inner surfaces of the thigh and in the axillae. First there are red spots from which pustules are formed with greenish-yellow, almost watery contents. Later the skin

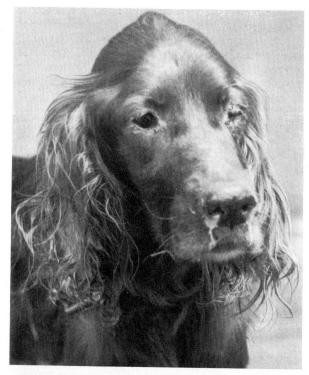

517

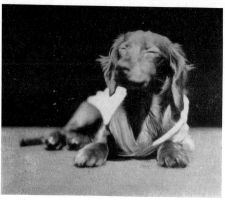

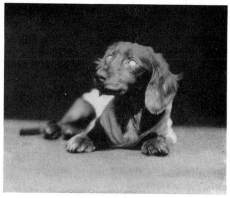

Fig. 517. Purulent nasal discharge in catarrhal distemper. In addition there is a bilateral purulent blepharitis and conjunctivitis.

Fig. 518a. Photophobia in distemper keratitis.

Fig. 518b. Parenchymatous keratitis in distemper.

518a   518b

of the pustules breaks down and a clear spot remains. Intensive treatment of this form is not necessary. It is sufficient to powder the affected spots with wound powder.

The changes in the conjunctivae of the eyelids or of the eyes are regarded by many workers as a special form of the disease, but this "eye form" accompanies almost all the other forms (except the exanthematic form) and therefore cannot

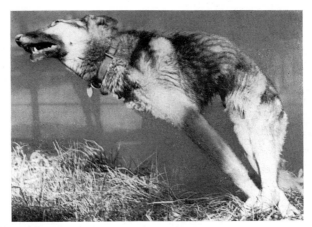

Fig. 519. Paralysis of the hindquarters in nervous distemper.

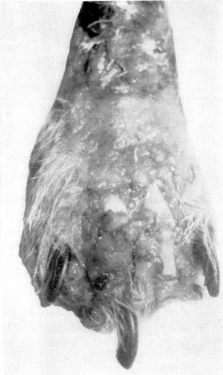

Fig. 520. Self-mutilation in distemper.

be regarded as a separate disease. The margins of the eyelids are stuck together
by a purulent exudate and must often be forcibly opened by the owner in the early
morning. The disease may spread to the cornea and to the interior of the eye,
causing cloudiness, ulceration and perforations (staphyloma, panophthalmia)
(Figs. 518a and b).

The **nervous form** of distemper is in a special category in that it does not show the disease of individual organ systems described in the secondary stage, but usually after about 14 days recovery seems to commence. The nervous form may then occur quite suddenly. The nervous symptoms may be very multifarious. There may be persistent rhythmical spasms (tonic-clonic cramps) with continuous spasms of the temporal muscles (Tick), of the lips and masticatory muscles (clicking of the teeth) and ultimately myoclonia of individual muscle groups of the limbs and of the trunk. Later paralyses occur. There is a slowly developing paresis which may ultimately pass into paralysis. At first, the animals show only uncertainty in the hindquarters when walking but later collapse on the hind legs (Fig. 519). In the final stages the animals can no longer get up and paralysis of the respiratory muscles and diaphragm ultimately leads to cessation of breathing and thus to death. In a third form of nervous distemper there are attacks of convulsions such as those seen in epilepsy (see p. 391). These convulsions may be accompanied by crying. In more severe nervous involvement, the nerve centres of the organs may be affected. There may be loss of hearing or smell, or blindness (amaurosis). Ultimately, forms of self mutilation are seen. The patients gnaw at places where puritus occurs so that the bones may be exposed. We have sometimes seen this on the ends of the limbs (Fig. 520).

Prognosis in the nervous forms should be very guarded. If the patients have a persistent temperature of over 39.7 °C (the critical temperature) in our experience the prognosis should be very unfavourable, whilst, when the temperature is lower than that, it should be cautious. If nervous distemper persists for any length of time there is marked cachexia and ultimately death. On the other hand, we have also seen cases in which, in spite of an apparently hopeless outlook, spontaneous cure occurred.

Bitches which contract distemper during pregnancy may have a miscarriage or the foetuses may be dead.

In an apparently healthy dog we often see a so-called **distemper dentition.** The surfaces of the incisors, canines and molars are brownish, rough and pitted, and show grooves and furrows. This is due to lack of formation of enamel (so-called hypoplasia) (see p. 242) and indicates an infection with distemper during teething. The degree of hypoplasia bears no relation to the severity of the distemper attack.

The diagnosis of distemper is extremely difficult, especially during the virus stage. It is often confused with tonsillitis (see p. 246).

About the course of distemper, nothing can be definitely laid down, because it can be extremely variable. We have seen dogs (especially large breeds such as Newfoundlands and St. Bernards) which died of a viraemia within 2–3 days and others which dragged on for weeks and seemed to be hopeless, but still recovered.

Convalescents must be specially cared for (maintenance and feeding) for a long time.

Treatment of distemper must be purely symptomatic. In the respiratory and catarrhal forms one uses the drugs mentioned on p. 220 for the respiratory passages and lungs. For the intestinal form the drugs recommended on p. 275 are used. It is especially important to recognise the disease during the viraemic stage and to treat it with suitable doses of serum. If a suitable quantity of serum is given at this stage the disease can be arrested before significant clinical symptoms appear. We inject 8–20 ml of distemper-hyper-immune serum and this dose seems to be effective. The hyper-immune serum may also be given during the secondary stage and often clinical improvement results. It is an open question as to how far this improvement is due to the specificity of the serum or to the albumin fraction in it. Non-specific protein therapy should be given during the secondary stage (see p. 138), and attempts should be made to control the secondary bacterial infection with antibiotics. Sulphonamide treatment should not be used because in our experience there is a clinical impression that the nervous stage may be provoked by it. It is noteworthy that Voss (Kleint.-Prax. **1**, 76, 1950) obtained good results with prednisone in various forms of the secondary stage. He combined the glucocorticoid with a broad spectrum antibiotic. The good effects of high doses of vitamin C, calcium and glucose during the secondary stage may be mentioned. These are given as a mixed injection of 500 mg of ascorbic acid and 5 ml of calcium thiosulphate in 20 ml of 40 % glucose solution. Some workers recommend 1 g ascorbic acid by intravenous injection daily.

In the nervous form, the tonic-clonic muscle spasms (chorea) cannot be influenced by drugs. If they increase, euthanasia must be considered. If they persist to the same marked degree, the owner usually becomes accustomed to and accepts the condition and improvements occur, but complete disappearance may take up to 2 years. When there are symptoms of paralysis one may use the strychnine treatment described on p. 389 and the measures there mentioned. Attacks of masticatory spasms and convulsions accompanied by crying are treated with a combination of snake venom and barbiturate.

Prophylaxis depends upon an effective immunisation procedure. At present most of the available distemper vaccines are composed of attenuated living virus propagated in tissue culture. The level of immunity depends to some extent upon the degree of attenuation of the vaccine virus, a good level of immunity resulting only if the virus retains the ability to multiply in the dog following injection. Over-attenuated strains may fail to provoke an effective immunity. The age for immunisation depends upon the level of maternal antibodies present in the puppy. If this is high then the virus will be neutralised before it has time to multiply. To cover this situation one of three methods may be adopted:

(1) Immunisation is delayed until the maternal antibodies have waned at around 11 weeks of age. This delay, however, will mean that quite a proportion of the puppies in a litter will be at risk from the time their maternal antibody falls until the time of vaccination.

(2) Double vaccination may be practised, where a first dose of vaccine is given at 8 weeks of age and repeated at 11 weeks. Puppies not responding to the first dose should be fully protected by the second injection.

(3) The puppies may be vaccinated with a measles vaccine, which is antigenically similar to distemper vaccine but to which maternal antibodies are not produced. One disadvantage of this method is that bitches vaccinated with measles vaccine as pups will pass on maternal antibodies to measles virus to their pups, thus invalidating the whole procedure.

Unless the vaccinated dog is exposed to contact with natural infection, the immunity level will fall off progressively over the following years. For this reason it is recommended that a booster dose of vaccine should be given 18 months to 2 years after the primary immunisation.

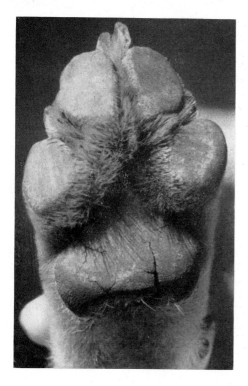

Fig. 521. Hardpad Disease. The skin of the pads is hard and a few days later was completely detached.

Most distemper vaccines are now combined with Canine Viral Hepatitis and Leptospirosis vaccines in a single injection.

Hardpad Disease is a form of distemper also caused by the classical distemper virus, but as the clinical picture differs in certain points from distemper, this disease will be described separately.

Clinical picture. Usually the biphasic temperature curve cannot be detected and the symptoms seen in the eyelids and nose in distemper are also absent. Very often intractable diarrhoea occurs. In the course of the disease hyperkeratoses develop on the pads, which are cracked and later hardened and become flattened and levelled off with a well-marked margin (Fig. 521). As the disease progresses the horny layer of the pads becomes completely detached. Hyperkeratosis can also be detected in the nose which is also fissured and scales off. Unfortunately, during the examination of a dog affected with distemper, hyperkeratosis is given too little attention. Sometimes the owner supplies the information that the patient "clatters" as it walks along. As the disease progresses, disorders of the central nervous system appear which are identical with those seen in distemper, but the temperature remains around 39.5 °C in many cases.

The prognosis should be extremely guarded after the appearance of nervous symptoms.

Treatment consists initially in giving a suitable amount of distemper hyper-immune serum. If nervous symptoms are apparent, injections of serum are useless.

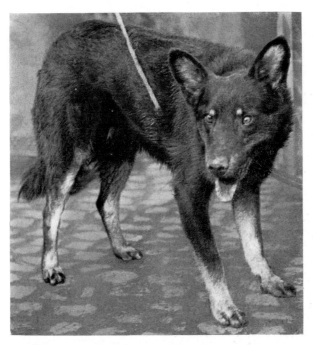

Fig. 522. Rabies. The dog stares aimlessly anywhere. The toe joints are gnawed and show hairless places. There is also convergent squint. (Photo by Prof. Dr. K. VÖHRINGER, Halle.)

Symptomatic treatment should be given according to the principles described for distemper.

Rabies is caused by a filterable virus. It is a disease of the central nervous system which affects all domesticated animals and man. Carnivores are especially affected and therefore the law pays special attention to the behaviour of dogs. Nevertheless, PITZCHKE (Mhefte Vet. Med. **11**, 511, 1956) was able to confirm that rabies of the dog has declined in our country whilst it is on the increase in cats and wild animals (fox, badger, marten, deer, etc.).

The virus occurs in a concentrated form in the central nervous system of animals affected and also in the saliva, blood, but only exceptionally in the milk. Natural infection is due to a bite in most cases. The virus (neurotropic) passes to the nerve tracts and hence to the brain from which it spreads peripherally.

Clinical picture. The incubation period may be extremely variable. Among other things, it depends on the distance of the site of infection from the central nervous system, on the virulence of the virus, and on the general condition of the patient. An incubation period of 2–8 weeks may be expected.

Three stages of classical rabies can be distinguished, but under natural conditions these merge into one another, so that the stages become indistinct.

The melancholy stage begins with a change in psychical behaviour. Good-natured dogs become capricious and morose, whilst ill-natured dogs may become

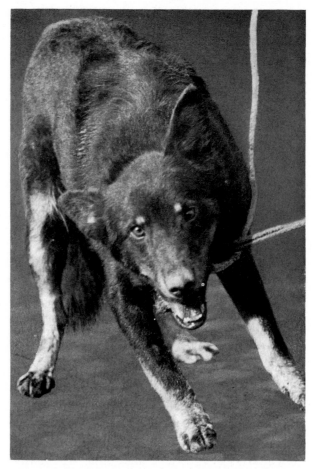

Fig. 523. Rabies. The dog strangles itself on its lead. (Photo by Prof. Dr. K. VÖHRINGER, Halle.)

more amenable. In addition, there is photophobia. The animals seek out dark places and corners. Typical of this stage also is the so-called "snapping at flies", a purposeless biting at the air. This is expressed by jumping up or colliding with objects as a result of acoustic stimuli. The reflexes are exaggerated. Particular changes in the pupils (alternating miosis and mydriasis) may be detected. The so-called "perverse appetite" makes the animal ingest objects that it would otherwise not swallow (fabrics, wood, stones, earth, faeces, etc.). The normal food is refused. During swallowing of indigestible objects, difficulties in swallowing may occur. The animal readily attempts to drink but only succeeds in swallowing a small amount. As a result of the difficulties in swallowing, there is a slowly-increasing flow of saliva. The nerves altered by the virus in the region of the bite appear to irritate because the site is constantly gnawed or lacerated (auto-mutilation) (Fig. 522). This stage lasts about ½–3 days and leads to the **stage of frenzy.**

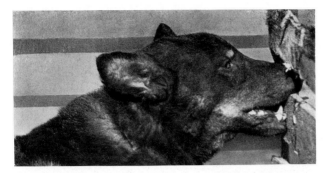

Fig. 524. Rabies. The dog tries to bite through the battens of its cage.

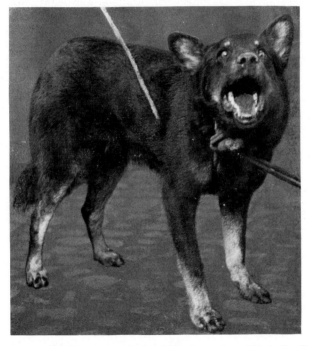

Fig. 525. Rabies. Hoarse howling in paralysis of the lower jaw. (Photo by Prof. Dr. K. Vöh-
RINGER, Halle.)

In this, the symptoms already described intensify. The animal seeks opportunities
to break out and escape (urgent desire to roam about). It may cover great distances
and may not find its way home again. During this time desire to bite and attack
is especially marked, but barking and snarling are completely absent (Fig. 523).
If the dog has no chance to break out during the attacks of frenzy, which alternate
with the intervals of depression, it bites the bars of its cage, its chain or objects

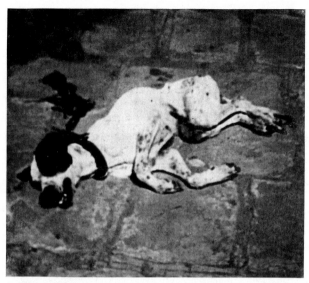

Fig. 526. Rabies. Complete paralysis. (Photo by Prof. Dr. B. NATSCHEFF, Sofia.)

held in front of it (for example, a red hot iron) (Fig. 524). At this stage paralyses of the eye muscles set in (nystagmus, strabismus) and these give the dog an innocent, artful, facial expression. The commencing symptoms of paralyses indicate the third stage. Nerves of the swallowing muscles seem to be especially affected. Salivary secretion increases.

The stage of depression sets in after the previous stage has lasted ½–8 days. The paralyses of individual muscle groups increase and the typical picture of paralysis of the lower jaw, the tongue and the eyes (trigeminal nerve) appears. The animal merely howls (Fig. 525). The paralyses spread to the muscles of the limbs and body and this ultimately leads to total paralysis and the death of the animal (Fig. 526).

Silent or Dumb Rabies is distinguished from the classical rabies described by the transition of the separate stages into one another, or by the fact that the stage of frenzy is not specially marked. There may be an immediate transition from the melancholic to the paralytic stage.

Silent rabies is manifested by apathy, little tendency to bite or howl, inappetence and a rapidly advancing paralysis. Sometimes there are also cases which are clinically little different from those already described. A dog brought to the clinic because of the sudden appearance of a tendency to bite showed a special tendency to bite the toes of shoes. It could be induced to bite a stick held in front of it only after exciting it to bite for a long time. After 8 days it died in convulsions and Negri bodies were detected. In addition, reference may be made to the case reported by VÖHRINGER (Mhefte Vet. Med. **10**, 320, 1955) in which the symptoms of rabies were so little evident on the first day of treatment that only a disorder of the gastro-intestinal tract was diagnosed.

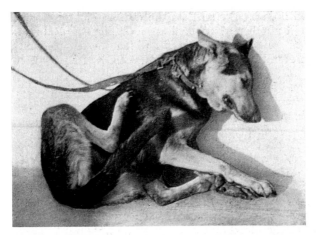

Fig. 527. Aujeszky's disease. Marked itching at the site of the bite. (Photo by Prof. Dr. B. NAT-SCHEFF, Sofia.)

The duration of the disease is about 3–7 days but cases have been reported which died in 2 to 27 days. The disease usually, but not invariably, results in death. Therefore there is no justification for the criterion that a dog, which has bitten a man but remains alive, was not infected with rabies.

Diagnosis may be very easy if the foregoing description of the clinical picture is applied. But lack of a preliminary report may make a clinical diagnosis doubtful. Therefore, if there is the slightest suspicion, one should arrange that the animal in question is kept under strict observation for several days.

Treatment of a rabid dog is forbidden. To prevent an epidemic drastic police regulations are imposed (quarantine, restraint by leads or muzzles, the capture or shooting of stray dogs, etc.). An obligatory protective inoculation of all dogs in a specified region cannot eradicate the disease in our country because a reservoir of infection exists in cats and wild animals.

Pseudorabies (Aujeszky's disease) is rare in the dog. The mode of infection is not yet known with certainty, but infection by the mouth is easy whilst it is only occasionally transmitted by the bite of infected dogs. The virus can be detected in the blood but not in the saliva.

Clinical picture. The incubation period is 3–6–10 days. The disease sets in with apathy, inappetence and photophobia. Sometimes there are expressions of pain (howling, groaning). An ever increasing irritation of certain parts of the body causes the animal to rub and gnaw at these parts (automutilation) (Fig. 527). Meanwhile, attacks of frenzy and destructiveness may occur. Alternating miosis and mydriasis of the pupils may be seen. The desire to attack and the paralysis of the lower jaw seen in rabies are absent. The patient may die within 1–1½ days.

No treatment is known.

Infectious Inflammation of the Liver [Canine Viral Hepatitis (C.V.H.), Rubarth's disease] is caused by a virus which is identical with the cause of encephalitis of foxes. Young dogs 2–3 months old are especially affected. They may be simultane-

30*

ously infected with distemper so that the clinical picture is confused. Probably only quite a small number of affected animals show clinical signs of the disease. This fact emerges from many reports in which the complement-fixation test is positive in a considerable number of dogs that are healthy, or were not previously clinically ill.

Clinical picture. The incubation period is 3–5 days. Then the temperature rises to 41.0 °C and this influences the general condition of the dog to a remarkable degree (apathy, inappetence). Often a tonsillitis with enlargement of the mandibular lymph glands can be detected. The mucosae of the head region react with serous inflammation. In most cases palpation in the region of the xiphoid cartilage (liver) causes pain. Sometimes there are also cramps. Oedema of the head, neck and body are also described. In some cases we found vomiting and haemorrhagic diarrhoea. The serous conjunctivitis and rhinitis became purulent. According to FREUDIGER (Schweiz. Arch. Tierhlk. **99**, 487, 1957) there is often a milky opacity of the cornea. When this symptom occurs it is regarded as diagnostic.

Investigation of the blood and urine plays an important part in the diagnosis. In the initial stages a leucopaenia always seems to occur, which is later replaced by a leucocytosis. The blood sedimentation rate is increased, coagulability is decreased and the a_2-globulin increased. There is also albuminuria. Serological examination of the blood is of no value for early diagnosis because complement-fixing antibodies cannot be detected before the 7th day of the disease. One can consider the diagnosis to be correct if the complement-fixation test is at first negative and becomes positive later in the course of the disease.

The course may be acute or very acute, so that usually any therapeutic measures are too late. When the course is subacute or chronic (2–4 weeks) the disease is only rarely recognised because of difficulties in differentiating it from distemper.

Treatment is symptomatic in every case. Special attention should be given to treatment designed to relieve and protect the liver (see p. 320). This can be carried to the extent that the patient has only sweetened water during the first days of the disease. Among antibiotics good results are ascribed to chloramphenicol and preparations of the tetracycline group. To increase the coagulability of the blood, vitamin K is injected. In the early stages serum treatment with hepatitis serum or with combined bivalent homologous sera (duo serum) is given in carefully controlled dosage. We agree here with the opinion of Freudiger that the albumin fraction in the sera may sometimes have an injurious effect on the badly-damaged liver.

As a prophylactic measure active immunisation against the infective agent causing hepatitis can be achieved with a live or killed vaccine which is usually combined with Distemper and Leptospirosis vaccines (see p. 462).

Tuberculosis is an infectious disease caused by **Mycobacterium tuberculosis,** which in the dog causes the most varied symptoms and usually has a chronic course. Recently, an increase in cases of tuberculosis has been detected in this clinic. How far this is to be ascribed to better diagnosis is an open question. It is impossible to decide whether the dog is a source of infection of man or vice versa. FREUDIGER and KUSLYS (Schweiz. Zschr. Tuberc. **12**, 247, 1955) found the bovine type of tuberculosis in 3 tuberculous dogs, and in a summary of the literature in the same paper, among 271 infected dogs there were 193 with the human type, 68 with the bovine type and 1 with the avian type. In two cases the typing was atypical. In the dog the points of entry of the infection are the respiratory and

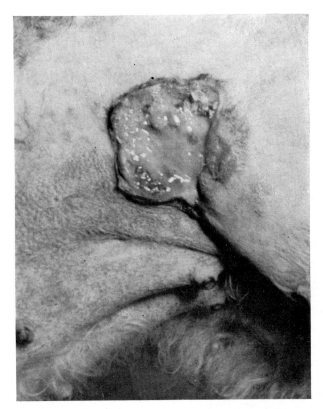

Fig. 528. Tuberculosis of the skin in the femoral fold of a Bedlington terrier.

digestive organs, as well as the skin. In his material PALLASKE (Berl. Münch. tierärztl. Wschr. **70**, 1–7 and 28–31, 1957) found the primary focus to be in the respiratory organs in 64.8 % of cases, in the digestive organs in 31.5 % and in the skin in 3.7 %. Tuberculosis may occur at any age but very young and quite old dogs do not seem to be affected so often.

Clinical picture. In most cases the history is not very informative. The animals are apathetic, often emaciated and show intractable respiratory disorders or diarrhoea and loss of appetite. The coat is rough and lustreless. The turgor of the skin may be decreased. Fistulae may appear on the outer surface or there may be wounds which show no tendency to heal (Fig. 528). Otitis that resists treatment indicates the possibility of a tuberculous infection. Palpation of the lymph glands may reveal enlargement of individual glands. In emaciated dogs, abdominal palpation may reveal enlargement of individual mesenteric lymph glands and possibly deposits may be detected in the liver and spleen. Enlargements of individual lymph glands indicate in many cases a tubercular infection. Percussion may possibly detect fluid in the thorax. Use should be made of auscultation to detect pathological respiratory sounds, although this does not provide definite

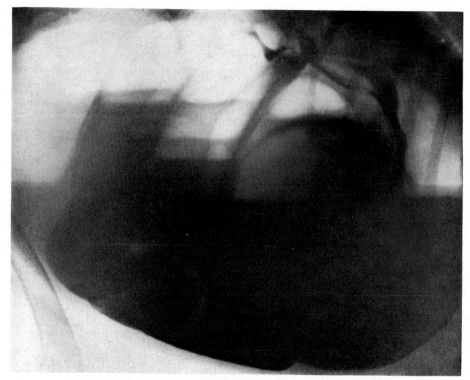

Fig. 529. Intestinal tuberculosis (diagnosed postmortem) in a German Shepherd. Marked accumulation of gas and fluid in the dilated loop of the intestine (mirror-image). In the stomach granules of bone. Clinical diagnosis: compression ileus due to tumours (enlarged lymph glands).

evidence of tuberculosis. Very often there is very pronounced coughing which is little influenced by the usual drugs. Collections of fluid in the thorax and also in the pericardium affect the respiration and activity of the heart. Sometimes the existence of acropachia (see p. 436) may indicate tubercular infection. If the digestive tract is infected, this can cause intractable diarrhoea and meteorism. Abdominal ascites often develops as a secondary expression of obstruction (Fig. 529). X-ray examination of the thorax may provide certain information about pulmonary tuberculosis. Differential diagnosis must exclude other diseases such as streptotrichosis, cancer, etc., and often this is impossible. "Marbling" or "cloudiness of the lungs" raises the possibility of tubercular disease (Fig. 530).

Often these investigations do not produce a definite result so that in addition allergic tests must be used. We regard the subcutaneous thermal reaction as very useful. Old or synthetic tuberculin can be used. We have found that the best time for tuberculinisation is the early hours of the morning. The diagnostic rise of temperature occurs within 2–8 hours of the subcutaneous injection of 0.2 ccm of tuberculin and is regarded as being positive if it exceeds 1 °C and becomes febrile. Nevertheless, in very emaciated dogs the reaction may not occur (Fig. 531).

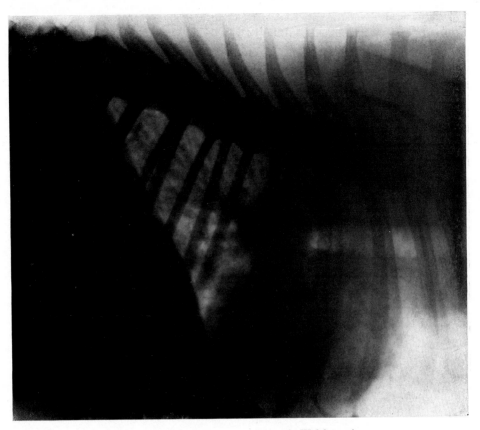

Fig. 530. Lung tuberculosis in a male Welsh terrier.

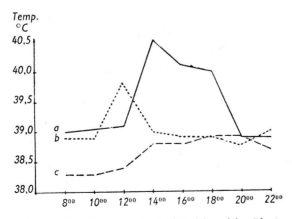

Fig. 531. Course of the temperature in a normal reaction. (a) positive (the temperature has risen more than 1 °C to become febrile); (b) doubtful (the temperature has also become febrile); (c) negative (the rise of temperature is not significant).

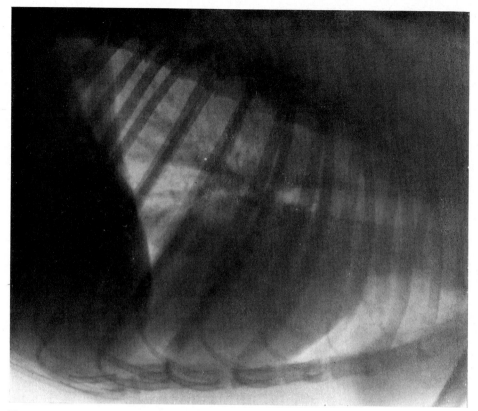

Fig. 532. Tuberculosis of the lung in a 3-year-old Welsh terrier (Fig. 530). Condition after 6 months
with treatment with INH (Isonicotinic acid hydrazide).

The dose of tuberculin should always be taken from an ampoule that has been
properly stored and freshly opened, because tuberculin may undergo certain
changes when it is exposed to the air. Very often there is a discrepancy between
the thermal reaction and the subsequent postmortem findings. We feel that a
positive result of a thermal reaction combined with a clinical diagnosis of tuberculosis is more valid than a negative postmortem, as in relatively early infections
no macroscopic lesion may be visible.

The haemagglutination test of Middlebrook and Dubos is to be assessed very
cautiously. This reaction fails especially in quite early cases, in which the antibodies are still absent, and also in severe cases in which no more antibodies are free
because of flooding of the body with antigens. We do not consider haematological
examination to be of much value in diagnosis. The findings (leucocytosis, accelerated
blood sedimentation rate, etc.) are too general to be accepted as specific for this
disease. Among other diagnostic methods are the microscopic examination of
sputum and discharges, the cultivation of the causative agent and animal inoculation.

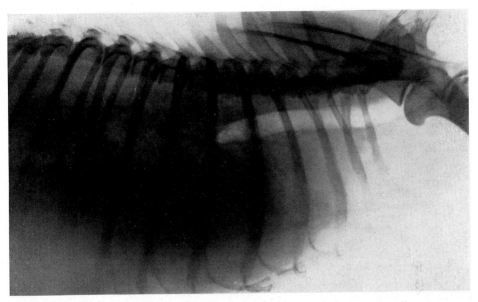

Fig. 533. Tuberculosis of the lung in a 3-year-old Welsh terrier. After cessation of the treatment with INH sudden deterioration occurred which led to collapse.

Treatment is possible with tuberculostatics. Our experience in the dog is based on the use of isonicotinic acid hydrazide. The dose for the dog is 10 mg/kg body weight per day and treatment must be continued for weeks or months (Fig. 532). We have not so far seen a cure with this drug. On the contrary, after the drug is withheld the symptoms flare up again and then finally there is a breakdown which can no longer be arrested (Fig. 533). The patient is always a source of infection for human contacts. For these reasons one should refuse treatment of a tuberculous dog and advise euthanasia. Exceptionally, one will start treatment in cases in which a member of the family is himself infected in order not to risk the psychical worry that he has infected his dog and thus caused its death.

Localised forms of tuberculosis of the skin can be surgically treated.

Streptotrichosis is a bacterial disease caused by *Nocardia canis* or *Streptothrix canis*. Infection is presumably through skin wounds.

The clinical picture may be very variable. Sometimes the predominant feature is pleurisy or peritonitis (Fig. 534). Sometimes a fistulous swelling appears on the skin. Differential diagnosis from tuberculosis by means of a tuberculin test, or examination of fluid taken by puncture or of the discharge of the fistula for tubercle bacilli or streptothrix threads, should not be omitted. Typical of streptotrichosis are small whitish-yellow soft granules in the discharge.

Treatment of the cutaneous form is by surgical removal of the foci. EIKMEIER (Dtsch. tierärztl. Wschr. **64**, 303, 1957) has cured cases of streptotrichosis of the peritoneum and skin with a combination of high doses of penicillin and streptomycin. Decisive factors in this treatment are probably the high dosage and ad-

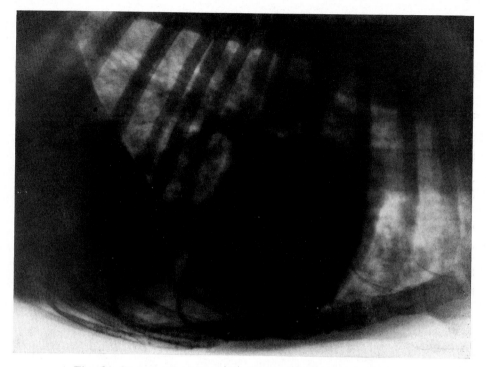

Fig. 534. Streptotrichosis in the lungs of an 8-year-old male Alsatian.

ministration for 10 days with subsequent repetition for 6 days after an interval of 10 days.

Salmonellosis may or may not produce clinical signs in the dog. Very often in clinically healthy dogs, when a bacteriological examination of the faeces is done, Salmonellae (mostly *S. typhimurium* and *S. enteritidii* GÄRTNER) are found. In other animals disorders of the general condition occur which especially affect the digestive tract. Chronic diarrhoea, which resists the usual treatment, may be catarrhal or haemorrhagic. There may also be vomiting, inappetence and a febrile temperature. When the intestinal infection persists for a long time, a profound anaemia may develop which may be serious and resistant to treatment. Sometimes there is jaundice, and nervous symptoms have been described by various authors.

Treatment is given with chloramphenicol for several days. Continuous examination of the faeces is necessary. Possibly an examination of the environment should be done to find the source of infection.

Anthrax is rare in the dog. It occurs most often on the lips (after ingestion of infected material) in the form of cutaneous anthrax. Sometimes there is haemorrhagic diarrhoea and the appetite may be decreased.

Treatment is given with anthrax serum (15–30 m*l*) and penicillin must be given at the same time for 4–5 days. Care should be taken to support the circulation.

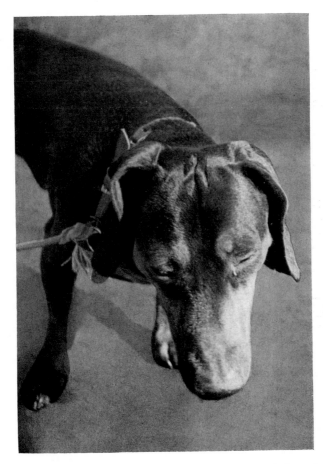

Fig. 535. Tetanus. Contraction of the temporal muscles and photophobia.

Tetanus is occasionally seen in the dog. *Clostridium tetani* is anaerobic and neurotropic.

The clinical symptoms commence after an incubation period of a few days to weeks. Very often we were able to diagnose tetanus after the site of infection had already healed up (Scar tetanus). There are muscular contractions to some extent. Local tetanus (restricted to the muscles of the head) seems to occur in the dog. Contraction of the temporal muscles causes the ears to be drawn together over the head and also protrusion of the eyeballs. Affection of the jaw muscles prevents passive or active opening of the mouth. The patient cannot take in food. Fluids are drunk if the whole mouth can be immersed in the fluid. The patient is very sensitive to mechanical and acoustic stimuli, causing accentuation of the muscle spasm. In generalised tetanus the limbs also are affected and the dog takes up the well-known "saw-horse" attitude. Ultimately, contraction of the thoracic muscles and of the diaphragm may cause respiratory failure leading to the death of the animal. Consciousness is fully maintained during the disease.

The course of the disease may be very variable. Prognosis must always be guarded because pneumonia may be a complication.

Treatment is by giving high doses of penicillin (about 50,000 units per kg body-weight) for 6–7 days. The patient should be protected from any external stimuli until the muscle spasms abate and should be kept in a quiet, darkened room. Tranquillisers and muscle relaxants are useful.

Botulism (*Clostridium botulinum*) has a very short incubation period, after which there are changes in the eyes, the digestive apparatus and the nervous system. There is always a conjunctivitis, which may be followed by ulcerative keratitis, iritis or haemorrhage into the anterior chamber of the eye. Miosis and strabismus are also seen. Digestive symptoms include complete loss of appetite, difficulty in swallowing food forcibly given and marked obstipation. Changes in the nervous system begin with an inability to move the eyes. Then follows a paralysis of the muscles of the neck and shoulder (the head can no longer be held up) and a progressive loss of co-ordination of the muscles of the limbs. The course of the disease ends in a coma-like state with respiration that is scarcely perceptible. Death finally results from asphyxia but many cases recover.

Treatment can only be symptomatic. It is very important to empty the alimentary canal (with high pressure enemas) (see p. 36), obstipation is treated with castor oil (30–50 ml). We have no experience of the use of botulinus toxoid. Prophylaxis (giving only fresh meat in the diet) is of great importance.

Leptospirosis may be caused by *Leptospira icterohaemorrhagica* or *L. canicola*. Infection with *L. icterohaemorrhagica* corresponds to Weil's disease of man. The reservoir of infection is in rats. Dogs should therefore be kept away from stagnant water which may be infected with the urine of rats. Dogs bitten by rats can also be infected.

The source of infection with *L. canicola* is chiefly the dog itself. Clinical illness only occurs in a proportion of infected dogs, there being many carriers of the disease. The intact and injured skin and mucosae (chiefly the mucosa of the mouth) are the main portals of infection, followed by the alimentary route. Leptospira are excreted in the urine and saliva. There is no especial breed incidence but male dogs are infected more often than bitches. This would appear to be due to the propensity of the male to sniff and lick places on which other dogs have previously urinated. In densely populated areas leptospirosis may become epidemic whilst in the country it is only sporadic. Cases are most numerous in the autumn and early spring. We most often see the clinical signs of leptospirosis in dogs between 2 and 3 years old, whilst older and old dogs often show latent infection.

Clinical picture. Icteric, uraemic and gastrointestinal forms of the disease are seen. The incubation period is on the average 5–20 days.

The icteric form is almost exclusively caused by *L. icterohaemorrhagica*. It begins with high fever (up to about 40 °C) and this may fall to normal on the second day or may even become subnormal. Jaundice is evident from about the 4th day onwards. Usually, the mucosae of the eyelids and mouth first become coloured. Later (on the 6–7th day) jaundice of the lower abdomen and inner surface of the thighs is evident. The mucosae may often show a tendency to bleed. This is revealed when the edges of the gums are vigorously rubbed with the pads of the fingers.

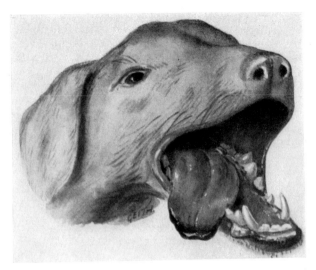

Fig. 536. Commencing necrosis of the tip of the tongue in leptospirosis.

The areas of the liver and kidneys are sensitive to pressure. The urine is brownish (bile pigments) and changes to green when exposed to the air. The urine has a high content of albumin and kidney cells with casts, leucocytes and erythrocytes in the sediment. During the disease, apathy, inappetence and gastrointestinal disorders such as vomiting and diarrhoea (which may be haemorrhagic) occur. After about 10–14 days of the disease the patient is completely emaciated and death soon occurs. Recovery does occur, but is rare.

The uraemic form also begins with a one-day rise of temperature. In addition, there is marked apathy increasing later to somnolence. Inappetence and intractable vomiting are seen and diarrhoea in all its variants may be added to these. The history usually records polydipsia. The patients show a tight, tense gait and the back may be arched (like the arched back of a cat). Pressure on the region of the loins causes pain. The mucosae are coloured a dirty red. This is especially evident on the mucosae of the cheeks and on the edges of the tongue, passing into a brownish coloration (Fig. 536), and the margins of the gums where they meet the teeth are brown. In many cases slight erosions of the mucosa of the mouth can be detected which later develop into extensive ulcers and penetrate deeply and contain a greyish-green necrotic deposit with a tendency to bleed. These ulcers usually develop first in the mucosa of the cheeks at the level of the canine and carnassial teeth, especially if these teeth have a deposit of tartar on them. Signs of ulceration appear on the edges of the tongue which may lead to necrosis of the whole marginal area. Ultimately, only a stump of the tongue remains. The tonsils are also affected in most cases. The mouth emits a gangrenous or uraemic odour (fetor of the mouth). The intractable vomiting and diarrhoea, which are sometimes watery, and a usually persistent polyuria (though anuria is also seen) cause de-hydration. This, together with the existing emaciation, cause a loss of elasticity of the skin (exsiccosis). Folds of skin pulled up remain standing or sink down only very slowly. The episcleral blood vessels are markedly injected and because they are full of blood they become sinuous. The pulse is irregular (jerky), wiry, or full and bounding. The blood urea nitrogen may be increased 5–10 times as a sign of renal insufficiency. Examination of the urine reveals a high degree of kidney damage. It contains abundant albumin, bile pigments and indican. The sediment contains kidney cells, casts, leucocytes and erythrocytes. This acute uraemic form lasts for about 6–10 days. The mortality may be very high. Patients that recover have a chronic nephritis, which should be borne in mind in the subsequent veterinary supervision of such an animal.

The symptoms of the gastrointestinal form are similar to those of the uraemic form. The uraemic symptoms are rather subdued and the gastrointestinal ones predominate. Vomiting and diarrhoea especially occur and the vomit and faeces may contain blood. This results in such symptoms as exsiccosis, circulatory troubles and kidney damage. During convalescence and subsequently, special attention must be paid to the kidneys because in this form also chronic nephritis follows the disease. We have not encountered the trembling of the muscles and the stiffening of the hindquarters described by GRATZL (Zentralbl. Vet. Med. 4, 945, 1957). The highest percentages of cures occur in the gastrointestinal form.

In chronic leptospirosis usually the symptoms are not well defined. Lassitude, inappetence, polydipsia and polyuria occur. Sometimes long continued gastrointestinal affections can be the expression of leptospirosis, the disease lasting more than 3 weeks, during which time the nutritional condition of the patients deteriorates remarkably and they become cachectic.

Diagnosis rests not only on the clinical picture, but also on determining the causative agent and on serological examination. In the early stages the causative agent can be found in the blood plasma by dark ground illumination. This can be done only by experienced workers whose wide experience enables them to differentiate clearly the spirochaetes from pseudospirillae, filarias, etc.

The spirochaetes can be found in the urine on the 7–10th day of the disease, at the earliest, by dark ground illumination. This technique is important for the identification of Leptospira carriers because leptospiruria may persist for months after clinical cure. Nevertheless, it must be stated that according to the investigations of ZISCH (Thesis, Vienna, 1951) there are dogs affected by leptospirosis in whose urine Leptospira can never be found. The agglutination-lysis test is little used for early diagnosis, because agglutination is not positive until the 12–14th day of the disease (RANDALL, J. Amer. vet. med. Ass. 112, 136, 1948). Examination of the urine by dark ground illumination and the agglutination-lysis test are recommended.

Treatment. Antibiotics have revolutionised the treatment of leptospirosis. We use streptomycin and inject 50 mg per kg weight on 3–6 successive days. Often a combination of streptomycin and penicillin is to be recommended. Streptomycin seems to remove the leptospiruria, but penicillin alone does not always do this. On the second or third day of treatment with sufficiently high dosage, a significant improvement of the patient's condition occurs. If this does not happen, one should immediately change the treatment to the tetracyclines. Nevertheless, symptomatic treatment should not be discontinued. Intravenous injection of 10 % sodium chloride solution (see p. 264) is especially important and can have a beneficial effect on the intractable vomiting. Treatment to protect the liver (see p. 320) should be given in every case. As to diet, no food should be given on the first

2–3 days, except possibly water sweetened with sugar. Later, only lean meat cut up small with small quantities of rice water are given. The patient is kept in a warm, well-ventilated room. The risk of transmission from affected dogs to man seems to be slight. As a prophylactic against the various forms of leptospirosis, leptospirosis vaccine (see p. 462) is used.

Toxoplasmosis is carried by the protozoan *Toxoplasma gondii*. It seems to be extremely widely distributed. According to Hoare (cited by SCHNELLNER and VOLL-BRECHTSHAUSEN, Tierärztl. Umschau **10**, 307, 1957) spontaneous infections have so far been found in 45 mammalian, 70 avian and 5 cold-blooded species. This indicates that the dog is not the sole carrier of the infection to man, as has been supposed in many quarters. The toxoplasms are distributed in the body in the blood and lymphatics. Infection is chiefly alimentary, e.g., by eating infected prey, such as rodents.

Unfortunately, not much can be said about the clinical picture of toxoplasmosis, because our experience of it is still quite limited. The incubation period is one to a few weeks. Gastrointestinal disorders, bronchopneumonia and general emaciation are described. In pregnant bitches, abortions have been noted. Nervous symptoms are very often described. These consist of aggressiveness, epileptiform convulsions, sudden paraplegias and meningo-encephalitic symptoms. According to Schnellner and Vollbrechtshausen, toxoplasmosis should be borne in mind in any case of unexplained encephalitis.

Diagnosis is by Sabin and Feldman's serological dye-reaction, but with this the question arises whether a high titre must be interpreted as being positive only for toxoplasmosis. CATEL (Münch. med. Wschr. **99**, 973, 1957) specifies a titre of 1 : 1024 and higher as suggestive of toxoplasmosis. SCHNELLNER and VOLLBRECHTS-HAUSEN endorse this opinion, whilst PIEKARSKI (Verhdl. Dtsch. Ges. Inn. Med. 1954, 60, Contress) maintains that a titre above 1 : 250 probably indicates a toxoplasma infection.

Treatment. No effective therapeutic methods are known. GROULADE (Bull. Acad. med. France **29**, 49, 1956) was able to obtain good effects on the nervous symptoms with sulphonamides (first given parenterally and then orally for 20 days). A combination of the drug Pyrimethamine in a dose of 1 mg/kg with the sulphonamide Sulphadiazine 50 mg/kg is the most effective treatment available.

19. Toxicology

A wide variety of poisons is given to dogs with malicious intent or through carelessness. Malicious poisoning is rare and most cases of poisoning are the result of ignorance that substances are poisonous to the dog or of overdosing with certain drugs. Therefore only a few risks of poisoning which have a special interest will be discussed.

Arsenical poisoning is caused by arsenious acid or its metallic salts. It can occur when the dog ingests rat poisons containing arsenic or by arsenic treatment with doses that are too high. The lethal dose by the mouth is 0.1–0.2 g, whilst parenterally 0.02 g suffices to cause death.

The clinical picture of acute arsenical poisoning is one of salivation, retching and vomiting (the vomit often mixed with blood), marked sensitivity to pain when the abdomen is palpated, polydipsia, and colicky pains. These symptoms are at first accompanied by obstipation, which later changes to enteritis with the passage of haemorrhagic foul-smelling faeces. Sometimes haematuria develops. The circulation is severely damaged. Respiration is accelerated and this is accompanied by general weakness, giddiness and collapse. Death may occur after a few hours or after some days with coma. In diagnosis a clue can be gained from the garlic-like odour of the breath due to the formation of arsenic hydride (arseniuretheal hydrogen, arsine).

Chronic arsenical poisoning (arsenical fumes disease) causes slow cachexia. Prominent features of the clinical picture are apathy, inappetence, coughing, respiratory difficulties, affections of the skin, general weakness and possibly paralyses.

The treatment of acute cases is by giving apomorphine hydrochloride (2–3 mg subcutaneously) in order to stimulate the vomiting of any residue of the poison still in the stomach. Sulphur treatment with sodium thiosulphate (5–15 ml) or dithioglycerin is an important antidote. Dithioglycerin (2 mg per kg bodyweight) is given intramuscularly for 3–4 days. Administration of large amounts of animal charcoal should not be omitted. To combat the circulatory collapse (paralyses of the capillaries) vasopressive agents are given.

Lead Poisoning causes the so-called "saturnism". It may result from licking the painted walls of kennels (red lead, white lead, litharge) or by ingesting objects containing lead (lead shot or lead weights) which may remain in the stomach as foreign bodies for months and cause chronic lead poisoning, as reported by PETIT et al. (J. Amer. vet. med. Ass. **128**, 205, 1956).

The clinical symptoms are salivation, vomiting, colic, obstipation, enteritis, and nervous symptoms, which may consist of epileptiform fits, opisthotonus and attacks of mania. In addition, the lead absorbed (as complex compounds) can cause severe damage to the kidneys, liver and heart muscle. The nervous system also shows inflammatory changes (polyneuritis, paralysis of the upper pharynx and the vocal cords, etc.). In chronic poisoning the so-called "blue line" appears on the gingiva. The patients become emaciated and develop skin lesions (pruritus, pustular eruption), changes in the blood picture (anaemia) and a chronic polyneuritis.

Sulphur treatment is given exactly as for arsenical poisoning. The circulation should be supported. Administration of large quantities of magnesium sulphate is to be recommended as this has a purgative effect and also converts the lead into harmless lead sulphate. In addition, injections of glucose (nephritis) and doses of the vitamin B complex (polyneuritis) are to be recommended. The administration of calcium disodium versenate intravenously, in doses of 1 ml of a 25 % solution diluted with 10 ml of 5 % glucose saline and repeated at 3–4 day intervals, is the treatment of choice. The injection should be made slowly to avoid shock reaction.

Coumarin and Warfarin poisoning are possible because these substances are often used as rat poisons. Poisoning occurs by ingestion of poison baits (pieces of meat) or by eating poisoned rodents. They are anticoagulants because they inhibit the formation of prothrombin in the liver. They increase capillary permeability and thus cause large haemorrhages into the tissues.

The clinical picture is one of marked liability to haemorrhage. Slight injuries may lead to the formation of extensive haematomata. Bleeding from the nose and blood in the vomit or faeces are often seen. The mucosae are pale or cyanotic, and the pulse is rapid and weak. Because of their general bodily weakness the animals lie down. A fall of the temperature until it is subnormal indicates the approach of death, which soon follows with collapse.

Treatment is usually difficult because acute poisoning leads to death in a few hours. High doses of vitamin K and transfusions with glucose saline or "Macrodex" may be tried.

Insecticide poisoning with DDT (Dichlorodiphenyl-trichlorethane) and BHC (gamma benzene hexachloride), which are present in many insecticides, may occur, especially when such products are used without veterinary advice. DDT and BHC are poisonous if there is a possibility of their absorption due to previous solution in fats. Therefore dogs in which these compounds are used to destroy ectoparasites should be fed a fat-free diet before and during treatment.

The clinical picture consists chiefly of nervous symptoms. These begin with restlessness, muscle spasms, clonic cramps, mydriasis and finally paralyses.

Treatment consists of the immediate removal of remains of the powder on the coat, in order to prevent further intake of the poison. The alimentary canal is cleaned out with emetic enemas (see p. 36). Injections of calcium may be given. The convulsions are treated with pentobarbitone given slowly intravenously. Fats and milk are contraindicated.

Poisoning with E-compounds (".605", "Wofatox") occurs when these compounds are carelessly used to kill vermin.

The clinical picture begins with restlessness, sudden jumping up and lying down again. There are vomiting and colicky pains, enteritis and sometimes also convulsions. The pulse is hard and rapid. Miosis occurs which disappears just before death. Sometimes there is oedema of the mucosae of the head region, so that respiration may be difficult. In coma the muscles are completely relaxed and there is rattling respiration.

Treatment is given with atropine. Doses of up to 50 mg can be given though these would normally cause toxic reactions. The injections are continued at intervals of 3–4 hours until the miosis is converted into mydriasis. To support the heart action combined injections of strophanthin and glucose are recommended. The blood may be detoxicated by injections of "Macrodex". To cleanse the alimentary canal emetic enemas (see p. 36) together with medicinal charcoal are given.

Poisoning with Filix mas (Malefern extract) is possible as this is a constituent of anthelmintics and lay administration may result in an overdose.

The symptoms are vomiting, inappetence, salivation and diarrhoea due to irritation of the mucosa of the stomach and intestine. If the poison is absorbed, restricted movements, ataxia and possibly also disorders of vision occur.

Treatment is restricted chiefly to giving mucilaginous substances and animal charcoal. The vitamin B complex could also be given.

Ethylene Glycol poisoning is seen in the dog. It occurs because the antifreeze used in car radiators has a sweetish taste and therefore dogs like to drink it. Eikmeier and Sandersleben (Mhft. Thkd. **8**, 189, 1956) were able to detect this form of poisoning in dogs. It attacks the brain and kidneys.

Clinical picture. In the early stages the brain is affected. There is restlessness, timidity, disturbance of equilibrium, dizziness, and loss of consciousness and deep coma occur. Death may follow after convulsions with a fall of temperature due to paralysis of the vital centres. A few hours after the early nervous symptoms, renal insufficiency may be evident, i.e., oliguria or anuria, haematuria, albuminuria and oxaluria.

No treatment is known. One should try to maintain the action of the kidneys (with glucose and strophanthin). The antifreeze in the alimentary canal can be expelled by emetic enemas (p. 36) or these may form chemical combinations with it.

Iodine poisoning is caused by licking ointments containing iodine, or by absorption of iodine (iodoform) from extensive wounds, or by internal administration of iodine (Lugol's solution).

The symptoms are disorders of the digestive tract (inappetence, vomiting, coprostasis) and of the nervous system. There may be signs of excitement especially in the early stages, followed by apathy and loss of consciousness. The kidneys are also damaged and there is renal insufficiency. A fall of temperature to subnormal and weakness of the heart indicate impending death. In chronic iodine poisoning inappetence and vomiting also occur. An important symptom is the development of skin lesions (iodine exanthema) shown by alopecia, the formation of scales and reddening of the skin. Catarrh of mucous membranes is also typical. Hyperactivity of the thyroid gland causes emaciation (iodine cachexia).

Treatment consists in the immediate withdrawal of any iodine treatment. The antidote is sodium thiosulphate (5–15 ml). In addition, in acute cases the alimentary canal can be washed out with an emetic enema (see p. 36) and potassium bromide can be given to quieten the patient. If the temperature falls, stimulants are given.

Phenol poisoning. "Lysol", creolin, resorcin, etc., cause poisoning if they are absorbed through the skin when used in the treatment of mange, demodicosis, etc.

Clinical picture. The skin is reddened and tender and there is an exudate from it. If there has been marked absorption of the poison, or if it has been taken in by the mouth, the nervous system is damaged, so that apathy, weakness or paralyses occur. Sometimes tetanic convulsions are seen. Vomiting is part of the clinical picture. Another typical symptom is mydriasis, which is distinguished from mydriasis caused by atropine, by the fact that there is practically no drying up of the eyes. Noteworthy also is the increasing green coloration of the urine when it is exposed to the air (hydroquinone).

In treatment one should try to remove the phenol as quickly as possible. Parts of the skin that have been treated with these compounds are washed and purgatives (Glauber's salts) are given internally. The disorders of function are treated symptomatically with special attention to the circulation.

Phosphorus poisoning is possible when dogs are able to ingest poison baits. The lethal dose is 0.05–1 g of the substance.

The clinical picture is governed by symptoms related to the alimentary canal. Inappetence, salivation, vomiting, colicky spasms and diarrhoea occur. If the phosphorus is able to act on the body for a long time, thickenings of the joints occur. The liver shows fatty degeneration and this results in jaundice. Albuminuria and lipuria result from renal damage. There is always injury to the blood vessels which causes a marked tendency to haemorrhage into the connective tissues, especially seen in the mucosae. Sometimes the breath may have the odour of garlic.

Treatment attempts to remove any phosphorus from the digestive tract with pressure enemas (see p. 36) to which medicinal charcoal has been added. Fats and liquid foods containing fat (milk, eggs, etc.) are contraindicated. One % copper sulphate solution, given in teaspoonful doses several times a day, acts as an antidote (by the formation of non-poisonous copper phosphide). The liver function must be strengthened by suitable liver-protective treatment (see p. 320). Treatment designed to maintain the work of the heart will also stimulate the activity of the kidneys. Vitamin K and calcium can be given to prevent leakage from the blood vessels.

Strychnine poisoning may occur on the one hand when strychnine is given in the wrong concentration (a 1 % instead of 0.1 % solution), or when the dosage is too high (when an estimate only of the patient's bodyweight is made), or when it is given for too long (cumulative effect). On the other hand, poisoning is possible through substances containing strychnine used to exterminate moles.

The symptoms are tonic-clonic muscular spasms. The patient lies on its side with the limbs stretched out in the "saw-horse attitude" and the head drawn back (opisthotonus). The extensor spasms may be sparked off by muscular convulsions in which the patient is thrown about. The irritation of the spinal cord may extend up to the higher centres, so that dyspnoea and cessation of respiration occur.

Treatment, when poison baits have been ingested, is immediate removal of these by giving apomorphine hydrochloride (2–3 mg subcutaneously) or by emetic enemas (see p. 36). If the poisoning has been caused by faulty injections, one must try to prevent the onset of convulsions. This also applies to poisoning by the mouth. For this purpose we use rectal administration of 10 % chloral hydrate solution. The moment the spasms and liability to them cease, the rectum is washed out with pure water in order to remove any chloral hydrate which may now be toxic. To eliminate any possible paralysis of the respiratory centre Leptazol (see p. 78) or Lobeline (0.002–0.01 g subcutaneously) is injected. The injection of Lobeline can be repeated 15 minutes later.

Prontosil rubrum in its tablet form, even in small doses, may cause poisoning which may be lethal. This kind of poisoning is mostly caused by the laity who give their dogs prontosil tablets for trifling affections (e.g. preputial catarrh). We saw a sheep dog die after ingesting one tablet and we were able to cause similar symptoms in a sheep dog bitch to which the approved dose was erroneously given parenterally twice at an interval of about 3 hours. The animal died within 5 hours.

Clinical picture. The symptoms of poisoning begin with disorders of visual accommodation. The patient can no longer estimate short distances correctly. It stumbles over steps, pavements or its jumps are short, etc., and this causes motor restlessness leading to impulsive roaming, walking in circles, etc. The gait is fumbling (circus movements) (Fig. 537). The patients are usually hypersensitive to mechanical and acoustic stimuli (hyperaesthesia). The nervous symptoms may increase until there are epileptiform attacks, combined with opisthotonus. There is superficial and accelerated respiration (hyperpnoea).

Treatment is given with high doses of vitamin B (200 mg), and vitamin B complex, 2–6 dragees daily for several days. In addition, the intravenous administration of methylene blue (6–15 ml of the 1–2 % solution) has proved effective. The methylene blue acts by formation of methaemoglobin, which is reduced to the

31*

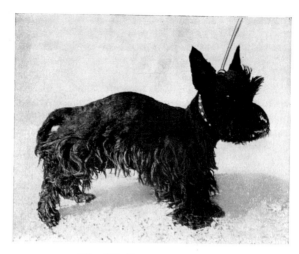

Fig. 537. Prontosil poisoning.

leuco-compound, thus converting the methaemoglobin into haemoglobin. The disorders of accommodation usually cannot be remedied.

Thallium poisoning occurs after ingestion of poison baits. Immediately vomiting and diarrhoea occur, which later may become haemorrhagic. Typical of thallium poisoning are a rash and falling out of the hair. The cutaneous rash occurs mostly in the region of the natural body openings. Incrustations occur on the lips and eyelids and when these are carefully softened with oil, bleeding spots are left behind. The anus and genital openings are often affected in the same way. Ultimately, pustules appear all over the body starting from the lower abdomen and the inner surfaces of the thighs. A little later alopecia accompanies these affections of the skin; occurring chiefly on the neck, the back and the sides of the thorax.

Treatment should in the first place remove from the gastrointestinal tract any poison present by means of emetic enemas (see p. 36) and medicinal charcoal may be added to these. The sulphur treatment described on p. 479 should also be used. As thallium also damages the kidneys, treatment for nephritis should be given. Special attention should be paid to support of the heart and circulation.

Index